Colorectal Cancer

Editor

TRACI L. HEDRICK

SURGICAL ONCOLOGY CLINICS OF NORTH AMERICA

www.surgonc.theclinics.com

Consulting Editor
TIMOTHY M. PAWLIK

April 2022 • Volume 31 • Number 2

ELSEVIER

1600 John F. Kennedy Boulevard ● Suite 1800 ● Philadelphia, Pennsylvania, 19103-2899

http://www.theclinics.com

SURGICAL ONCOLOGY CLINICS OF NORTH AMERICA Volume 31, Number 2
April 2022 ISSN 1055-3207, ISBN-13: 978-0-323-84900-5

Editor: John Vassallo (j.vassallo@elsevier.com)
Developmental Editor: Diana Ang

Surgical Oncology Clinics of North America (ISSN 1055-3207) is published quarterly by Elsevier Inc., 360 Park Avenue South, New York, NY 10010-1710. Months of publication are January, April, July, and October. Business and Editorial Offices: 1600 John F. Kennedy Blvd., Ste. 1800, Philadelphia, PA 19103-2899. Customer Service Office: 3251 Riverport Lane, Maryland Heights, MO 63043. Periodicals postage paid at New York, NY and additional mailing offices. Subscription prices are $325.00 per year (US individuals), $776.00 (US institutions) $100.00 (US student/resident), $363.00 (Canadian individuals), $803.00 (Canadian institutions), $100.00 (Canadian student/resident), $470.00 (foreign individuals), $803.00 (foreign institutions), and $205.00 (foreign student/resident). Foreign air speed delivery is included in all *Clinics* subscription prices. All prices are subject to change without notice. **POSTMASTER**: Send address changes to *Surgical Oncology Clinics of North America*, Elsevier Health Science Division, Subscription Customer Service, 3251 Riverport Lane, Maryland Heights, MO 63043. **Customer Service: 1-800-654-2452 (US and Canada). 314-447-8871 (outside US and Canada). Fax: 314-447-8029. E-mail: journalscustomerservice-usa@elsevier.com (for print support); journalsonline support-usa@elsevier.com (for online support).**

Reprints. For copies of 100 or more, of articles in this publication, please contact the Commercial Reprints Department, Elsevier Inc., 360 Park Avenue South, New York, New York 10010-1710. Tel. 212-633-3874; Fax: 212-633-3820; E-mail: reprints@elsevier.com.

Surgical Oncology Clinics of North America is covered in *MEDLINE/PubMed (Index Medicus)* and *EMBASE/ Excerpta Medica, Current Contents/Clinical Medicine,* and *ISI/BIOMED.*

Contributors

CONSULTING EDITOR

TIMOTHY M. PAWLIK, MD, MPH, MTS, PhD, FACS, FRACS (Hon.)
Professor and Chair, Department of Surgery, The Urban Meyer III and Shelley Meyer Chair for Cancer Research, Professor of Surgery, Oncology, Health Services Management and Policy, Surgeon in Chief, The Ohio State University, Wexner Medical Center, Columbus, Ohio, USA

EDITOR

TRACI L. HEDRICK, MD, MSc, FACS, FACRS
Associate Professor of Surgery, Chief, Division of General Surgery, Vice Chair, Clinical Affairs, Department of Surgery, University of Virginia Health, Charlottesville, Virginia, USA

AUTHORS

MARYLISE BOUTROS, MD, FRCS(C)
Associate Professor, Department of Surgery, McGill University, Division of Colon and Rectal Surgery, Jewish General Hospital, Montreal, Quebec, Canada

DANIEL I. CHU, MD, MSPH
Department of Surgery, Division of Gastrointestinal Surgery, The University of Alabama at Birmingham, Birmingham, Alabama, USA

LISA A. CUNNINGHAM, MD
Assistant Professor, Department of Surgery, The Ohio State University Medical Center, Columbus, Ohio, USA

ALESSANDRA GASIOR, DO
Assistant Professor, Pediatric and Adult Colorectal Surgery, Director of Transitional Care, The Ohio State University Medical Center, Nationwide Children's Hospital, Columbus, Ohio, USA

AMANDA GONG, BS
Department of Surgery, University of Arizona Medical Center, Tucson, Arizona, USA

EMRE GORGUN, MD, FACS, FASCRS
Department of Colorectal Surgery, Digestive Disease and Surgery Institute, Cleveland Clinic, Cleveland, Ohio, USA

ANGELITA HABR-GAMA, MD, PhD
Angelita & Joaquim Gama Institute, Hospital Alemão Oswaldo Cruz, Colorectal Surgery Division, University of São Paulo School of Medicine, Sao Paulo, Brazil

SUE J. HAHN, MD
Assistant Professor of Surgery, Icahn School of Medicine at Mount Sinai, New York, New York, USA

TRACI L. HEDRICK, MD, MSc, FACS, FACRS
Associate Professor of Surgery, Chief, Division of General Surgery, Vice Chair, Clinical Affairs, Department of Surgery, University of Virginia Health, Charlottesville, Virginia, USA

JESSICA HOLLAND, MD, FRCS(C)
Department of Surgery, McGill University, Montreal, Quebec, Canada

ROBERT H. HOLLIS, MD, MSPH
Department of Surgery, Division of Gastrointestinal Surgery, The University of Alabama at Birmingham, Birmingham, Alabama, USA

MATTHEW F. KALADY, MD
Professor of Surgery, Chief, Division of Colorectal Surgery, Medical Director, Clinical Cancer Genetics Program, Department of Surgery, The Ohio State University Medical Center, Columbus, Ohio, USA

TSUYOSHI KONISHI, MD, PhD
Associate Professor, Department of Colon and Rectal Surgery, Division of Surgery, The University of Texas MD Anderson Cancer Center, Houston, Texas, USA

DAVID W. LARSON, MD, MBA, FACS
Professor of Surgery, Department of Surgery, Division of Colon and Rectal Surgery, Mayo Clinic, Rochester, Minnesota, USA

NAJJIA N. MAHMOUD, MD
Emilie and Roland T. DeHellebranth Professor of Surgery, Chief, Division of Colon and Rectal Surgery, Department of Surgery, University of Pennsylvania Health System, Philadelphia, Pennsylvania, USA

VALENTINE NFONSAM, MD, MS, FACS
Department of Surgery, University of Arizona Medical Center, Tucson, Arizona, USA

ILKER OZGUR, MD
Department of Colorectal Surgery, Digestive Disease and Surgery Institute, Cleveland Clinic, Cleveland, Ohio, USA

RODRIGO OLIVA PEREZ, MD, PhD
Angelita & Joaquim Gama Institute, Hospital Alemão Oswaldo Cruz, Hospital Beneficência Portuguesa, Sao Paulo, Brazil

FELIPE F. QUEZADA-DIAZ, MD
Colorectal Surgeon, Colorectal Unit, Department of Surgery, Complejo Asistencial Doctor Sótero del Río, Santiago, Puente Alto, RM, Chile

GUILHERME PAGIN SÃO JULIÃO, MD
Angelita & Joaquim Gama Institute, Hospital Alemão Oswaldo Cruz, Hospital Beneficência Portuguesa, Sao Paulo, Brazil

SHINICHIRO SAKATA, MBBS, PhD, FRACS
Department of Surgery, Division of Colon and Rectal Surgery, Mayo Clinic, Rochester, Minnesota, USA

EBRAM SALAMA, MD, MBA
Department of Surgery, McGill University, Montreal, Quebec, Canada

J. JOSHUA SMITH, MD, PhD, FACS
Colorectal Surgeon, Associate Attending Surgeon, Colorectal Service, Department of Surgery, Memorial Sloan Kettering Cancer Center, New York, New York, USA

PATRICIA SYLLA, MD, FASCRS
Professor of Surgery, Icahn School of Medicine at Mount Sinai, New York, New York, USA

BRUNA BORBA VAILATI, MD
Angelita & Joaquim Gama Institute, Hospital Alemão Oswaldo Cruz, Hospital Beneficência Portuguesa, Sao Paulo, Brazil

PRIYANKA VIJ, MD
Department of Surgery, University of Arizona Medical Center, Tucson, Arizona, USA

EMILY WUSTERBARTH, BS
Department of Surgery, University of Arizona Medical Center, Tucson, Arizona, USA

Y. NANCY YOU, MD, MHSc
Professor, Department of Colon and Rectal Surgery, Division of Surgery, The University of Texas MD Anderson Cancer Center, Houston, Texas, USA

VICTOR M. ZAYDFUDIM, MD, MPH, FACS
Associate Professor of Surgery, Section of Hepatobiliary and Pancreatic Surgery, Division of Surgical Oncology, Director of Health Services Research, Department of Surgery, University of Virginia, Charlottesville, Virginia, USA

Contributors

PERAM SALDANA, MD, MBA
Department of Surgery, McGill University, Montreal, Quebec, Canada

J. JOSHUA SMITH, MD, PhD

Contents

Najjia N. Mahmoud

> The preoperative assessment of patients with colorectal cancer (CRC) re-
> quires a multimodal approach, including endoscopic evaluation and clin-
> ical, radiographic, and biochemical assessment. In addition to providing
> a diagnosis, histologic review of biopsy specimens imparts valuable infor-
> mation about tumor grade and other important prognostic features that
> can help determine treatment. A thorough history and physical examina-
> tion rounds out the initial evaluation and provides the surgeon and other
> treating physicians with vital additional information for detailed operative
> planning. Colon and rectal cancer, although closely related histologically,
> are considered, and often treated, very differently, depending on stage,
> based solely on location.

Valentine Nfonsam, Emily Wusterbarth, Amanda Gong, and Priyanka Vij

> Colorectal cancer (CRC) is the third leading cause of cancer-related
> deaths in the United States, and the incidence of early-onset CRC
> (EOCRC, <50 years old) has been steadily increasing over the past 30
> years. This article provides a comprehensive review of EOCRC traits,
> including incidence rates and patterns, tumor biologic differences
> compared to late-onset CRC, dietary risk factors, relationship between
> CRC and the microbiome, and patient survival outcomes associated
> with EOCRC. These factors carry importance in determining diagnostic,
> prognostic, disease monitoring, and treatment planning practices for
> EOCRC in the future. They also serve as guides for optimizing CRC
> screening recommendations.

Robert H. Hollis and Daniel I. Chu

> Health care disparities are defined as health differences between groups
> that are avoidable, unnecessary, and unjust. Racial disparities in colorectal
> cancer mortality, particularly for Black patients, are well-described. Dis-
> parities in preventative measures, early detection, effective treatment,
> and posttreatment services contribute to these differences. Underlying
> these issues are patient, provider, health care system, and policy-level fac-
> tors that lead to these disparities. Multilevel interventions designed to

address each level of care can provide an effective means to mitigate these disparities.

In recent decades, rectal cancer management has become increasingly challenging for multiple reasons. Proper imaging using dedicated magnetic resonance, standardization of total mesorectal excision, and incorporation of neoadjuvant treatment regimens have contributed to a significant decrease in local recurrence rates. The observation of complete tumor response to radiation or chemoradiation led to the proposal of organ-preservation strategies with avoidance of immediate surgery and close surveillance (Watch and Wait strategy) in selected patients. The purpose of this article is to review the current evidence related to the selection criteria and outcomes in patients enrolled in this Watch and Wait strategy.

Efforts toward standardization of surgical techniques have facilitated adoption of oncologic resections for colorectal cancer with associated improvement in outcomes. With the introduction of laparoscopy, total mesorectal excision (TME) and complete mesocolic excision (CME) techniques were progressively adapted to the minimally invasive surgery (MIS) approach with significant benefits with regards to patient recovery and comparable oncologic outcomes when performed by surgeons beyond their learning curve. Anastomotic complications and functional disturbances following TME remain significant. Recent innovations include intracorporeal anastomosis, which avoids midline extraction sites, and transanal TME, which lowers conversion rates and facilitates sphincter preservation for low rectal tumors.

Local excision and endoluminal surgery are organ preservation techniques, which are more widely accepted and practiced in colorectal cancer management. Although endoluminal surgery is considered challenging, it will continue to progress and gain more popularity over time. Increased education, research, and availability of the tools to perform these procedures will help more endoscopists be adept over time. Owing to the ability to avoid intraabdominal surgery, endoluminal surgery can be the next big step for minimally invasive surgery. Through research and development, fully flexible endorobotic platforms with stable camera positioning and precision will become a reality and push endoluminal surgery forward.

This article reviews the oncological principles of rectal cancer surgery, beginning with an overview of the pertinent rectal and pelvic anatomy, followed by a discussion of the historical evolution in surgical management. Evidence supporting current practices with respect to proximal, distal, and circumferential margins are reviewed. Finally, operative approaches to restorative proctectomies and abdominoperineal resections are highlighted.

Metastatic colorectal cancer (mCRC) is incurable in patients with unresectable disease. For most patients, the primary treatment is palliative systemic chemotherapy. Genomic profiling is used to detect specific genetic mutations that may offer selected patients a modest survival benefit with targeted therapy. Patients with mCRC with KRAS/NRAS/BRAF wild-type left-sided tumors may benefit from epidermal growth factor receptor (EGFR) inhibition with either cetuximab or panitumumab, in conjunction with chemotherapy. EGFR inhibitors can extend survival by 6 months compared with chemotherapy alone. The vascular endothelial growth factor (VEGF) inhibitor bevacizumab can serve as an alternative to EGFR inhibitors in right-sided tumors or second-line therapy. Many patients will have RAS mutations, and targeted therapies will not provide any benefit. The PRIME trial demonstrated that the addition of panitumumab to FOLFOX was associated with reduced overall survival. Patients with BRAF mutations do not benefit from targeted therapy unless a BRAF inhibitor supplements treatment. Triple combination therapy with cetuximab, the BRAF inhibitor encorafenib, and the MEK kinase inhibitor binimetinib has extended overall survival by about 3 months compared with chemotherapy alone. Finally, for the minority patients with microsatellite instability (MSI) high/mismatch repair (MMR) deficient tumors, either due to Lynch syndrome or sporadic mutations, immunotherapy is recommended as first-line treatment. The KEYNOTE-177 trial demonstrated that therapy with single-agent pembrolizumab improved progression-free survival by 8 months compared with FOLFOX or FOLFIRI and with or without EGFR inhibition. At this time, targeted therapy should only be used in patients with unresectable metastatic disease.

The management of patients with metastatic colorectal cancer (CRC) has evolved significantly over the last decade owing to advances in aggressive multimodality chemotherapy options, targeted therapy, development of sophisticated operative techniques, and adjunct radiotherapy options. Patients with synchronous CRC require complex decision-making with multidisciplinary collaboration to develop individualized treatment strategies taking into account tumor biology and patients' individual goals and objectives. We will outline important considerations with regard to treatment options for patients with synchronous metastatic CRC to facilitate

The treatment of locally advanced rectal cancer is challenging and requires a multidisciplinary approach. Neoadjuvant treatment has improved local control by the combination of radiotherapy, surgery, and chemotherapy. However, neoadjuvant treatment has not yet been shown to improve overall survival and is associated with toxicities and late sequelae that impair the quality of life of patients. Currently, different types of neoadjuvant strategies have raised the question about which one is the optimal strategy for rectal cancer treatment. In this article, we explore the different neoadjuvant treatment regimens currently available, their associated benefits and toxicities, and novel approaches in this area.

Curative-intent surgical resection of colon cancer involves optimal approaches to the peri-tumoral tissue, the mesocolon, and the draining lymph nodes. The key corresponding concepts that will be discussed are complete mesocolic excision (CME), central vascular ligation (CVL) or D3 dissection, and circumferential resection margin (CRM). We aim to describe these techniques and delineate evidence surrounding their technical feasibility, pathologic detail, as well as long-term oncologic impact. CME with CVL and D3 dissection are overlapping concepts both emphasizing anatomy-based resection of tumor and regional lymph nodes that does not breach the embryonic visceral fascia and ensures complete lymph node dissection up to the mesenteric root. Completeness of the mesocolic plane, number of harvested nodes, and CRM are surgical pathologic parameters that impact oncologic outcome. Attention to these details has been associated with improved outcomes in retrospective observational trials and the choice of open or minimally invasive approaches must be determined by surgeon's technical experiences.

Approximately 5% of all colorectal cancers develop within a hereditary colorectal cancer syndrome. Patients and families with these syndromes have an increased risk of colorectal and extracolonic cancers that develop at an early age. Recognition and diagnosis of these conditions are crucial to management and risk reduction. Surgeons must be aware of the unique aspects of the timing and extent of surgery (both therapeutic and prophylactic) within these syndromes, particularly for the most common syndromes, Lynch syndrome and familial adenomatous polyposis.

SURGICAL ONCOLOGY CLINICS OF NORTH AMERICA

SERIES OF RELATED INTEREST

Surgical Clinics of North America
http://www.surgical.theclinics.com
Thoracic Surgery Clinics
http://www.thoracic.theclinics.com
Advances in Surgery
http://www.advancessurgery.com

THE CLINICS ARE AVAILABLE ONLINE!
Access your subscription at:
www.theclinics.com

Foreword

Colorectal Cancer

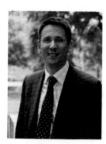

Timothy M. Pawlik, MD, MPH, MTS, PhD, FACS, FRACS (Hon.)
Consulting Editor

This issue of the *Surgical Oncology Clinics of North America* focuses on the management of Colorectal Cancer. Globally, colorectal cancer is the third most commonly diagnosed malignancy and the second leading cause of death. In the United States, more than 100,000 new cases of colon cancer and 40,000 cases of rectal cancer are diagnosed on an annual basis.[1] In turn, more than 53,000 people will die from colorectal cancer this year. The annual incidence rates of colorectal cancer have declined since the late 2000s, likely due to the widespread uptake of colorectal screening with colonoscopy. However, incidence rates of colorectal cancer among younger adults have increased, with younger patients (20–39 years) experiencing the steepest increase.[2] Although inherited susceptibility is associated with the most striking increase in risk, the majority of colorectal cancer cancers still remain sporadic rather than familial. As such, colorectal cancer is a heterogeneous disease with different patient populations having distinctive molecular profiles. A greater understanding of these molecular underpinnings of colorectal cancer has led to an increase in the use of personalized treatment approaches, as well as the use of targeted therapies. Recently, even the role of surgical therapy has been questioned with some data suggesting that nonoperative management of select patients with rectal cancer may be appropriate. For those patients who do require surgery, there have been important technological advances in the operative treatment of colorectal cancer. Amid the evolution of the multidisciplinary management of colorectal cancer, the surgeon remains a central actor on the treatment team. As such, I am grateful to have Dr Traci Hedrick as the guest editor of this important issue of *Surgical Oncology Clinics of North America*. Dr Hedrick is an associate professor with the University of Virginia School of Medicine. Dr Hedrick received both her undergraduate and her medical degrees from the University of Kentucky. She completed her general surgery training and a two-year postgraduate research fellowship at the University of Virginia followed by a fellowship in colon and rectal surgery at the University of Pennsylvania. Dr Hedrick has won numerous

Surg Oncol Clin N Am 31 (2022) xiii–xiv
https://doi.org/10.1016/j.soc.2022.02.002
1055-3207/22/© 2022 Published by Elsevier Inc.

surgonc.theclinics.com

national awards for her research, and she serves as the co-director of the Enhanced Recovery after Surgery Program at the University of Virginia, which has been featured by the American College of Surgeons, the *Wall Street Journal* and, *US News and World Report*. She has made many national and international research presentations of her research and has numerous peer-reviewed publications within the field of colorectal surgery. As such, I can think of no one more qualified to lead this issue on colorectal cancer in *Surgical Oncology Clinics of North America*.

The issue covers a wide range of topics germane to colorectal cancer. In particular, an impressive team of experts details the preoperative staging and evaluation, nonoperative management of rectal cancer, local excision and endoscopic strategies, as well as the general surgical principles to treat colorectal cancer. In addition, other important subjects are covered, including early-onset colorectal cancer, hereditary syndromes, and health care disparities relative to colorectal cancer diagnosis, treatment, and outcomes.

I wish to thank Dr Hedrick for her work to identify such a wonderful group of leaders in the field of colorectal surgery to contribute to this issue of *Surgical Oncology Clinics of North America*. The authors have done a masterful job to feature the latest important data that surgeons who care for patients with colorectal cancer should know. I am convinced that this issue of *Surgical Oncology Clinics of North America* will serve faculty and trainees well. Again, I would like to thank Dr Hedrick and all the contributing authors for an outstanding issue of the *Surgical Oncology Clinics of North America*.

Timothy M. Pawlik, MD, MPH, MTS, PhD, FACS, FRACS (Hon.)
Department of Surgery
The Urban Meyer III and Shelley Meyer Chair for Cancer Research
Departments of Surgery, Oncology, and Health Services Management and Policy
The Ohio State University Wexner Medical Center
395 West 12th Avenue, Suite 670
Columbus, OH 43210, USA

E-mail address:
tim.pawlik@osumc.edu

REFERENCES

1. Available at: https://www.cancer.org/content/dam/cancer-org/research/cancer-facts-and-statistics/colorectal-cancer-facts-and-figures/colorectal-cancer-facts-and-figures-2020-2022.pdf. Accessed January 14, 2022.
2. Siegel RL, Fedewa SA, Anderson WF, et al. Colorectal cancer incidence patterns in the United States, 1974-2013. J Natl Cancer Inst 2017;109(8). https://doi.org/10.1093/jnci/djw322.

Preface

Colorectal Cancer

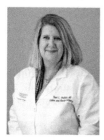

Traci L. Hedrick, MD, MSc, FACS, FACRS
Editor

Although the incidence and mortality rates of colorectal cancer (CRC) are decreasing, the number of people over the age of 65 is expected to double by the year 2060. As CRC prevalence increases with age, the number of people diagnosed with CRC is expected to increase dramatically over the ensuing decades.[1] Described as the "silver tsunami," this trend will result in a substantial increase in the number of CRC patients, particularly those with accompanying comorbidities and complex surgical needs.[2] Paradoxically, there has also been a significant rise in the incidence of early-onset CRC. CRC rates are expected to increase by 90% for individuals aged 20 to 34 years in the ensuing decade.[1,2] This concerning trend has left clinicians and researchers fervently searching for possible causes and mitigation strategies.

CRC screening rates steadily improved in the United States to a peak of nearly 70% at the start of the year 2020.[3] However, the COVID-19 pandemic brought about a reduction in CRC screening and early diagnosis leading to the proliferation of more advanced disease.[4] The impact of COVID-19 has yet to be fully realized but will inevitably have far-reaching effects on the trajectory of CRC for years to come.[5] This is particularly true for disadvantaged groups, who have borne the greatest burden of the pandemic.[6] Despite improvements in CRC screening and treatment resulting in improved CRC survival, certain disadvantaged groups also experience higher incidence of CRC with worsened mortality rates.[7] In the current issue, we explore the cause, implications, and possible strategies to address these tragic racial, social, and financial disparities as they pertain to the diagnosis and management of CRC.

The management paradigm of CRC has evolved significantly over the last century since Miles' original description of the extralevator abdominoperineal resection with an accompanying 41% mortality rate.[8] Innovative endoscopic and transanal techniques along with advancements in novel therapeutic agents have led to substantial improvements in oncologic and patient-reported outcomes with increasing rates of

Surg Oncol Clin N Am 31 (2022) xv–xvi
https://doi.org/10.1016/j.soc.2022.02.001
1055-3207/22/© 2022 Published by Elsevier Inc.

sphincter preservation. In the current issue, we learn from the world's experts, who are leading this innovative renaissance.

As history demonstrates, controversy frequently lies in the shadow of innovation. Two particularly controversial topics in the surgical treatment of CRC focus on the technical aspects of the mesenteric excision: (1) the complete mesocolic excision and extent of lymphadenectomy for colon cancer, and (2) the minimally invasive total mesorectal excision (laparoscopy, robotics, transanal) for rectal cancer. We delve into both of these important topics, hearing from highly skilled surgeons in the technical and practice aspects of each of these evolving techniques.

In the current issue of *Surgical Oncology Clinics of North America*, we sought to highlight the most important surgical aspects of CRC management. I am inspired by and thankful to my esteemed colleagues, who contributed their expertise to the current issue, and I hope you will gain valuable information to improve your practice.

Traci L. Hedrick, MD, MSc, FACS, FACRS
Division of General Surgery
Department of Surgery
University of Virginia Health
PO Box 800709
Charlottesville, VA 22901, USA

E-mail address:
TH8Q@hscmail.mcc.virginia.edu

REFERENCES

1. CDC. Expected New Cancer Cases and Deaths in 2020. 2016. Available at: https://www.cdc.gov/cancer/dcpc/research/articles/cancer_2020.htm. Accessed November 12, 2018.
2. Bluethmann SM, Mariotto AB, Rowland JH. Anticipating the "silver tsunami": prevalence trajectories and comorbidity burden among older cancer survivors in the United States. Cancer Epidemiol Biomarkers Prev 2016;25(7):1029–36.
3. CDC. Use of Colorectal Cancer Screening Tests. 2021. Available at: https://www.cdc.gov/cancer/colorectal/statistics/use-screening-tests-BRFSS.htm. Accessed September 1, 2021.
4. Morris EJA, Goldacre R, Spata E, et al. Impact of the COVID-19 pandemic on the detection and management of colorectal cancer in England: a population-based study. Lancet Gastroenterol Hepatol 2021;6(3):199–208.
5. Malagon T, Yong JHE, Tope P, et al. Predicted long-term impact of COVID-19 pandemic-related care delays on cancer mortality in Canada. Int J Cancer. 2022 Apr 15;150(8):1244–54.
6. Shiels MS, Haque AT, Haozous EA, et al. Racial and ethnic disparities in excess deaths during the COVID-19 pandemic, March to December 2020. Ann Intern Med. 2021 Dec;174(12):1693–9.
7. Carethers JM. Racial and ethnic disparities in colorectal cancer incidence and mortality. Adv Cancer Res 2021;151:197–229.
8. Miles WE. A method of performing abdomino-perineal excision for carcinoma of the rectum and of the terminal portion of the pelvic colon (1908). CA Cancer J Clin 1971;21(6):361–4.

Colorectal Cancer
Preoperative Evaluation and Staging

Najjia N. Mahmoud, MD

KEYWORDS

- Colorectal cancer • Rectal cancer • Colon cancer • TNM Stage
- Microsatellite instability (MSI) • Colonoscopy • Carcinoembryonic antigen (CEA)

KEY POINTS

- A CT scan of the chest, abdomen and pelvis with oral and IV contrast should be routinely ordered before surgery.
- The preoperative colonoscopy report should be very specific about location of the lesion. If it is not, then review of the CT scan or preoperative colonoscopy with tattoo is needed to localize the cancer.
- A focused physical examination can help direct the operation.
- Specific assessment of inherited risk is an important part of establishing the liklihood of a germline mutation and assessing whether further genetic risk assessment should take place.

INCIDENCE AND EPIDEMIOLOGY

Colorectal cancer is a widespread clinical entity—affecting more than 1 million individuals globally on an annual basis.[1-3] Colorectal cancer remains the third most common nonskin cancer in the United States after lung cancer in both genders, with an annual incidence of 42.9 per 100,000 people. This condition accounts for 8% of cancer-related deaths in the United States alone.[4] Marked geographic variations exist, with industrialized countries bearing significantly higher incidences, thought to be attributed to a complex interplay of diet, environment, and genetic predisposition.[2,3] The prevalence and incidence vary worldwide, with Australia and New Zealand having the highest incidence, followed by North America and Europe. Africa and South-Central Asia have the lowest incidence. Males are affected slightly more than females, and African Americans have the highest incidence in the United States, and at a younger age.

Colorectal cancer displays a strong correlation with increasing age, the maximum rate at age greater than 75 years and the lowest less than 40 years. It has been

Division of Colon and Rectal Surgery, Department of Surgery, Hospital of the University of Pennsylvania, Philadelphia, PA 19104, USA
E-mail address: najjia.mahmoud@pennmedicine.upenn.edu

Surg Oncol Clin N Am 31 (2022) 127–141
https://doi.org/10.1016/j.soc.2021.12.001
1055-3207/22/© 2021 Elsevier Inc. All rights reserved.

estimated that annually there are roughly 100,000 new cases of colon cancer and more than 40,000 cases of rectal cancer in the United States.[5–7] Fortunately, both the incidence and mortality of colorectal cancer have declined steadily in the past 3 decades—largely due to more effective screening programs and improvements in treatment modalities.[5–7] However, despite these measurable gains, there remain significant disparities in incidence and mortality, particularly among African Americans.[8–10] Overall, the lifetime risk of developing colorectal cancer in the United States is approximately 5% with a likelihood increasing notably after age 50 years. It is estimated that up to 90% of cases occur in individuals older than 50 years.[11]

The overall incidence rate of CRC has declined significantly in the past 4 decades. Colonoscopy allows for the detection and removal of polyps in the colon before they develop into cancer and represents our most validated screening modality. Polypectomy or "secondary prevention" has been credited with lowering the incidence rates of CRC in adults older than 50 years. In contrast, for patients younger than 50 years, there has been an increase in the incidence of CRC.[12] CRC incidence assayed by Surveillance, Epidemiology, and End Results (SEER) data from 1974 to 2013 shows that adults aged 20 to 39 years were noted to have a 2.4% annual increase in CRC incidence. Going forward from that time, between 2012 and 2016, there was a 3.3% annual decline in rates of CRC among those greater than age 65 years, coinciding with increased and widespread screening. Simultaneously, for those younger than 50 years, there was a 2.2% annual increase in incidence of CRC, with the greatest increase in rates seen among patients between ages 20 and 34 years.[13] Among adults younger than 50 years, CRC is now the second most common cause of cancer among men, and the fourth most common among women.[14] Rectal cancer is increasing at a higher rate than colon cancer, with an increased annual incidence rate of 3.2% in adults aged 20 to 39 years and 2.3% per year beginning in the 1990s in adults aged 40 to 49 years.[15] Recent estimates suggest that by 2030, the incidence rate of colon cancer among this group (ages 20–39 years) will increase by 90%, and the incidence rate of rectal cancer in this group will increase by 124.2%.[13] It is estimated that by 2030, roughly 1 in 10 colon cancers and 1 in 4 rectal cancers will be diagnosed in patients younger than 50 years.[13] Although CRC mortality rates have decreased among older adults, mortality among those younger than 50 years seems to be gradually increasing, with an estimated 1.9 deaths per 100,000 as of 2018.[16]

Once the diagnosis of colon cancer is made, the goal of preoperative evaluation is to establish the location of the tumor, assess for metastatic disease, and identify patient and tumor factors that may affect outcome or change the medical or surgical approach to treatment. The primary importance of staging in both colon and rectal cancer is to rule out additional pathology and distant metastatic disease (stage IV), which can affect treatment approach. This differs from rectal cancer in which specific locoregional staging is mandatory and stage dictates a potentially different treatment paradigm entirely for nonmetastatic disease.

CLINICAL PRESENTATION AND HISTORY

Colorectal cancer presents in 3 common ways: asymptomatic findings detected during routine screening; symptoms like weight loss, fatigue/anemia, and rectal bleeding or other change in bowel habits that lead to further investigation; and emergently, with perforation or obstruction.

Early cancers are often asymptomatic, which underscores the importance of routine screening. It is estimated that about 30% of all cancers are diagnosed by endoscopy in the absence of symptoms.[17] Unfortunately, overall compliance with colonoscopy screening in the United States is still quite low—less than 50% for most average-risk adults. Rates of screening can vary widely between states and regions. The Centers for Disease Control and Prevention estimates that when all screening modalities are examined collectively, including fecal occult blood testing alone within 1 year, flexible sigmoidoscopy within 3 years, or colonoscopy within 10 years, the highest rates of screening are in the Northeast at 75% and the lowest are in the West with maximal screening compliance rates of 54%.[18] When symptoms do occur, patients commonly present with crampy abdominal pain (obstructive symptoms), gastrointestinal bleeding, iron deficiency anemia, change in bowel habits, or vague nonspecific symptoms such as lethargy, weight loss, and loss of appetite.[5,19,20] Symptoms can differ depending on tumor location and size (anemia for right-sided cancers and obstruction for left-sided ones, eg). Late findings can include palpable abdominal mass, weight loss, intestinal obstruction, and perforation.

Abdominal pain in the setting of colon cancer is often poorly localized and nonspecific. Patients may describe a vague visceral discomfort, which changes to crampy, colicky pain as luminal narrowing occurs. Rectal bleeding is a common finding, and its clinical manifestation can be varied, therefore taking a careful history is important. Patients with distal, left-sided lesions will often present with bright red blood in the stools, whereas more proximal lesions will cause occult bleeding that results in iron deficiency anemia.[3,19] This anemia can ultimately result in weakness, shortness of breath and other cardiopulmonary symptoms, and generalized fatigue. Similarly, changes in bowel habits will be affected by tumor location within the colon. Patients may report changes in the caliber, frequency, and consistency of their stools; these are more notable with left-sided lesions, which are more likely to cause narrowing of the colon lumen and impede passage of solid stool. As the luminal diameter tends to be wider in the proximal colon, and stool more liquid, alterations in stools generally coincide with very large, exophytic or advanced lesions or cancers that obstruct the ileocecal valve.

Approximately 20% to 25% of colon cancer will present with metastatic disease at the time of diagnosis; therefore, it is also critical to evaluate these patients for signs and symptoms associated with metastatic disease. On the whole, widely advanced cancers can result in constitutional symptoms such as unintentional weight loss, cachexia, weakness, and anorexia.[3]

Colorectal cancer typically spreads via lymphatic, intraperitoneal extension, or hematogenous spread, and the most common sites include the liver, lungs, and peritoneal surfaces. Rectal cancer, in particular, when present within 5 cm of the anus can spread hematogenously to the lungs (10%) without hepatic involvement via the internal iliac venous channels. Spread to the central nervous system and bones is less likely but possible. Common sites of intraperitoneal spread include the so-called "drop" metastases to the ovaries and spread to the omentum. Although symptoms of liver metastasis are uncommon, some patients may develop right upper quadrant pain, abdominal distention, anorexia, weakness, or jaundice when the burden of liver metastases is large. Direct local invasion of colorectal cancers into adjacent structures such as the small intestine, bladder, abdominal wall, or pelvic structures can result in bowel obstruction, abscesses and perforation, pneumaturia, fecaluria, or enterocutaneous or rectovaginal fistula. A Virchow node (left supraclavicular node) and Sister Mary Joseph node (umbilical implant) are other uncommon findings that have been associated with the distant spread of colorectal cancer.[3] Patients who present with symptoms are at higher risk of having advanced disease at diagnosis than those for whom the primary is detected by routine screening. For example, in one study of more than 1000 patients with colorectal cancer, only 217 were found during screening.

Those that came to attention via symptoms were twice as likely to have a transmural tumor, twice as likely to present with stage III disease, more than 3 times as likely to have distant spread at diagnosis, and have double the risk of recurrence.[21]

PREOPERATIVE EVALUATION

The evaluation of a patient with a new diagnosis of colorectal cancer should begin with a complete history and physical examination.[22] The history should focus on the duration and severity of symptoms with emphasis on obstructive symptoms, weight loss, anemia, and abdominal pain and rectal bleeding. Information should also be obtained about any family history of colorectal cancer or other cancers known to be associated with inherited syndromes. Finally, details regarding the patient's overall health will provide initial insight into their readiness for any surgical intervention. A focused physical examination can elucidate important signs such as a palpable mass, distant adenopathy, tenderness, or distention.[22] The evaluation of rectal cancer includes a digital rectal examination, and either a proctoscopy or flexible sigmoidoscopy in the office to establish the precise location of the cancer. Distance from the anal verge, distance above the anorectal ring, fixation to underlying tissue, degree of obstruction, sphincter involvement, size, morphology, and location in the rectum (anterior, posterior, left, and so forth) need to be carefully evaluated and recorded in the chart at the time of office visit. Subsequent therapeutic options heavily depend on these details.

Assessment of Inherited Risk

The vast majority (85%) of colorectal cancers are sporadic in nature; however, there are significant nonhereditary risk factors that have been identified. Modifiable risk factors associated with colon cancer include a low-fiber high-fat diet; obesity; smoking; and heavy alcohol consumption. The primary risk factor for colorectal cancer is increasing age; however, a personal history of colorectal cancer, polyps, or inflammatory bowel disease will substantially increase risk. Approximately 5% to 10% of colorectal cancers can be linked to discrete inherited syndromes. Familial adenomatous polyposis and Lynch syndrome are the most common. It is therefore important to identify these risk factors because they serve as the basis for the established screening strategies and can help inform choice of procedure. Taking a careful family history including siblings, parents, and grandparents is important. Putting the neoplasm in the context of the patient's medical history can change the operative strategy greatly. For example, a patient with inflammatory bowel disease (Crohn or ulcerative colitis) who is found to have a colorectal cancer has additional medical and surgical considerations that must be addressed. A patient who meets criteria for Lynch syndrome or is a known carrier of a germline mutation in DNA mismatch repair (MMR) genes will need counseling on the choice between subtotal colectomy with ileorectal anastomosis versus segmental colectomy with yearly surveillance. Additional procedures such as total abdominal hysterectomy and bilateral salpingo-oophorectomy should be coordinated in patients with Lynch syndrome who meet criteria and are appropriately counseled.

Colonoscopy

If not completed at the time of diagnosis, a thorough endoscopic examination of the entire colon is critical because it provides added information about synchronous cancers or polyps and a chance to remove or mark them preoperatively. The rate of synchronous cancers is about 5% with synchronous polyps occurring more frequently.[23] It is important to endoscopically resect those polyps that are amenable for both prevention and diagnosis.[5] Colonoscopy allows for the localization and biopsy of the primary tumor; however, it is important to keep in mind that the flexible scope may not provide an exact measurement of distance. Therefore, it is important to assess known landmarks and whenever possible to mark the location of the cancer with an endoscopic tattoo, particularly in the case of a small tumor or malignant polyp. Tattoo localization is very important in the era of minimally invasive surgery, particularly for smaller lesions that may not be easily palpated at the time of surgery or if a minimally invasive approach is planned. It is not unusual for the endoscopist to resect a large polyp only to find an occult cancer within it requiring formal resection on pathology. In these cases, rapid re-evaluation of the colon via colonoscopy with marking is essential. Typically, if the colon can be rescoped within 2 weeks, a healing ulcer can be identified and tattooed, if needed.

Several agents for endoscopic marking have been evaluated. Only India ink and SpotEx have been widely accepted. Both agents are colloid suspensions of fine carbon particles. India ink is suspended in a 0.9% solution of saline at a 1:100 dilution and sterilized by autoclaving or passing through a Millipore filter. SpotEx is also composed of highly purified, fine carbon particles and is the only US Food and Drug Administration-approved marking solution for endoscopic tattooing. Both have been tested extensively and are safe and durable.[24] Identification of the endoscopic tattoo can be made for years after the initial tattoo was placed. Other agents that have been used include methylene blue, hematoxylin, and toluene blue. Methylene blue has limited durability. Mucosal ulceration is a problem with the other agents. Technique of injection has been studied extensively. Four-quadrant injection of 2 to 4 mL ink at or near the level of the lesion allows for accurate identification even if the lesion is on the mesenteric aspect of the colon lumen.[24] Submucosal injection limits intraperitoneal spread that can make intraoperative identification confusing or difficult. Some advocate for placing a tattoo both proximally and distally to the tumor or polyp to help identify the extent or length of the lesion, but this is typically not necessary. Clear documentation of technique in the report is mandatory and will limit misunderstandings. Additional benefits of tattoo placement may include increased nodal harvest by virtue of the ability to see and enumerate lymph nodes that take up the colloid carbon particles. There is a significant increase in the number of specimens with greater than 12 lymph nodes harvested after tattoo placement.[25,26]

If a colonoscopy cannot be completed, then a computed tomographic (CT) colonography ("virtual colonoscopy") or barium enema may be attempted instead. It can, however, be technically challenging to both bowel prep a patient who is nearly obstructed and to reflux contrast in a way that makes these studies accurate, meaningful, and safe. For cases of obstructing cancers that inhibit adequate endoscopic or radiographic assessment preoperatively, a full colonoscopy should be performed 3 to 6 months after surgery when safe to do so.[5]

Carcinoembryonic Antigen

Preoperative evaluation should include routine laboratory studies, including a complete blood cell count and a basic metabolic profile. The serum carcinoembryonic antigen (CEA) level is the only other mandatory basic laboratory test needed in an otherwise healthy patient and provides prognostic information.[27] CEA is a glycoprotein primarily involved in intercellular adhesion[28]; it is produced by columnar and goblet cells and can be found in normal colonic mucosa. In addition, it can be found in low levels in the circulation of healthy individuals but is overexpressed in a variety of malignancies and in about 80% of colorectal cancers. Elevated serum levels may be identified in heavy smokers, in benign conditions such as pancreatitis and inflammatory bowel disease, as well as in other malignancies both in and outside of the gastrointestinal tract[28]; therefore, CEA is not a sensitive or specific screening tool for colorectal cancer.[3,29] However, it is an important tool in CRC surveillance after surgical resection because its elevation may herald the existence of metastatic disease.[30]

Patients with preoperative serum CEA greater than 5 ng/mL have a worse prognosis, stage for stage, than those with lower levels. Elevated preoperative CEA levels have been shown to be associated with poorer survival and increased recurrence in several studies; however, contradictory studies do exist.[29,31–35] Therefore, there is currently insufficient evidence to support the use of elevated preoperative serum CEA levels as an absolute indication for adjuvant chemotherapy.[5,34]

Current American Society of Clinical Oncology and National Cancer Institute guidelines recommend that serum CEA levels be obtained preoperatively in patients with demonstrated colorectal cancer for posttreatment follow-up and assessment of prognosis. Elevated preoperative CEA levels that do not normalize following surgical resection imply the presence of persistent disease.[34]

Radiographic Evaluation

Preoperative radiographic imaging is fundamental for initial staging of newly diagnosed colorectal cancers.[5] CT scan of the chest, abdomen, and pelvis with oral and intravenous contrast is the most common staging study and is indicated for both colon and rectal cancers. The CT scan of the chest, if performed separately, may be noncontrast. CT provides valuable preoperative information about liver or lung metastasis in a cost-effective manner. This test should be done with both oral and intravenous contrast if there is no contraindication (anaphylaxis to contrast or renal insufficiency) to maximize accuracy of visualization of the abdominal viscera as well as highlight vascular structures and better determine the relationships between lymphatics, ureters, and vessels.[36] In addition, cross-sectional imaging also facilitates more precise tumor location and delineates the extent of any extracolonic invasion of adjacent organs or the abdominal wall, all of which are extremely important for operative planning.[37] CT scan has a sensitivity ranging from 75% to 90% for detecting distant metastasis; however, the ability to accurately detect nodal involvement or small subcentimeter peritoneal metastasis is poor.

As imaging technology has improved, so has the sensitivity of CT scans for identifying liver metastases. However, there are studies that suggest that contrast-enhanced MRI is particularly valuable in evaluating smaller suspicious liver lesions (especially in the presence of fatty liver changes) with sensitivities up to 97%.[3,37] In routine clinical practice, MRI should be reserved for the evaluation of suspicious liver lesions not clearly characterized on CT scan and for operative planning before liver metastectomy.

PET/CT scan has emerged as a useful imaging modality in the evaluation of many cancers. However, for colorectal cancers, the routine use of PET/CT remains controversial. Although it has been shown to be more sensitive in the detection of liver metastases as well as extrahepatic disease when compared with routine CT scan, other studies suggest that it does not add significant information that makes a distinct difference in determining treatment.[19,38–40] The strongest evidence for use of PET/CT in the management of colorectal cancer is in the evaluation of patients with recurrent disease.[39–41] PET/CT is often more helpful as an adjunct to conventional imaging studies in patients suspected of having metastasis, especially those with a rising CEA level.[42,43] Additionally, in patients with potentially resectable metastatic disease, PET/CT has been shown in a randomized trial to reduce the number of unnecessary laparotomies.[44]

Pelvic MRI has become the dominant modality for the preoperative locoregional staging of rectal cancer. While endorectal ultrasonography may have advantages in determining T stage in distal rectal cancers (particularly determining T1 from T2 tumors), evaluation of mesorectal nodal metastases, establishment of the status of the circumferential radial margins, and determining the relationship between the tumor and structures such as the prostate/vagina and sphincter mechanism is superior with MRI. High-resolution T2-weighted imaging (T2WI) is used because of its superior tissue contrast resolution, and is an established aspect of rectal cancer MRI examination protocols. T2WI uses a thin-section (3-mm) T2-weighted fast spin-echo sequence performed orthogonal to the tumor in the sagittal, axial, and coronal planes. The high-resolution T2WI sequences can accurately distinguish the layers of the rectal wall, tumor penetration into the wall, and the relationship between the tumor margin and the outer edge of the mesorectal envelope.[45] In low rectal cancers, additional sequences can be added to optimally depict the levator muscles, sphincter complex, intersphincteric plane, and the relationship to the rectal wall, improving visualization and operative planning and augmenting physical examination.[45] MRI T staging is based mainly on differences in T2 signal intensity among the tumor, submucosa, muscular layer, and mesorectum. The accuracy of MRI for T staging has been reported as up to 95%. Most staging failures occur in the differentiation between T2 and borderline T3 lesions or failure to distinguish mesorectal fascia tumor invasion from desmoplastic changes.[45] Synoptic Reporting Standards for Rectal MRI are outlined in **Box 1**, below.

American Joint Committee on Cancer Staging

Stage is the strongest predictor of survival for patients with colorectal cancer. The TNM (tumor, nodes, metastasis) staging system supported by the American Joint

---

Box 1
Synoptic Reporting Standards for Rectal MRI[60]

- Assessment of the safety of the TME surgical plane (radial margin, involvement of any adjacent structures such as the vagina or prostate)
- Height from puborectalis sling and anal verge; craniocaudal length
- Relationship to peritoneal reflection and seminal vesicles
- Presence/absence of extramural venous invasion
- Presence/absence of vascular mediate tumor deposits (N1c)
- Morphology (annular/semiannular/mucinous infiltrating border [smooth/nodular])
- Maximum extramural depth spread
- Presence/absence malignant lymph nodes (smooth border/uniform signal are likely benign irrespective of size)
- Minimum distance to mesorectal fascia or intersphincteric plane greater than 1 mm (MRI CRM clear)
- In final assessment, TNM stage
- In final assessment, assessment of potential resection margin involvement/safety of the TME plane (classified as potentially involved if tumor less than 1 mm to the mesorectal fascia/intersphincteric plane)

Abbreviations: CRM, circumferential resection margin; TME, total mesorectal excision; TNM, tumor, node, metastases.

Committee on Cancer/Union Internationale Contre le Cancer (AJCC/UICC) is the recommended staging system for this disease.[46] The TNM system is universally used and understood across health systems and internationally. This system is data driven and is continuously reviewed to maintain relevance and accuracy. The TNM system is based on pathologic inspection of surgical resection specimens. The T refers to depth of invasion of the primary tumor, including extension into other structures. The N refers to tumor involvement of regional lymph nodes and the lymphatic system. The M refers to metastatic disease. This system, which is summarized in **Table 1**, consists of 3

Table 1
TNM classification and staging of colorectal cancer (AJCC eighth edition)

Primary tumor staging (T)	
T0	No evidence of primary tumor
Tis	Carcinoma in situ
T1	Tumor invades submucosa
T2	Tumor invades muscularis propria
T3	Tumor invades through the muscularis propria into the pericolonic tissue
T4a	Tumor penetrates to the surface of the visceral peritoneum (serosa)
T4b	Tumor invades and/or is adherent to other organs or structures
Regional lymph node staging (N)	
N0	No regional lymph node metastasis
N1a	Metastasis in 1 regional lymph node
N1b	Metastasis in 2–3 regional lymph node
N1c	Tumor deposits in subserosa, mesentery, or nonperitonealized pericolic or perirectal tissues without regional nodal metastases
N2a	Metastasis in 4–6 regional lymph nodes
N2b	Metastasis in 7 or more regional lymph nodes
Distant metastasis staging (M)	
M0	No distant metastasis
M1a	Metastasis confined to 1 organ or site
M1b	Metastasis in more than 1 organ/site or the peritoneum

Stage	T	N	M
0	Tis	N0	M0
I	1–2	N0	M0
IIA	T3	N0	M0
IIB	T4a	N0	M0
IIC	T4b	N0	M0
IIIA	T1–T2	N1–N1c	M0
	T1	N2a	M0
IIIB	T3–T4a	N1–N1c	M0
	T2–T3	N2a	M0
	T1-2	N2b	M0
IIIC	T4a	N2a	M0
	T3–T4a	N2b	M0
	T4b	N1–N2	M0
IVA	Any T	Any N	M1a
IVB	Any T	Any N	M1b

categories: tumor depth of invasion, nodal involvement, and distant metastasis. Based on the clinical and pathologic data, the combination of these categories forms the final stage, which correlates with the overall prognosis. Recent analysis of survival outcomes in a large group of patients with invasive colon cancer from the SEER population-based database has led to the revision of the CRC TNM staging system in the eighth edition of the AJCC Cancer Staging Manual.[46] These changes include the following:

- Stage II is further subdivided into IIA (T3N0), IIB (T4aN0), and IIC (T4bN0)
- Satellite tumor deposits in the pericolonic adipose tissue are classified as N1c
- Several stage III groups have been revised based on survival outcomes
- N1 and N2 subcategories are further subdivided according to the number of involved nodes to reflect prognosis
- T4 lesions are subdivided as T4a (tumor penetrates the surface of the visceral peritoneum) and T4b (tumor directly invades adjacent organs or structures)
- M1 is subdivided into M1a (single metastatic site) and M1b (metastasis to more than one organ or the peritoneum)

The completeness of resection, or suspected completeness, should also be noted by the surgeon in the operative report:

- R0—complete tumor resection with negative margins
- R1—incomplete tumor resection with microscopic involvement of the margin
- R2—incomplete tumor resection with gross residual disease that was not resected

In addition to the aforementioned components of the TNM staging system, there are several other histologic criteria that should be routinely reported. These include histologic grade, tumor deposits, lymphovascular invasion, perineural invasion, and margin status (distal, proximal, and radial). Each of these features provides important prognostic information.

Histologic Grade

Histologic grade has consistently been shown to be a stage-independent prognostic factor and is determined by the degree of differentiation in the colon tumor. Although most systems stratify cancers into 4 grades, ranging from well differentiated (grade 1) to undifferentiated (grade 4),[47] histologic assessment is often affected by interobserver variability. Consequently, the AJCC has recommended a 2-tiered system for reporting: low grade (well and moderately differentiated) and high grade (poorly differentiated and undifferentiated).[27,47,48] This system serves to capture the actionable differences that may make a therapeutic difference. In other words, poor differentiation drives different therapeutic choices in both colon and rectal cancers, therefore specifically identifying it is most important.

There are histologic variants such as mucinous adenocarcinomas and signet ring cell adenocarcinomas that may also affect overall prognosis. Mucinous adenocarcinomas are characterized by extracellular mucin in greater than 50% of the tumor volume. When compared with conventional invasive adenocarcinomas, mucinous adenocarcinomas typically behave more aggressively, especially in patients without microsatellite instability (MSI). Signet ring cell adenocarcinomas are uncommon and carry a worse prognosis when compared with conventional adenocarcinomas.[19] These tumors are characterized histologically by greater that 50% tumors cells with signet ring features—a prominent intracytoplasmic mucin vacuole that pushes the nucleus to the periphery.[48]

Lymph Node Evaluation

Lymph node metastasis remains the single most important prognostic factor in the outcome of colon cancers.[13] The identification of at least 12 lymph nodes has been identified as a key quality indicator in the resection of colon cancers.[7] Although there are physiologic factors that influence lymph node yield, the completeness of surgical resection and thorough examination by the pathologist are also paramount. Numerous studies have shown that increasing the number of lymph nodes examined is associated with improved survival in stage II and stage III patients, primarily by providing a more accurate stage and allowing those with more advanced disease to qualify for chemotherapy.[49] Tumor deposits that are found in the pericolonic fat that do not show any evidence of residual lymph node are not counted as lymph nodes replaced by tumor and are designated as N1c. The number of these nodules should be reported because they confer a poor prognosis and alter the course of therapy postresection.[7,50]

Rectal cancers are not held to the same "12 lymph node" standards as colon cancer. Lymph node quantification in rectal cancer, particularly those treated with chemotherapy and radiation, is not as clearly defined because of the effect of treatment on the mesorectal tissue. Shrinkage and eradication of lymphatic tissue and fibrosis secondary to radiation creates an environment in which lymph node harvest is difficult. Correlation between number of lymph node harvested and outcomes is not as linear or meaningful in rectal cancer, therefore it is not used as a quality metric as it is in colon cancer. However, as mentioned earlier, the proxy for a quality rectal cancer resection is, instead, intactness of the mesorectal envelope and lack of defects in the fascia propria.[51]

Margin Status

Surgical resection with curative intent requires removal of the affected colon and rectum along with the feeding vessels and associated lymphatics, which will vary based on the location of the primary tumor. To minimize the risk of local anastomotic recurrence, a segment of normal bowel of 5 to 10 cm on the proximal and distal sides of the tumor should be achieved.[5,47,51] The radial margin is characterized by the adventitial margin closest to the deepest portion of the tumor. The visceral peritoneum is not considered a surgical margin; therefore, for sections of the colon that are completely peritonealized, the sole radial margin is the resected mesenteric margin.[47] Consequently, the reporting of this margin has limited utility for colon cancers but is critical for rectal cancers. In the case of rectal cancer, the quality of the mesorectum, degree of intactness of the fascia propria, and exact quantification of the circumferential radial margin status is essential. A positive circumferential resection margin confers a 6 times higher rate of local recurrence (5% vs 33%). The distal margins in rectal cancer are more flexible and liberally considered. A radiated rectal cancer with a distal negative margin greater than or equal to 2 mm is generally considered adequate and has been shown to be associated with good rates of recurrence-free survival.[52]

Other Prognostic Features

The presence of lymphovascular and perineural invasion has been shown to be significantly associated with poorer prognosis.[27,47,53–56] Tumor budding refers to small clusters of undifferentiated cancer cells ahead of the invasive front of the lesion. Although this is not a routinely examined pathologic parameter, there is increasing evidence that the quantitative assessment of tumor budding (with higher budding conferring a more aggressive neoplasm) reflects clinical aggressiveness of colon cancers. This has also been shown by some to be a poor prognostic feature.[47,53]

DNA Mismatch Repair/Microsatellite Instability

A germline mutation in one of the DNA MMR genes (*MLH1, MSH2, MSH6, PMS2*) is genetically characteristic of Lynch syndrome. In sporadic colon cancers, MMR defects occur in approximately 20% of cases and are generally caused by hypermethylation of *MLH1*.[3,57] Patients with dropout of *MLH1* on immunohistochemistry (IHC) can be accurately identified as either a sporadic or germline mutation by staining for *BRAF*. If *BRAF* is mutated as well, then a sporadic mutation is 96%.[58]

The presence of MMR proteins in tumor tissue can be assessed with IHC and should be done routinely in all cases of colorectal cancer in an effort to align pathology with prognosis and therapy.

MSI is another indicator of DNA repair defects caused by defective MMR proteins. MSI is typically assessed by PCR amplification of repeated single nucleotide units of DNA, or microsatellites, in tumor tissue. Tumors are characterized as MSI-high (MSI-H) or MSI-low (MSI-L) based on the number of microsatellite sequences that appear. If the tumor has 2 or more mutated sequences, it is termed MSI-H, whereas if only 1 sequence is mutated it is classified as MSI-L. Finally, if no mutation is present, then the tumor is microsatellite stable (MSS).[48,59] Recent studies demonstrate that stage II patients with MSI-H tumors did not have the same survival benefit from 5-fluorouracil-based adjuvant chemotherapy as those who had MSI-L and MSS tumors.[3,41,60–63] Because PCR-based testing is relatively slow and labor intensive, and because it correlates so well with IHC, almost all MMR protein status is determined via IHC now. Because of differences in chemosensitivity, establishment of MMR status is quite important.

SUMMARY

Colorectal tumor staging has evolved over time, but not dramatically. Refinements in our understanding of the influence of tumor genetics, and the evolution of the use of technologies like MRI for rectal cancer staging, have changed the way we evaluate and consider colon and rectal cancers in the last 10 years. CT scanning for assessment of distant disease, a good history and physical examination, and colonoscopic assessment for location still dominate our staging paradigm. The staging of colorectal cancer is a multidisciplinary endeavor. Coordination and cooperation between surgery, gastroenterology, medical oncology, pathology, and radiology are key features of successful staging of colorectal cancer and the first key step toward accurate diagnosis and treatment.

DISCLOSURE

The author has nothing to disclose.

REFERENCES

1. Cunningham D, Atkin W, Lenz HJ, et al. Colorectal cancer. Lancet 2010;375: 1030–47.
2. Haggar FA, Boushey RP. Colorectal cancer epidemiology: incidence, mortality, survival, and risk factors. Clin Colon Rectal Surg 2009;22:191–7.
3. Cappell MS. Pathophysiology, clinical presentation, and management of colon cancer. Gastroenterol Clin North Am 2008;37:1–24, v.

4. US Preventive Services Task Force, Bibbins-Domingo K, Grossman DC, Curry SJ, et al. Screening for Colorectal Cancer: US Preventive Services Task Force Recommendation Statement. JAMA 2016;315(23):2564–75. https://doi.org/10.1001/jama.2016.5989.

5. Chang GJ, Kaiser AM, Mills S, et al. Practice parameters for the management of colon cancer. Dis Colon Rectum 2012;55:831–43.

6. Aarons CB, Mahmoud NN. Current surgical considerations for colorectal cancer. Chin Clin Oncol 2013;2:14.

7. Engstrom PF, Arnoletti JP, Benson ABr, et al. NCCN Clinical Practice Guidelines in Oncology: colon cancer. J Natl Compr Canc Netw 2009;7:778–831.

8. Engstrom PF, Arnoletti JP, Benson ABr, et al. NCCN Clinical Practice Guidelines in Oncology: rectal cancer. J Natl Compr Canc Netw 2009;7:838–81.

9. Govindarajan R, Shah RV, Erkman LG, et al. Racial differences in the outcome of patients with colorectal carcinoma. Cancer 2003;97:493–8.

10. Tammana VS, Laiyemo AO. Colorectal cancer disparities: issues, controversies and solutions. World J Gastroenterol 2014;20:869–76.

11. Winawer SJ, Stewart ET, Zauber AG, et al. A comparison of colonoscopy and double-contrast barium enema for surveillance after polypectomy. National Polyp Study Work Group. N Engl J Med 2000;342:1766–72.

12. Murphy CC, Lund JL, Sandler RS. Young-Onset Colorectal Cancer: Earlier Diagnoses or Increasing Disease Burden? Gastroenterology 2017;152:1809–12.

13. Bhandari A, Woodhouse M, Gupta S. Colorectal cancer is a leading cause of cancer incidence and mortality among adults younger than 50 years in the USA: a SEER-based analysis with comparison to other young-onset cancers. J Investig Med 2017;65:311–5.

14. Murphy CC, Singal AG, Baron JA, et al. Decrease in Incidence of Young-Onset Colorectal Cancer Before Recent Increase. Gastroenterology 2018;155:1716–9.

15. Siegel RL, Fedewa SA, Anderson WF, et al. Colorectal Cancer Incidence Patterns in the United States, 1974-2013. J Natl Cancer Inst 2017;109(8):djw322.

16. Done JZ, Fang SH. Young-onset colorectal cancer: A review. World J Gastrointest Oncol 2021;13(8):856–66.

17. Moiel D, Thompson J. Early detection of colon cancer-the Kaiser Permanente Northwest 30-year history: how do we measure success? Is it the test, the number of tests, the stage, or the percentage of screen-detected patients? Perm J 2011;15:30–8.

18. Joseph DA, King JB, Miller JW, et al. Prevalence of colorectal cancer screening among adults–Behavioral Risk Factor Surveillance System, United States, 2010. MMWR Morb Mortal Wkly Rep 2012;61(Suppl):51–6.

19. Fleshman JW, Wolff BG. The ASCRS textbook of colon and rectal surgery. New York: Springer; 2007.

20. Majumdar SR, Fletcher RH, Evans AT. How does colorectal cancer present? Symptoms, duration, and clues to location. Am J Gastroenterol 1999;94:3039–45.

21. Amri R, Bordeianou LG, Sylla P, et al. Impact of screening colonoscopy on outcomes in colon cancer surgery. JAMA Surg 2013;148:747–54.

22. Lynch ML, Brand MI. Preoperative evaluation and oncologic principles of colon cancer surgery. Clin Colon Rectal Surg 2005;18:163–73.

23. Mulder SA, Kranse R, Damhuis RA, et al. Prevalence and prognosis of synchronous colorectal cancer: a Dutch population-based study. Cancer Epidemiol 2011;35:442–7.

24. Luigiano C, Ferrara F, Morace C, et al. Endoscopic tattooing of gastrointestinal and pancreatic lesions. Adv Ther 2012;29:864–73.

25. Dawson K, Wiebusch A, Thirlby RC. Preoperative tattooing and improved lymph node retrieval rates from colectomy specimens in patients with colorectal cancers. Arch Surg 2010;145:826–30.
26. Bartels SA, van der Zaag ES, Dekker E, et al. The effect of colonoscopic tattooing on lymph node retrieval and sentinel lymph node mapping. Gastrointest Endosc 2012;76:793–800.
27. Compton CC, Fielding LP, Burgart LJ, et al. Prognostic factors in colorectal cancer. College of American Pathologists Consensus Statement 1999. Arch Pathol Lab Med 2000;124:979–94.
28. Au FC, Stein BS, Gennaro AR, et al. Tissue CEA in colorectal carcinoma. Dis Colon Rectum 1984;27:16–8.
29. Fletcher RH. Carcinoembryonic antigen. Ann Intern Med 1986;104:66–73.
30. McCall JL, Black RB, Rich CA, et al. The value of serum carcinoembryonic antigen in predicting recurrent disease following curative resection of colorectal cancer. Dis Colon Rectum 1994;37:875–81.
31. Wiratkapun S, Kraemer M, Seow-Choen F, et al. High preoperative serum carcinoembryonic antigen predicts metastatic recurrence in potentially curative colonic cancer: results of a five-year study. Dis Colon Rectum 2001;44:231–5.
32. Huh JW, Oh BR, Kim HR, et al. Preoperative carcinoembryonic antigen level as an independent prognostic factor in potentially curative colon cancer. J Surg Oncol 2010;101:396–400.
33. Kirat HT, Ozturk E, Lavery IC, et al. The predictive value of preoperative carcinoembryonic antigen level in the prognosis of colon cancer. Am J Surg 2012;204:447–52.
34. Locker GY, Hamilton S, Harris J, et al. ASCO 2006 update of recommendations for the use of tumor markers in gastrointestinal cancer. J Clin Oncol 2006;24:5313–27.
35. Park IJ, Choi GS, Lim KH, et al. Serum carcinoembryonic antigen monitoring after curative resection for colorectal cancer: clinical significance of the preoperative level. Ann Surg Oncol 2009;16:3087–93.
36. Mauchley DC, Lynge DC, Langdale LA, et al. Clinical utility and cost-effectiveness of routine preoperative computed tomography scanning in patients with colon cancer. Am J Surg 2005;189:512–7 [discussion: 517].
37. Sahani DV, Bajwa MA, Andrabi Y, et al. Current status of imaging and emerging techniques to evaluate liver metastases from colorectal carcinoma. Ann Surg 2014;259:861–72.
38. Furukawa H, Ikuma H, Seki A, et al. Positron emission tomography scanning is not superior to whole body multidetector helical computed tomography in the preoperative staging of colorectal cancer. Gut 2006;55:1007–11.
39. Pelosi E, Deandreis D. The role of 18F-fluoro-deoxy-glucose positron emission tomography (FDG-PET) in the management of patients with colorectal cancer. Eur J Surg Oncol 2007;33:1–6.
40. Whiteford MH, Whiteford HM, Yee LF, et al. Usefulness of FDG-PET scan in the assessment of suspected metastatic or recurrent adenocarcinoma of the colon and rectum. Dis Colon Rectum 2000;43:759–67 [discussion: 767–70].
41. Edge SB, Byrd DR, Compton CC, et al. AJCC cancer staging manual. New York: Springer; 2010.
42. Gollub MJ, Schwartz LH, Akhurst T. Update on colorectal cancer imaging. Radiol Clin North Am 2007;45:85–118.

43. Flamen P, Hoekstra OS, Homans F, et al. Unexplained rising carcinoembryonic antigen (CEA) in the postoperative surveillance of colorectal cancer: the utility of positron emission tomography (PET). Eur J Cancer 2001;37:862–9.
44. Ruers TJ, Wiering B, van der Sijp JR, et al. Improved selection of patients for hepatic surgery of colorectal liver metastases with (18) F-FDG PET: a randomized study. J Nucl Med 2009;50:1036–41.
45. Deborah S, Keller MS. Staging of Locally Advanced Rectal Cancer Beyond TME. Clin Colon Rectal Surg 2020;33(5):258–67.
46. Amin MB, Greene FL, Edge SB, et al. The Eighth Edition AJCC Cancer Staging Manual: Continuing to build a bridge from a population-based to a more "personalized" approach to cancer staging. CA Cancer J Clin 2017;67(2):93–9.
47. Compton CC. Colorectal carcinoma: diagnostic, prognostic, and molecular features. Mod Pathol 2003;16:376–88.
48. Fleming M, Ravula S, Tatishchev SF, et al. Colorectal carcinoma: Pathologic aspects. J Gastrointest Oncol 2012;3:153–73.
49. Chang GJ, Rodriguez-Bigas MA, Skibber JM, et al. Lymph node evaluation and survival after curative resection of colon cancer: systematic review. J Natl Cancer Inst 2007;99:433–41.
50. Ueno H, Hashiguchi Y, Shimazaki H, et al. Peritumoral deposits as an adverse prognostic indicator of colorectal cancer. Am J Surg 2014;207:70–7.
51. Rullier A, Laurent C, Capdepont M, et al. Lymph nodes after preoperative chemoradiotherapy for rectal carcinoma: number, status, and impact on survival. Am J Surg Pathol 2008;32(1):45–50.
52. Nelson H, Petrelli N, Carlin A, et al. Guidelines 2000 for colon and rectal cancer surgery. J Natl Cancer Inst 2001;93:583–96.
53. Quirke P, Steele R, Monson J, et al, MRC CR07/NCIC-CTG CO16 Trial Investigators., NCRI Colorectal Cancer Study Group. Effect of the plane of surgery achieved on local recurrence in patients with operable rectal cancer: a prospective study using data from the MRC CR07 and NCIC-CTG CO16 randomised clinical trial. Lancet 2009;373(9666):821–8.
54. Aarons CB, Shanmugan S, Bleier JI. Management of malignant colon polyps: current status and controversies. World J Gastroenterol 2014;20:16178–83.
55. Bujanda L. Malignant colorectal polyps. WJG 2010;16:3103.
56. Hassan C, Zullo A, Risio M, et al. Histologic risk factors and clinical outcome in colorectal malignant polyp: a pooled-data analysis. Dis Colon Rectum 2005;48:1588–96.
57. Tominaga K, Nakanishi Y, Nimura S, et al. Predictive Histopathologic Factors for Lymph Node Metastasis in Patients With Nonpedunculated Submucosal Invasive Colorectal Carcinoma. Dis Colon Rectum 2005;48:92–100.
58. Coppede F, Lopomo A, Spisni R, et al. Genetic and epigenetic biomarkers for diagnosis, prognosis and treatment of colorectal cancer. World J Gastroenterol 2014;20:943–56.
59. Gausachs M, Mur P, Corral J, et al. MLH1 promoter hypermethylation in the analytical algorithm of Lynch syndrome: a cost-effectiveness study. Eur J Hum Genet 2012;20:762–8.
60. Kurzawski G, Suchy J, Debniak T, et al. Importance of microsatellite instability (MSI) in colorectal cancer: MSI as a diagnostic tool. Ann Oncol 2004;15(Suppl 4):iv283–4.
61. Benatti P, Gafa R, Barana D, et al. Microsatellite instability and colorectal cancer prognosis. Clin Cancer Res 2005;11:8332–40.

62. Ribic CM, Sargent DJ, Moore MJ, et al. Tumor microsatellite-instability status as a predictor of benefit from fluorouracil-based adjuvant chemotherapy for colon cancer. N Engl J Med 2003;349:247–57.
63. Adamina M, Buchs NC, Penna M, et al, St.Gallen Colorectal Consensus Expert Group. St.Gallen consensus on safe implementation of transanal total mesorectal excision. Surg Endosc 2018;32(3):1091–103.

Early-Onset Colorectal Cancer

Valentine Nfonsam, MD, MS*, Emily Wusterbarth, BS, Amanda Gong, BS, Priyanka Vij, MD

KEYWORDS

• Colorectal cancer • Microbiome • Disease monitoring • Prognosis

INTRODUCTION

Colorectal cancer (CRC) is the third most common cancer in the world and is a leading cause of morbidity and mortality.[1] In the United States, it is associated with the third highest number of new cancer diagnoses and cancer-related deaths each year.[2] Although CRC is often thought to be a disease of the elderly population, the incidence in this age group has been declining over the past 30 years.[3] This decline has been largely attributed to improved and more robust screening practices, including routine colonoscopies in patients aged 50 years, or the traditional screening age. Despite these gains made in older patients, the percentage of young patients diagnosed with early-onset CRC (EOCRC) has been steadily increasing since the 1990s.[4] The cut-off age for EOCRC is not strictly defined but is generally denoted as all CRCs diagnosed in patients younger than 50 years. There are a large number of studies on hereditary causes of young-onset CRC, such as Familial Adenomatous Polyposis and Lynch Syndrome. However, 3 of 4 individuals with EOCRC have no familial history at all.[5] Recently, owing to the trends of increasing sporadic cases, the American Cancer Society has lowered the recommended age for initial polyp screenings for average-risk individuals from age 50 to 45 years.[6] These worrying trends have also inspired countless studies aimed at uncovering the unique characteristics and clinicopathologic mechanisms underlying EOCRC as well as the factors contributing to the sharp increase in cases.

Studies have revealed EOCRC as a distinct biologic disease from late-onset CRC (LOCRC) with its own molecular, genetic, and histopathologic characteristics.[7] EOCRC is known to demonstrate patterns of invasive, aggressive behavior and overexpresses specific genes when compared with LOCRC.[8] These unique features can be used to aid in early diagnosis, prognosis, and disease course monitoring that is specific to EOCRC. They can also serve as targets of current and future treatments. Risk factors that have been implicated in EOCRC development include genetic

Department of Surgery, University of Arizona Medical Center, Tucson, AZ, USA
* Corresponding author. Department of Surgery, University of Arizona Medical Center, 1501 North Campbell Avenue, Room 4410, Tucson, AZ 85724.
E-mail address: vnfonsam@surgery.arizona.edu

predisposition, aspects of environment, dietary effects, and likely differences in the gut microbiome. The latter is a novel area of interest that is largely understudied in the current literature. The goal of this article is to provide a broad overview of EOCRC addressing several of these associated characteristics and influencing factors. In addition, differences in patient survival outcomes between EOCRC and LOCRC are also discussed.

EPIDEMIOLOGY
Overall Incidence

According to the Surveillance, Epidemiology, and End Results (SEER) database, approximately 6.8% of new CRC cases are diagnosed in patients younger than 45 years and this age group accounts for about 3.4% of total CRC-related deaths. In the 45- to 54-year-old age group, 15.1% of new CRC cases are diagnosed and this group accounts for about 9.2% of CRC-related deaths.[9] Men carry a higher probability of developing CRC than women but this only translates to a modest, if any, increase in the likelihood of development of EOCRC.[2] The increase in new cases diagnosed between the less than 45 and 45 to 54 years age groups is likely a function of screening practices rather than a characteristic of the 45- to 54-year-old age group itself. Modalities such as fecal occult blood testing, sigmoidoscopy, and colonoscopy recommended at age 45 years have the potential to identify disease that has been present asymptomatically for months to years prior. Although these new case percentages still only account for a small proportion of total CRC cases, the trend in increasing incidence rates in the younger population is concerning. EOCRC in the United States has continued to increase at a rate of about 2% per year since 1994.[10] Colon cancer rates are predicted to increase by 90% for individuals aged 20 to 34 years and by 27.7% for individuals aged 35 to 49 years by 2030. Similarly, rectal cancers are also predicted to increase by 124.2% for individuals aged 20 to 34 years and by 46% for individuals aged 35 to 49 years.[11] These large percentage jumps represent an alarming increase in the burden of illness on our patient population, medical providers, and health care system as a whole. They also serve as motivation for continued research and optimization of EOCRC diagnosis and treatment protocol. Patterns of worldwide EOCRC incidence have been studied as well and data reported in several other countries seem to mirror trends in the United States. Siegel and colleagues analyzed cancer registry data across 36 countries and found a significant increase in EOCRC incidence to be present in 19 of those countries. Korea, New Zealand, Cyprus, and United Kingdom were countries with the highest reported percent increase in cases over 10 years. Incident rates ranged 3.3% to 4.2% on average annually in these populations. A significant portion of the 19 countries were high-income countries, raising concern for early exposure to certain risk factors in these environments.[12] However, it must be considered that incidence data and reporting mechanisms may be lacking in low-middle-income countries and numbers may not be accurately reflected.

Racial and Geographic Disparities

Incidence rates differ by race and geographic region in the United States. EOCRC is known to occur at a disproportionately higher rate in minorities and uninsured populations[13] and findings of racial disparities have been demonstrated in several retrospective studies.[14–16] Acuna-Villaorduna and colleagues reviewed the SEER database from 1973 to 2010 and found that although EOCRC is still most common in Non-Hispanic Whites, it occurs at a disproportionately higher rate in Non-

Hispanic Black and Hispanic patients compared with Non-Hispanic White patients. Specific percentages listed in this study were 12.7% in Non-Hispanic Blacks versus 16.5% in Hispanics versus 8.7% in Non-Hispanic Whites.[14] Furthermore, minority groups have a higher likelihood of CRC-related death compared with Whites.[17,18] In previously published studies by Hanna and colleagues and Ewongwo and colleagues, they surveyed tumor incidence by race in the American College of Surgeons—National Surgical Improvement Program (ACS-NSQIP) database, which includes patient data from institutions across the United States and Canada. Their findings showed that patients in the early-onset category were more likely to be Black and Hispanic than late-onset patients.[15,16] Hypotheses for the increased incidence in these groups include differential exposure to risk factors, lack of access to consistent care and screening, or delay in seeking care. Future studies are needed to explore these factors and underpin concrete causes. Clinicians should be aware that disparities exist and use this information in individualized risk stratification for CRC screening. Patients in these populations should also be made aware of their increased risk so they may make informed decisions about their care and engage in preventive measures such as regular screening and modifiable risk factor reduction.

Differences in incidence rates by geographic region have also been reported across the United States. In a study by Abualkhair and colleagues analyzing cancer incidence data from 2000 to 2015 in the SEER 18 database, researchers found EOCRC incidence was highest in the South and lowest in the West with about a 36% difference between the two. Kentucky and Louisiana specifically had the highest EOCRC rates.[19] Another study by Rogers and colleagues explored EOCRC "hotspots" or areas determined to have high numbers of EOCRC-related deaths in the United States.[20] Ninety-two percent of the hotspot areas were located in the South and 8% were located in the Midwest. In examining characteristics of these areas, hotspot individuals had overall greater exposure to EOCRC risk factors than individuals in other geographic areas. Hotspots had higher rates of smoking, higher rates of obesity and sedentary lifestyle, and decreased access to healthy foods—all of which are risk factors well associated with increased risk of CRC development.[21–23] In addition, these areas have increased poverty, lower rates of insurance, and fewer primary care physicians available to the population.[20] This highlights the importance of increasing access to care and health resources in these regions.

TUMOR BIOLOGY

Many studies have examined the molecular and genetic differences in EOCRC and LOCRC, and have found that EOCRC represents a distinct biological entity.[24] Its characteristic mucinous, poorly differentiated, signet ring histology has been described extensively as a hallmark of EOCRC in the literature.[7,25–27] Additional hallmarks include more distal tumor location and later TNM stage at presentation.[7] These features illustrate the aggressive nature of EOCRC and emphasize the need for early detection and treatment to prevent progression. Particular attention has been raised in recent years to differences in gene expression and epigenetics between EOCRC and LOCRC. Several genes have been profiled for expression in early-onset tumors and findings are detailed in the following sections.

Differential Gene Expression

MSH 6 and MUTYH

Lynch syndrome is one of the most common hereditary CRC syndromes caused by mutations in DNA mismatch repair (MMR) genes.[28] A retrospective study conducted at 2 Spanish centers in 2007 performed germline genetic testing on patients with EOCRC with Lynch syndrome to determine which specific MMR genes may be implicated in the development of EOCRC. They found that mutations in the MMR gene MSH6 were most common among patients with EOCRC. The study also shed light on certain base excision repair genes, specifically MUTYH, that are more common in EOCRC than in LOCRC. The authors concluded that it may be wise to include MSH6 and MUTYH as part of the genetic panel when treating and preventing EOCRC.[29] Many other studies have also investigated MUTYH. Riegert-Johnson and colleagues further explored MUTYH by researching the value of MUTYH testing in patients with early-onset microsatellite stable CRC, and found that MUTYH mutation testing may be a reasonable test in EOCRC that is associated with proficient DNA MMR.[30] Though Lynch syndrome and the MMR pathway are important in the etiology of EOCRC, Lynch syndrome only represents 15% to 20% of the cases in this group.[31] Therefore, many studies have aimed to examine EOCRC in patients without a diagnosis of Lynch syndrome.

KRAS, BRAF, TP53, and PI3KCA

The oncogenes KRAS, BRAF, TP53, and PI3KCA have been widely studied as important players in CRC carcinogenesis.[32,33] Kirzin and colleagues investigated these genes in the context of EOCRC to assess for any patterns of differential overexpression compared with LOCRC. According to the authors, no statistically significant difference was found in the expression of KRAS, TP3, and PI3KCA.[3] However, the profile for BRAF expression was significantly different in EOCRC patients. Specifically, early-onset patients lacked BRAF mutations, whereas almost 40% of late-onset patients had BRAF mutations.[3] BRAF mutations were further examined by Perea and colleagues who defined early-onset colorectal as cancer found in individuals younger than 45 years and studied a total of 88 patients. To prevent confounding, 6 patients with familial adenomatous polyposis were excluded. Mutational analysis and molecular classification were performed for the BRAF exon 15 and the authors also found that LOCRC patients had more frequent BRAF mutations.[34]

Another study by Berg and colleagues exploring the same 4 oncogenes showed slightly different results. These authors found the same statistically significant pattern for BRAF, with older patients having more BRAF mutations. However, they also found that EOCRC patients had more frequent TP53 mutations when compared with the late-onset patients.[35] Research conducted in the Filipino community had similar findings with regards to p53. They found that younger patients with CRC (average age 30.7 years) had greater expression of p53 compared with their older counterparts (average age 67 years).[36] The difference in findings in the aforementioned studies could simply be due to differing exclusion criteria and slightly different ages used to define EOCRC and LOCRC. Nonetheless, all the studies suggest that EOCRC lacks BRAF mutations, which is important for treatment planning. BRAF-targeted treatment likely will not benefit young patients in the same way it has proved promising in the LOCRC population.

SFRP4 and COMP

Jandova and colleagues extensively studied patterns of differential overexpression between EOCRC and LOCRC, and have identified several novel genes to be uniquely overexpressed in early-onset patients.[8] Two of the most important highly expressed genes, which have served as the premise for several studies, are secreted frizzled-related protein 4 (SFRP4) and cartilage oligomeric matrix protein (COMP). Both genes have potential as EOCRC-specific targets of treatment, prognostic indicators, or markers for disease monitoring that may be superior to our current standard. They have also been significant in piecing together some of the molecular mechanisms that are contributing to the aggressive nature of EOCRC. SFRP4 is a modulator in the WNT/β-catenin signaling pathway known to function in cell proliferation and differentiation.[37] It has been found to coexpress with epithelial-mesenchymal transition (EMT) factors which contribute to cancer's ability to invade and metastasize. EOCRC patients with overexpression of this gene have associated lower survival rates when compared with those without significant SFRP4 expression.[38] COMP is a gene that codes for a glycoprotein known to participate in extracellular matrix assembly. Expression of this gene in EOCRC correlates with the Ki67 proliferation marker, tying it to cancer growth.[39] Like SFRP4, it also coexpresses with EMT factors, and its expression is increased in more aggressive molecular subtypes of colon cancer. Expression also increases sequentially as the CRC stage progresses from I to IV.[40] Higher COMP expression is associated with poorer survival outcomes in EOCRC patients.[41] COMP has shown promise as a prognostic or disease monitoring marker, given its ability to be measured in the serum.[42] It may be superior in EOCRC to our current biomarker of CRC surveillance, carcinoembryonic antigen (CEA). Future studies are required to directly compare the measurement of serum COMP to CEA before superiority may be determined.

Epigenetics

It is known that epigenetic changes are an early event involved in many different types of cancer, including CRC. Epigenetics refers to those changes that do not involve a change in any actual sequence of the gene, as the nucleotide order remains unaltered.[43] Addition or removal of methyl groups ($-CH3$) or acetylation of histones are both epigenetic changes that have been implicated in cancer development. These changes result in silencing or overexpression of a gene, and depending on the gene involved, these changes can result in oncogenesis.[43] Of interest to our current topic is that certain epigenetic changes are seen more often in EOCRC compared with LOCRC. This is significant because depending on the degree of methylation involved, different chemotherapies and treatments are of greater use.

A study by Antelo and colleagues explored how the methylation pattern of long interspersed nucleotide element-1 (LINE-1) differed in EOCRC versus LOCRC, and found that EOCRC had significantly lower LINE-1 methylation than other groups.[31] A recent review from 2019 further corroborated these findings, suggesting that LINE-1 hypomethylation should be targeted when treating EOCRC and perhaps LINE-I hypomethylation can be used as a prognostic marker for these younger patients as well.[44] On the other hand, Alvaro and colleagues found that hypermethylation at a different site may also be underlying the molecular differences in EOCRC versus LOCRC. Specifically, they found that more than 70% of EOCRC in their analysis had hypermethylation in the MLH1 promoter.[45] Miyakura and colleagues also studied the methylation patterns of the MLH1 promoter in the peripheral blood lymphocytes of 87 patients with EOCRC. Their findings corroborated those of Alvaro and colleagues.[46]

In addition to epigenetic changes, other studies have attempted to localize where in the genome the majority of differences between EOCRC and LOCRC may lie. Mourra and colleagues compared the genomic profile from EOCRC and LOCRC and found that chromosome 14 had more DNA on the tumor suppressor loci in the LOCRC group, suggesting that the loss of tumor suppressor genes in the early-onset group may be coming largely from chromosome 14. In particular, they found 2 specific deletions on chromosome 14 in the early-onset group, namely between D14S63 and D14S292.[47] Further studies are underway to elucidate if these changes are heritable.

CLINICAL BEHAVIOR
Tumor Location and Stage at Presentation

Early-onset patients have unique features of presentation compared with patients with later-onset disease. EOCRC tumors are more likely to occur in the distal colon and rectum than LOCRC tumors.[3,4,48] This has been reported in several studies and is now considered a hallmark of early-onset disease. In one study by Chang and colleagues, 80% of early-onset tumors (defined as age 40 years or younger) were found in the left colon and rectum, whereas only 58% were found in this location in the late-onset group.[26] In another study by Willauer and colleagues, the amount of distal tumors were again higher in younger age groups (74%–82% of tumors in patients younger than 50 years), and the percentages of left-sided and rectal tumors were shown to decrease with older age.[48] The location at presentation is thought to be important in determining characteristics contributing to cancer formation and progression. It also paves the way for differential treatment strategies in younger versus older patients and has been discussed in the context of adjusting screening practices. Some have suggested flexible sigmoidoscopy be used as a screening technique as early as 40 to identify left colon and rectal tumors early in their course.[49]

Identifying these tumors early is important, given the higher likelihood of invasion and metastasis in EOCRC often leading to a later stage at presentation. Chang and colleagues reported 63% of early-onset cases presented in stage III or IV versus 52% in older patients. Tumors in the younger age group were also more likely to be a high grade (27% vs 14%) and have lymphatic invasion (46% vs 37%).[26] Another study examining the SEER database from 1991 to 99 found that 56% of early-onset cases presented in stage III or IV compared with 40.1% of late-onset cases.[50] Similar results have been reported in various other studies again raising the issue of optimal screening practices.[51,52] Patients in the early-onset group are known to delay seeking care with an average time of delay being about 6.2 months.[7] Screening guidelines must be structured to limit this delay while also appropriating screening resources wisely to avoid procedural waste and afford a substantial gain in life years. Developing an algorithm that determines screening age based on the presence of several EOCRC risk factors is one model that has been proposed, and this would likely represent the most judicious approach.

Diet and the Microbiome

Understanding dietary risk factors for EOCRC, and how such factors affect gut microbiome health, can aid physicians and researchers in improving patient education and overall care. It can provide patients with valuable information to minimize the risk of cancer development through engaging in preventive behaviors. Dietary factors can also factor into determining a patient-adjusted risk profile for proper CRC screening. CRC-associated dietary risk factors have been researched extensively and shown to match risk factors for EOCRC discussed below. A paucity of data exists exploring the gut microbiome in relationship to EOCRC, indicating an important area for future research. However, the microbiome has been tied to CRC development as a whole in a few novel studies.

Dietary Factors

Nonhereditary CRC diagnoses are associated with the adoption of Western dietary risk factors, including increased processed and red meat consumption, increased excessive animal protein and fat intake, and decreased fiber intake. A balanced dietary intake of protein, fat, and fiber decreases cancer risk by leading to the production of the metabolite butyrate. This short-chain fatty acid acts as a favorable source for anti-inflammatory and antineoplastic properties, decreasing the potential for CRC formation.[53]

In a study published in Cancer Causes and Control in 2012 by Rosato and colleagues, increased consumption of processed meats was recorded to have the second highest odds ratio (OR) associated with the development of EOCRC—second only to family history.[54] This same study found an insignificant OR describing association of EOCRC with increased red meat consumption. However, many other studies have reported that EOCRC correlates with an increase in both processed and red meat consumption.[5,55,56] In a study published by Archambault and colleagues, greater red meat consumption was specifically related to a higher likelihood of EOCRC compared with LOCRC.[55]

Another factor that has been implicated in CRC diagnosis is calcium intake. In a study of 10 cohorts of primary data from 5 countries, dietary intake was measured with a food frequency questionnaire. Of the 534,536 individuals, 0.93% developed sporadic CRC within the 6- to 16-year follow-up period, displaying an inverse relationship between calcium and milk intake, and CRC incidence.[57] Chang and colleagues completed a similar study that showed a low OR for EOCRC diagnosis with calcium supplement usage.[58] A recent publication from UCLA published in 2021 has shown the importance of the prebiotic fiber inulin in calcium absorption, relaying possible protection from EOCRC inflammation and neoplasia.[59]

In a literature review published by Li and colleagues in the Journal of Cancer in 2021, sugar-sweetened beverage consumption was shown to be a risk factor for CRC diagnosis.[60] Results were corroborated by another study published by Hur and colleagues in 2021, illustrating sugar-sweetened drinks to be a risk factor in EOCRC for women, with 2 or more servings per day doubling the risk of EOCRC.[58,61] Replacement of a sugar-sweetened beverage with milk had a lowered risk of EOCRC.[61] Furthermore, 2 studies published in 2021 provided evidence that a high intake of sugary beverages in adolescent years increases the risk for adenomas, but this same consumption of sugary beverage intake in adulthood is not associated with an increased risk of adenomas.[61,62]

Alcohol intake and its association with CRC have been the subject of several research projects. A study published by Ferrarri and colleagues in the International Journal of Cancer found a positive association between lifetime alcohol intake and CRC development. A total of 478,732 individuals were followed up for 6.2 years, after which 1833 CRC diagnoses were made. Of the patients who received CRC diagnoses, 1447 (69% of CRC cases) were lifetime alcohol consumers. Both lifetime and baseline (recent) alcohol consumers had a higher risk for rectum cancers than colon cancers.[63] Increased length of time and amount of alcohol consumption (more than 100g per week), particularly in conjunction with tobacco usage or obesity, has been implicated as a factor increasing EOCRC occurrence. According to The World Cancer Research Fund/American Institute for Cancer Research, every additional 10g in daily alcohol intake past 30g daily increases CRC risk by 7%.[64] Another study found the OR of alcohol use and EOCRC compared to LOCRC was 1.71. In an analysis of patients based on age, individuals with current usage of alcohol alone were associated with onset at 61.1 years, whereas the average age of nonusers was 67.7 years.[65]

Overall, alcohol usage has been implicated in a higher risk for developing CRC, specifically in early-onset populations, and can be targeted as a modifiable risk factor in preventive care. Intake of processed meats and sugar-sweetened drinks are also modifiable risk factors in cancer development while calcium intake may have some protective effect.

Gut Microbiome

The microbiome and its relationship to cancer development is a topic that has gained traction in recent years. The microbiomes of CRC patients have been shown to possess decreased microbial diversity and altered taxonomy of bacteria and viruses. In a comparison study of healthy and CRC patient stool samples to investigate the gut microbiome and microbial interactions, *Escherichia viruses*, *Salmonella viruses*, and bacteria that reside in the oral cavity, such as *Fusobacterium nucleatum*, *Fusobacterium hwasookii*, *Porphyromonas gingivalis*, and *Bacteroides fragilis*, were increased in CRC patients. However, select phages, such as *Enterobacteria phages*, butyrate-producing microbes, and anti-inflammatory microbes, were decreased in adenoma and CRC patients. The data also showed a negative association between healthy gut bacteria and viruses in CRC patients.[66]

   F nucleatum, a gram-negative obligate anaerobic species in the *Bacteroidaceae* family, has been reported to be present at higher levels in CRC tumor tissue compared with adjacent normal tissue.[67] Several studies have examined *F nucleatum* amount by age group, but statistically significant results correlating its presence to age have not been established.[68] Studies directly investigating *F nucleatum* and the microbiome as whole in EOCRC specifically are lacking. In a study conducted by Tahara and colleagues, the average age of the study population was more than 60 years and a trend was identified showing greater amounts of *F nucleatum* in patients older than 70 years.[69] This may indicate that *F nucleatum* is associated with LOCRC pathogenesis. In addition, the proportion of *F nucleatum* present by tumor location was reported by Mima and colleagues, and data showed higher proportions in right-sided tumors than left-sided tumors.[70] Since most EOCRC tumors occur distally, this again supports *F nucleatum* as a feature of the older disease. The *Bifidobacterium* genus has also been studied in relation to CRC and is thought to play a role in antitumor immunity. It is associated with the presence of signet ring cells, which are a prominent feature of EOCRC and may indicate a tie to the early-onset disease process.[71]

PATIENT OUTCOMES

Survival outcomes of patients with EOCRC and LOCRC have been compared in several populations and conflicting data exist in the literature depending on the outcome measures included. In 2 published studies by Hanna and Ewongwo, they specifically examined short-term surgical outcomes, which have not been well reported elsewhere. Outcomes included hospital length of stay, 30-day complications, 30-day mortality, 90-day mortality, and 30-day readmission rates. Two of our studies analyzing the ACS-NSQIP database did not find a difference between surgical outcomes of EOCRC and LOCRC patients.[15,16] However, in one of our current projects surveying the National Cancer Database from 2004 to 2017, we did find a decrease in 30-day (OR 0.37, confidence interval [CI] 0.34–0.40) and 90-day mortality (OR 0.47, CI 0.43–0.49) in the early-onset group. This retrospective review included more patients than the previous studies, which could account for the discrepancy in the results. However, further research on short-term outcomes is required before a clear consensus can be reached.

   Several other groups have examined long-term survival outcomes comparing EOCRC and LOCRC patients. Overall, the results in the literature are inconsistent and seem to depend on the exact age groups and survival measures included in the analysis. Mauri and colleagues performed a systematic review of 37 articles comparing such outcomes and reported that patients younger than 50 years carried a favorable prognosis when directly compared with those older than 50 years.[72]

This included improved stage-specific relative survival[73] and CRC-specific survival.[74] In examining age-specific survival data, Kolarich and colleagues found no significant difference in survival when comparing various age groups.[75] In another study by Zabrowski and colleagues, 5-year overall survival was improved in the early-onset group after surgical resection, whereas 5-year disease-free survival was 81% in both the younger and older age groups.[76] Improved overall survival in the younger-onset patient group is often attributed to decreased comorbidities and the use of more aggressive therapies in the younger population. Surgical resection may be pursued more readily in younger patients because of perceived better tolerance of treatment and more aggressive neoadjuvant or adjuvant treatment modalities may be used.[77] In the context of the invasive nature of EOCRC, adjuvant therapy is often favored to target potential micrometastases that may be present but undetectable by diagnostic methods.[78] However, aggressive adjuvant treatment in this early-onset group has been analyzed in several studies and does not correlate with any true survival benefit.[73,75,79,80] Similar findings were demonstrated with aggressive use of neoadjuvant therapies.[7] The absence of survival benefit does call for a more careful consideration of who should receive each treatment rather than an all-encompassing approach. Overtreatment is associated with greater exposure to the harsh side effects of chemotherapy and radiation, leading to potential lifelong complications in these patients. These risks and recent findings of the absence of true survival gain should serve as a guide for clinical practice moving forward.

REFERENCES

1. Ferlay J, Parkin DM, Steliarova-Foucher E. Estimates of cancer incidence and mortality in Europe in 2008. Eur J Cancer 2010;46(4):765–81.
2. Siegel RL, Miller KD, Fuchs HE, et al. Cancer Statistics, 2021. CA: a Cancer J clinicians 2021;71(1):7–33.
3. Kirzin S, Marisa L, Guimbaud R, et al. Sporadic early-onset colorectal cancer is a specific Sub-Type of cancer: a Morphological, molecular and genetics study. In: Cheah PY, editor. PLoS ONE 2014;9(8):e103159.
4. Siegel RL, Jemal A, Ward EM. Increase in Incidence of Colorectal Cancer Among Young Men and Women in the United States. Cancer Epidemiol Prev Biomarkers 2009;18(6):1695–8.
5. Stoffel EM, Murphy CC. Epidemiology and Mechanisms of the Increasing Incidence of Colon and Rectal Cancers in Young Adults. Gastroenterology 2020; 158(2):341.
6. Wolf AMD, Fontham ETH, Church TR, et al. Colorectal cancer screening for average-risk adults: 2018 guideline update from the American Cancer Society. CA: A Cancer J Clinicians 2018;68(4):250–81.
7. Collaborative R, Zaborowski AM, Abdile A, et al. Characteristics of Early-Onset vs Late-Onset Colorectal Cancer: A Review. JAMA Surg 2021;156(9):865–74.
8. Jandova J, Xu W, Nfonsam V. Sporadic early-onset colon cancer expresses unique molecular features. J Surg Res 2016;204(1):251–60.
9. Colorectal Cancer — Cancer Stat Facts. Available at: https://seer.cancer.gov/statfacts/html/colorect.html. Accessed August 15, 2021.
10. Siegel RL, Miller KD, Jemal A. Cancer statistics, 2018. CA: A Cancer J Clinicians 2018;68(1):7–30.
11. Bailey CE, Hu C-Y, You YN, et al. Increasing Disparities in Age-Related Incidence of Colon and Rectal Cancer in the United States, 1975-2010. JAMA Surg 2015; 150(1):17.

12. Siegel RL, Torre LA, Soerjomataram I, et al. Global patterns and trends in colorectal cancer incidence in young adults. Gut 2019;68(12):2179–85.

13. You YN, Xing Y, Feig BW, et al. Young-Onset Colorectal Cancer: Is It Time to Pay Attention? Arch Intern Med 2012;172(3):287–9.

14. Acuna-Villaorduna AR, Lin J, Kim M, et al. Racial/ethnic disparities in early-onset colorectal cancer: implications for a racial/ethnic-specific screening strategy. Cancer Med 2021;10(6):2080.

15. Hanna K, Zeeshan M, Hamidi M, et al. Colon cancer in the young: contributing factors and short-term surgical outcomes. Int J Colorectal Dis 2019;34(11):1879–85.

16. Ewongwo A, Hamidi M, Alattar Z, et al. Contributing factors and short-term surgical outcomes of patients with early-onset rectal cancer. Am J Surg 2020;219(4):578–82.

17. Wang W, Chen W, Lin J, et al. Incidence and characteristics of young-onset colorectal cancer in the United States: An analysis of SEER data collected from 1988 to 2013. Clin Res Hepatol Gastroenterol 2019;43(2):208–15.

18. Rahman R, Schmaltz C, Jackson CS, et al. Increased risk for colorectal cancer under age 50 in racial and ethnic minorities living in the United States. Cancer Med 2015;4(12):1863.

19. Abualkhair WH, Zhou M, Ochoa CO, et al. Geographic and intra-racial disparities in early-onset colorectal cancer in the SEER 18 registries of the United States. Cancer Med 2020;9(23):9150.

20. Rogers CR, Moore JX, Qeadan F, et al. Examining factors underlying geographic disparities in early-onset colorectal cancer survival among men in the United States. Am J Cancer Res 2020;10(5):1592. Available at: /pmc/articles/PMC7269786/. Accessed September 29, 2021.

21. Marchand L Le, Wilkens LR, Kolonel LN, et al. Associations of Sedentary Lifestyle, Obesity, Smoking, Alcohol Use, and Diabetes with the Risk of Colorectal Cancer. Cancer Res 1997;57(21).

22. Tsoi KKF, CYY Pau, Wu WKK, et al. Cigarette Smoking and the Risk of Colorectal Cancer: A Meta-analysis of Prospective Cohort Studies. Clin Gastroenterol Hepatol 2009;7(6):682–8.e5.

23. Giovannucci E, Ascherio A, Rimm EB, et al. Physical activity, obesity, and risk for colon cancer and adenoma in men. Ann Intern Med 1995;122(5):327–34.

24. Boardman LA, Johnson RA, Petersen GM, et al. Higher Frequency of Diploidy in Young-Onset Microsatellite-Stable Colorectal Cancer. Clin Cancer Res 2007;13(8):2323–8.

25. Davis DM, Marcet JE, Frattini JC, et al. Is it time to lower the recommended screening age for colorectal cancer? J Am Coll Surg 2011;213(3):352–61.

26. Chang DT, Pai RK, Rybicki LA, et al. Clinicopathologic and molecular features of sporadic early-onset colorectal adenocarcinoma: An adenocarcinoma with frequent signet ring cell differentiation, rectal and sigmoid involvement, and adverse morphologic features. Mod Pathol 2012;25(8):1128–39.

27. Myers EA, Feingold DL, Forde KA, et al. Colorectal cancer in patients under 50 years of age: A retrospective analysis of two institutions' experience. World J Gastroenterol 2013;19(34):5651–7.

28. Jasperson KW, Vu TM, Schwab AL, et al. Evaluating Lynch syndrome in very early onset colorectal cancer probands without apparent polyposis. Fam Cancer 2010;9(2):99.

29. Giráldez MD, Balaguer F, Bujanda L, et al. MSH6 and MUTYH Deficiency Is a Frequent Event in Early-Onset Colorectal Cancer. Clin Cancer Res : official J Am Assoc Cancer Res 2010;16(22):5402.

30. Riegert-Johnson DL, Johnson RA, Rabe KG, et al. The Value of MUTYH Testing in Patients with Early Onset Microsatellite Stable Colorectal Cancer Referred for Hereditary Nonpolyposis Colon Cancer Syndrome Testing. Genet Test 2008;11(4): 361–5. Available at: https://www.liebertpub.com/gte.

31. Antelo M, Balaguer F, Shia J, et al. A High Degree of LINE-1 Hypomethylation Is a Unique Feature of Early-Onset Colorectal Cancer. PLoS ONE 2012;7(9):45357.

32. Yokota T. Are KRAS/BRAF Mutations Potent Prognostic and/or Predictive Biomarkers in Colorectal Cancers? Anti-Cancer Agents Med Chem 2012;12(2):163.

33. Baviskar T, Momin M, Liu J, et al. Target Genetic Abnormalities for the Treatment of Colon Cancer and Its Progression to Metastasis. Curr Drug Targets 2020;22(7): 722–33.

34. Perea J, Rueda D, Canal A, et al. Age at Onset Should Be a Major Criterion for Subclassification of Colorectal Cancer. J Mol Diagn 2014;16(1):116–26.

35. Berg M, Danielsen SA, Ahlquist T, et al. DNA Sequence Profiles of the Colorectal Cancer Critical Gene Set KRAS-BRAF-PIK3CA-PTEN-TP53 Related to Age at Disease Onset. PLoS ONE 2010;5(11):e13978.

36. Uy GB, Kaw LL, Punzalan CK, et al. Clinical and molecular biologic characteristics of early-onset versus late-onset colorectal carcinoma in Filipinos. World J Surg 2004;28(2):117–23.

37. Ford CE, Jary E, Ma SSQ, et al. The Wnt Gatekeeper SFRP4 Modulates EMT, Cell Migration and Downstream Wnt Signalling in Serous Ovarian Cancer Cells. In: Samant R, editor. PLoS ONE 2013;8(1):e54362.

38. Nfonsam LE, Jandova J, Jecius HC, et al. SFRP4 expression correlates with epithelial mesenchymal transitionlinked genes and poor overall survival in colon cancer patients. World J Gastrointest Oncol 2019;11(8):589–98.

39. Nfonsam VN, Jecius H C, Janda J, et al. Cartilage oligomeric matrix protein (COMP) promotes cell proliferation in early-onset colon cancer tumorigenesis. 1:3. doi:10.1007/s00464-019-07185-z

40. Wusterbarth E, Chen Y, Jecius H, et al. Cartilage Oligomeric Matrix Protein, COMP may be a better prognostic marker than CEACAM5 and correlates with colon cancer molecular subtypes, tumor aggressiveness and overall survival. J Surg Res 2021;270:169–77.

41. Nfonsam VN, Nfonsam LE, Chen D, et al. COMP gene coexpresses with EMT genes and is associated with poor survival in colon cancer patients. J Surg Res 2019;233:297–303.

42. Papadakos KS, Darlix A, Jacot W, et al. High Levels of Cartilage Oligomeric Matrix Protein in the Serum of Breast Cancer Patients Can Serve as an Independent Prognostic Marker. Front Oncol 2019;9(OCT):1141.

43. Babaei K, Khaksar R, Zeinali T, et al. Epigenetic profiling of MUTYH, KLF6, WNT1 and KLF4 genes in carcinogenesis and tumorigenesis of colorectal cancer. BioMedicine 2019;9(4):1–9.

44. Strum WB, Boland CR. Clinical and Genetic Characteristics of Colorectal Cancer in Persons under 50 Years of Age: A Review. Dig Dis Sci 2019;64(11):3059–65.

45. Álvaro E, Cano JM, García JL, et al. Clinical and Molecular Comparative Study of Colorectal Cancer Based on Age-of-Onset and Tumor Location: Two Main Criteria for Subclassifying Colorectal Cancer. Int J Mol Sci 2019;20(4). https://doi.org/10.3390/IJMS20040968.

46. Miyakura Y, Sugano K, Akasu T, et al. Extensive but hemiallelic methylation of the hMLH1 promoter region in early-onset sporadic colon cancers with microsatellite instability. Clin Gastroenterol Hepatol 2004;2(2):147–56.
47. Najat M, Guy Z, Bruno B, et al. High frequency of chromosome 14 deletion in early-onset colon cancer. Dis colon rectum 2007;50(11):1881–6.
48. Willauer AN, Liu Y, Pereira AAL, et al. Clinical and molecular characterization of early-onset colorectal cancer. Cancer 2019;125(12):2002.
49. Weinberg BA, Marshall JL. Colon Cancer in Young Adults: Trends and Their Implications. Curr Oncol Rep 2019;21(1):1–7.
50. O'Connell JB, Maggard MA, Liu JH, et al. Do Young Colon Cancer Patients Have Worse Outcomes? World J Surg 2004;28(6):558–62.
51. Saraste D, Järås J, Martling A. Population-based analysis of outcomes with early-age colorectal cancer. Br J Surg 2020;107(3):301–9.
52. Liang JT, Huang KC, Cheng AL, et al. Clinicopathological and molecular biological features of colorectal cancer in patients less than 40 years of age. Br J Surg 2003;90(2):205–14.
53. Yang J, Yu J. The association of diet, gut microbiota and colorectal cancer: what we eat may imply what we get. Protein & Cell 2018;9(5):474.
54. Rosato V, Bosetti C, Levi F, et al. Risk factors for young-onset colorectal cancer. Cancer Causes & Control 2012;24(2):335–41.
55. Archambault AN, Lin Y, Jeon J, et al. Nongenetic Determinants of Risk for Early-Onset Colorectal Cancer. JNCI Cancer Spectr 2021;5(3). https://doi.org/10.1093/JNCICS/PKAB029.
56. Hofseth LJ, Hebert JR, Chanda A, et al. Early-onset colorectal cancer: initial clues and current views. Nat Rev Gastroenterol Hepatol 2020;17(6):352–64.
57. Cho E, Smith-Warner SA, Spiegelman D, et al. Dairy Foods, Calcium, and Colorectal Cancer: A Pooled Analysis of 10 Cohort Studies. JNCI: J Natl Cancer Inst 2004;96(13):1015–22.
58. Chang VC, Cotterchio M, De P, et al. Risk factors for early-onset colorectal cancer: a population-based case–control study in Ontario, Canada. Cancer Causes & Control 2021;32(10):1063–83.
59. Yoon LS, Michels KB. Characterizing the Effects of Calcium and Prebiotic Fiber on Human Gut Microbiota Composition and Function Using a Randomized Crossover Design—A Feasibility Study. Nutrients 2021;13(6):1937.
60. Li Y, Guo L, He K, et al. Consumption of sugar-sweetened beverages and fruit juice and human cancer: A systematic review and dose-response meta-analysis of observational studies. J Cancer 2021;12(10):3077–88.
61. Hur J, Otegbeye E, Joh H-K, et al. Sugar-sweetened beverage intake in adulthood and adolescence and risk of early-onset colorectal cancer among women. Gut 2021. https://doi.org/10.1136/GUTJNL-2020-323450.
62. Joh H-K, Lee DH, Hur J, et al. Simple Sugar and Sugar-Sweetened Beverage Intake During Adolescence and Risk of Colorectal Cancer Precursors. Gastroenterology 2021;161(1):128–42.e20.
63. Ferrari P, Jenab M, Norat T, et al. Lifetime and baseline alcohol intake and risk of colon and rectal cancers in the European prospective investigation into cancer and nutrition (EPIC). Int J Cancer 2007;121(9):2065–72.
64. Scherübl H. Alcohol Use and Gastrointestinal Cancer Risk. Visc Med 2020;36(3):175–81.
65. Rueda M, Robertson Y, Acott A, et al. Association of tobacco and alcohol use with earlier development of colorectal pathology: should screening guidelines be modified to include these risk factors? Am J Surg 2012;204(6):963–8.

66. Gao R, Zhu Y, Kong C, et al. Alterations, Interactions, and Diagnostic Potential of Gut Bacteria and Viruses in Colorectal Cancer. Front Cell Infect Microbiol 2021; 11:657867.
67. Mehta RS, Nishihara R, Cao Y, et al. Association of Dietary Patterns With Risk of Colorectal Cancer Subtypes Classified by Fusobacterium nucleatum in Tumor Tissue. JAMA Oncol 2017;3(7):921–7.
68. Mukherji R, Weinberg BA. The gut microbiome and potential implications for early-onset colorectal cancer 2020;9(3):CRC25.
69. Tahara T, Yamamoto E, Suzuki H, et al. Fusobacterium in Colonic Flora and Molecular Features of Colorectal Carcinoma. Cancer Res 2014;74(5):1311–8.
70. Mima K, Sukawa Y, Nishihara R, et al. Fusobacterium nucleatum and T Cells in Colorectal Carcinoma. JAMA Oncol 2015;1(5):653–61.
71. Kosumi K, Hamada T, Koh H, et al. The Amount of Bifidobacterium Genus in Colorectal Carcinoma Tissue in Relation to Tumor Characteristics and Clinical Outcome. Am J Pathol 2018;188(12):2839.
72. Mauri G, Sartore-Bianchi A, Russo A, et al. Early-onset colorectal cancer in young individuals. Mol Oncol 2019;13(2):109.
73. Kneuertz PJ, Chang GJ, Hu C-Y, et al. Overtreatment of Young Adults With Colon Cancer: More Intense Treatments With Unmatched Survival Gains. JAMA Surg 2015;150(5):402–9.
74. Wang R, Wang M-J, Ping J. Clinicopathological Features and Survival Outcomes of Colorectal Cancer in Young Versus Elderly: A Population-Based Cohort Study of SEER 9 Registries Data (1988–2011). Medicine 2015;94(35):e1402.
75. Kolarich A, George TJ, Hughes SJ, et al. Rectal cancer patients younger than 50 years lack a survival benefit from NCCN guideline–directed treatment for stage II and III disease. Cancer 2018;124(17):3510–9.
76. Zaborowski AM, Murphy B, Creavin B, et al. Clinicopathological features and oncological outcomes of patients with young-onset rectal cancer. Br J Surg 2020;107(5):606–12.
77. Abdelsattar ZM, Wong SL, Regenbogen SE, et al. Colorectal cancer outcomes and treatment patterns in patients too young for average-risk screening. Cancer 2016;122(6):929–34.
78. Adjuvant therapy for resected colon cancer in older adult patients - UpToDate. Available at: https://www-uptodate-com.ezproxy2.library.arizona.edu/contents/adjuvant-therapy-for-resected-colon-cancer-in-older-adult-patients?search=Adjuvant.therapy for resected colon cancer in older adult patients&source=search_result&selectedTitle=1~150&usage_type=default&display_rank=1. Accessed September 15, 2021.
79. Manjelievskaia J, Brown D, McGlynn KA, et al. Chemotherapy Use and Survival Among Young and Middle-Aged Patients With Colon Cancer. JAMA Surg 2017; 152(5):452–9.
80. Burnett-Hartman AN, Powers JD, Chubak J, et al. Treatment patterns and survival differ between early-onset and late-onset colorectal cancer patients: the patient outcomes to advance learning network. Cancer Causes & Control 2019;30(7):747–55.

Healthcare Disparities and Colorectal Cancer

Robert H. Hollis, MD, MSPH, Daniel I. Chu, MD, MSPH*

KEYWORDS

- Healthcare disparities • Racial disparities • Colorectal cancer • Colon cancer
- Rectal cancer

KEY POINTS

- Health care disparities in colorectal cancer continue to exist
- Disparities in colorectal cancer mortality may be attributable to gaps in prevention, detection, stage at presentation, treatment, and/or posttreatment surveillance.
- Underlying reasons for racial disparities in colorectal cancer can be tied to patient, provider, health care system, and policy-level factors.
- Interventions to address disparities in colorectal cancer need to be multilevel.

INTRODUCTION

In 2021 it is estimated that there will be 150,000 new diagnoses of colorectal cancer in the United States, and 53,000 patients will die from colorectal cancer.[1] The burden of new colorectal cancer diagnoses and subsequent mortality will not be equally shared among all individuals. Specific, often disadvantaged, groups of individuals will experience higher rates of new colon cancer and be at higher risk of subsequent mortality. Health care disparities are defined as differences in health outcomes that are associated with characteristics of persons often represented by social and/or economic disadvantages.[2] Common examples include differences in one's health by race, geography, sexual orientation, religion, income, or disability.

Efforts to eliminate these disparities and to remove the unfair burden carried by certain groups are synonymous with efforts to promote health equity. In this review, we will highlight (1) healthcare disparities that exist in the prevention, treatment, and outcomes of colorectal cancer, (2) potential reasons for why these health care disparities exist, and (3) potential interventions to address these disparities in the future. While many different types of disparities exist, this review will focus on racial disparities in colon and rectal cancer. More specifically, our focus will be on health care disparities experienced by Black patients in the United States given that this population

Department of Surgery, Division of Gastrointestinal Surgery, University of Alabama at Birmingham, 1720 2nd Avenue S, Birmingham, AL 35209, USA
* Corresponding author.
E-mail address: dchu@uabmc.edu

Surg Oncol Clin N Am 31 (2022) 157–169
https://doi.org/10.1016/j.soc.2021.11.002
surgonc.theclinics.com

has the highest incidence and mortality rate for colorectal cancer compared with other racial/ethnic groups.[3,4]

BACKGROUND
Disparities in Colorectal Cancer Incidence

Data from National Cancer Registries between 2012 and 2016 show that Black patients have an almost 20% higher incidence of colorectal cancer compared with non-Hispanic White (NHW) patients (age-adjusted incident rate for Blacks: 45.7 vs 38.6 per 100,000 for NHW).[5] These rates are even more pronounced in Black men who have an age-adjusted rate of colorectal cancer of 53.8 per 100,000 compared with 44.0 in NHW men.[5] Incidence rates of colorectal cancer over time by race are shown in **Fig. 1**. Notably, rates of colorectal cancer have been significantly declining over time with the uptake of screening colonoscopies. However, the rate of decline was not equally shared over time with patients with NHW experiencing earlier declines in the 2000s compared with Black patients.[5]

While earlier reports highlighted increased rates of new colorectal cancers in young Black patients less than age 50, the incidence rates are now similar to NHW for this age group.[5] The latest data from the Surveillance, Epidemiology, and End Results Program (SEER) in 2018 report overall incidence rates for Black patients at 39.8 per 100,000 patients versus 36.4 for patients with NHW.[6] The causes for disparities in colorectal cancer incidence are complex and may be related to variations in risk factors including socioeconomic factors, health behaviors (ie, tobacco use, physical activity), comorbidities (ie, obesity), the utilization of preventative screening measures, and less clear genetic susceptibilities.

Disparities in Colorectal Cancer Mortality

Compared with differences in incidence, there is a more striking 38% difference in mortality for Black patients than patients with NHW during years 2013 to 2017 (age-adjusted mortality rate for Blacks: 19.0 vs 13.8 per 100,000 for NHW).[5] This mortality rate was highest among Black men at 23.8 per 100,000.[5] SEER rates of mortality from colorectal cancers over time are shown in **Fig. 2**.[6] Similar to incidence rates, mortality rates have decreased over time. This change has been attributed to improvement in modifiable risk factors and preventative measures; however, differences in mortality still exist by race.

The latest data from the SEER Program show that Black patients have an age-adjusted mortality rate of 16.8 per 100,000 patients than 13.1 patients with NHW.[6,7]

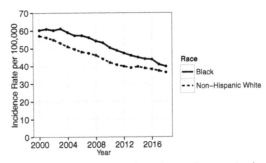

Fig. 1. Age-adjusted incidence rates by race for colorectal cancer in the United States over time. (*From* https://seer.cancer.gov/explorer)

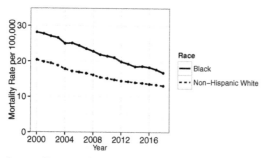

Fig. 2. Age-adjusted mortality rates by race for colorectal cancer in the United States over time. (*From* https://seer.cancer.gov/explorer)

Even in young patients with early-stage disease, Black patients have been shown to consistently have higher mortality rates compared with patients with NHW.[8] The causes for disparities in mortality parallel those factors influencing the incidence of colorectal cancer and likely include factors at the patient, provider, health care system, and policy-levels which in turn influence early detection and treatment.

Disparities in Colorectal Cancer Screening

Colorectal cancer screening allows for removal of polyps to reduce the development and thus the incidence of colorectal cancer as well as allows for the early identification of malignant lesions to reduce subsequent mortality.[9] This knowledge has led to a rapid uptake of colorectal cancer screening in the 2000s with a goal set by the Healthy People 2020 campaign to achieve 70% screening rates among eligible patients aged 50 to 75.[5] Using data from the National Health Interview Study (NHIS), 52% of eligible patients met colorectal cancer screening guidelines in 2008 and this increased to 66% by 2018.[10] Among Black patients the percent meeting screening guidelines increased from 48% in 2008% to 67% in 2018, while among White patients the percentage increased from 53% to 67%.[10] Compared with cancer screening for breast, cervical, and prostate cancer, colorectal cancer was the only screening that increased in use between 2000 and 2015.[11]

While overall screening rates for patients with colorectal cancer are improving, there are still specific populations of Black patients that fail to receive appropriate screening and remain at elevated risk. Notably, in 2018, data from the NHIS show that only 34% of the uninsured population is up-to-date with age-appropriate colorectal cancer screening.[10] Data from the Southern Community Cohort Study (SCCS) report further screening inequities. The SCCS included 47,596 patients between 2002 and 2009 with most patients receiving care in federally supported community health centers in the southeastern United States. The participants included 68% who were Black and 55% with annual household income <$15,000. The study showed that in this disadvantaged group of patients there were significantly lower rates of any colorectal cancer screening in Black (34%) compared with White patients (40%).[12] Data from the same cohort have shown that Black patients with increased risk due to a first-degree relative history of colorectal cancer are less likely to undergo high-risk age-appropriate or interval-specific screening protocols.[13] Black patients are also more likely to undergo endoscopy by lower quality providers with lower polyp detection rates (PDRs) and are at higher risk for the development of interval cancers.[14]

Many factors contribute to delayed screening. Key access issues include patient-related factors such as lack of knowledge, perceived benefits, and perceived susceptibility in addition to barriers in costs, time, availability, and transportation.[7,15] Focus groups among Black patients who have undergone colonoscopy screening shows that facilitators of successful screening include social/community support, religion, and having a recommendation for screening from their provider.[16] In a study of patients with nonadherence to colorectal screening guidelines in California, 19% of participants reported nonadherence due to the lack of physician recommendation, and Black patients had 1.5 times higher odds of lack of physician recommendation as the reason for nonadherence compared with White patients.[17]

While increased screening can be a viable means to reduce incidence and mortality in colorectal cancer, it will not explain all these disparities. In a simulation of outcomes in colorectal cancer between 1975 and 2007 whereby screening patterns for White patients were applied to Black patients, it was estimated that 42% of the disparity in colorectal cancer incidence and 19% of the disparity in mortality can be explained by differences in screening.[18] Following the detection of abnormal endoscopic findings, Black patients struggle more than White patients to achieve appropriate follow-up care.[19] These breakdowns in care from early detection to treatment can be directly attributable to delays in care with more advanced stage presentation. Furthermore, following treatment of colorectal cancer Black patients are 38% less likely to have appropriate surveillance screening colonoscopy interval at 1, 3, or 5 years.[20]

Disparities in Stage at Presentation

Stage at presentation has been shown to be one of the largest factors contributing to racial differences in mortality.[21] The National Cancer Institute Black/White Cancer Survival Study longitudinally followed patients diagnosed with colon cancer between years 1985 to 1986 to determine what features might explain the Black/White mortality disparity.[22] The authors found a 50% higher mortality among Blacks than Whites at 5-year follow-up, and adjustment for stage at presentation reduced this to a 20% difference in mortality (60% reduction).[23] Further adjustment for socioeconomic factors did not further reduce the mortality difference, suggesting that socioeconomic factors were a significant mediator for the stage difference. In this study Black/White mortality disparities were largely driven by mortality differences for stage II/III disease.[23] Later studies have suggested that disparities in stage IV disease mortality rates contribute up to 60% of overall Black/white mortality differences.[24] Thus, both higher stage at presentation and higher stage-specific mortality contribute to overall mortality differences.[25] Timely screening remains an important mechanism to prevent late-stage presentation and its impact on mortality.[26]

Disparities in Treatment

Differences in stage-specific survival are less likely to explain by screening strategies, and studies have increasingly focused on treatment differences between populations. In an analysis of factors contributing to disparities in colorectal cancer mortality in the California Cancer Registry between 1993 and 2004, the addition of treatment (surgery, chemotherapy, radiation) significantly reduced the Black–White differences in mortality even after controlling for demographics and stage at presentation.[27] The impact of treatment on mortality disparities may be due to the effectiveness of treatment, the receipt of treatment, the timeliness of treatment, and/or the quality of treatment received.

In the controlled setting of clinical trials, the effectiveness of treatment of both Black and White patients with colorectal cancer has been supported. For example, for patients with advanced stage colorectal cancer who were treated in the Southwest

Oncology Group randomized control trial of the addition of cetuximab or bevacizumab to 5-fluorouracil (5-FU), oxaliplatin, and leucovorin (FOLFOX) or 5-FU, irinotecan, and leucovorin (FOLFIRI) chemotherapy, there were no significant differences between Black and White patients in either overall survival at 7 years or response to treatment when matched on trial covariates.[28] Similar results have been found in earlier trials of 5-FU in early-stage colon cancer.[29] However, analysis of pooled data from 12 clinical trials of standardized adjuvant chemotherapy between 1977 and 2002 for early-stage colon cancer in North America found that Black patients had worse overall and recurrence-free survival yet similar timing to recurrence between races.[30] These findings suggest that the effectiveness of the chemotherapy was likely similar among groups given similar time to recurrence. However, the authors suggest that the differences in long term survival may be more attributed to other health care disparities impacting mortality outside of the clinical trial (ie, impact of social determinants of health and ability to receive salvage therapy).[30]

Patients must first receive therapy for it to be effective, and several studies have revealed that Black patients are less likely to undergo surgery for resectable cancers, receive adjuvant chemotherapy, or undergo radiation for rectal cancer.[15,31–33] While patient refusal has been identified as one reason for these disparities, this represents a small proportion of the reasons behind these differences and there are many factors that contribute to why a patient may refuse or not seek therapy.[34] The explanation behind differences in receipt of therapy is more likely related to a complex interplay of patient comorbidities, social determinants of health, and systemic level issues including structural racism.

The quality of therapy significantly varies between Black and White patients. Black patients are more likely to receive their treatment at minority-serving hospitals that are associated with lower rates of standard therapy delivery and higher mortality than nonminority serving hospitals.[35] For rectal cancer, Black patients have historically been less likely to undergo surgery with sphincter preservation surgery based on the SEER data from 1988 to 1999,[26] and are more likely to have rectal cancer surgery from lower volume surgeons.[32] Analysis from the National Cancer Data Base (NCDB) from years 1998 to 2006 showed that Black patients have higher rates of positive circumferential resection margins on rectal cancer specimens.[34] Multivariable models of colorectal cancer mortality show significant reductions in racial disparities when controlling for additional structural measures including hospital and provider characteristics and process measures such as lymph node harvest.[32] More recent data using data from 2006 to 2007 suggest the rate of concordant care among Black patients has now significantly improved over White patients (77% vs 73% in white patients); however, Black patients still had higher recurrence rates and mortality in 5-year follow-up.[36]

Treatment differences may only explain a small portion of the differences in colorectal mortality by race. When Black and White patients with colon cancer in the SEER database between years 1998 and 2009 were matched sequentially based on patient, tumor, and treatment factors, treatment explained only 0.1% of the 8.3% difference in 5-year survival seen between Black and White races.[37] When examining patients with colon and rectal cancer in the NCDB database for years 2004 to 2012, a 40% increased hazard of 5-year survival among Black patients than White patients was reduced to 7% after controlling for patient demographics, comorbidities, insurance, and tumor characteristics.[33] The addition of treatment factors only reduced the ratio of increased hazard for 5-year mortality to 6%. These findings suggest that while promoting equal treatment among races is essential for equitable care, we must look at additional factors outside of treatment to address the mortality disparity.

Factors Underlying Disparities in Colorectal Cancer

Race represents a social construct, and we must seek to understand the complex milieu of variables that race is serving as a surrogate for.[38] Potential factors that may be contributing to racial disparities in colorectal cancer mortality include patient, provider, health care system, and policy-level variables as shown in **Fig. 3**. Social determinants of health are known major contributors to racial disparities in colorectal cancer mortality.[25] Social determinants of health include not only socioeconomic factors such as a person's education, income, and health insurance but also other factors influencing health such as housing, transportation, and residential area.[38] When analyzing data from SEER-Medicare linked claims, data between 1992 and 2002, area-based measures of poverty and rurality were the single most explanatory factors for racial disparities in colorectal cancer mortality compared with the individual contribution of patient comorbidities, tumor characteristics, or treatment.[39] For colorectal cancers in the California Registry between 2000 and 2013, the top 3 contributors to racial disparities were the stage of cancer, marital status, and a composite measure of neighborhood socioeconomic status.[3]

Geographic disparities in colorectal cancer mortality exist and many contribute to or worsen racial differences in mortality. Variation in colorectal mortality across states in 2018 is illustrated in **Fig. 4**, and an example of within-state variation of colorectal mortality is shown in **Fig. 5**. Even the neighborhood in which a Black individual life has

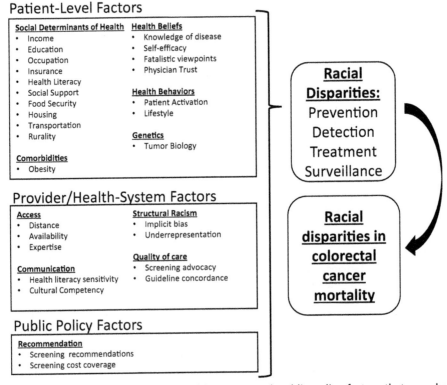

Fig. 3. Potential patient, provider/health-system, and public policy factors that may be contributing to health care disparities in colorectal cancer.

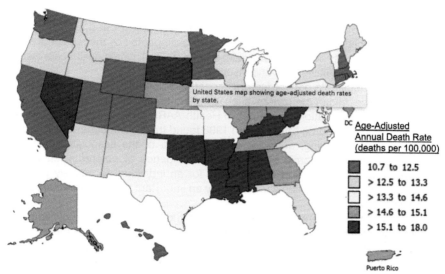

Fig. 4. Age-adjusted mortality rates for colorectal cancer between 2014 and 2018 within the United States. (*From* https://seer.cancer.gov/explorer)

been associated with their risk of presenting at advanced stage colorectal cancer.[40] Specifically, as the level of segregation increases, the rate of presenting at a late stage increases and as well as their risk of mortality.[40]

Up to half of the racial difference in mortality from colorectal cancer has been estimated to be attributable to health insurance; however, mixed findings have been shown in equal access health systems. In the Military Health System, Black patients with colon cancer had no difference in time to treatment compared with White patients, though Black patients were still more often diagnosed with a later stage

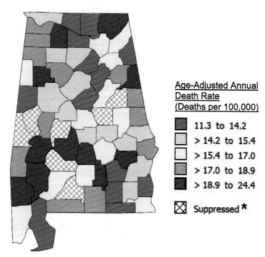

Fig. 5. Age-adjusted mortality rates for colorectal cancer between 2014 and 2018 for the State of Alabama. (*From* https://seer.cancer.gov/explorer Data from counties with counts fewer than 16 is suppressed for data stability and confidentiality.)

cancer.[41] Among patients with colorectal cancer identified in 6 separate integrated health systems, Black patients were still more likely to present at a later stage and had higher associated mortality. This difference was impacted by the receipt of surgical therapy even in this equal access health system.[42] To eliminate health care disparities, access must be viewed beyond insurance status.

Other more modifiable patient factors impacting colorectal cancer incidence and mortality include health behaviors such as diet, sedentary lifestyle and smoking.[43,44] In a study of National Institutes of Health-AARP Diet and Health data linked to state tumor registry data from 1995 to 1996 found that health behaviors including physical activity, smoking, and diet explained 36% of the association between neighborhood socioeconomic status and the incidence of colorectal cancers.[45] Additionally, patient activation or the ability for an individual to actively promote their own health care has been shown to play an important role in colorectal cancer screening.[46]

Beyond health behaviors, a patient's health attitudes, beliefs, and knowledge are important contributors to their decisions to seek care for preventative measures or treatment.[43] Fear, anxiety, and knowledge can present significant barriers to colorectal cancer screening.[7] Fatalistic beliefs are those in which one believes that their outcome from a condition is certain and that no intervenable action would impact that outcome. Data from the Cancer Care Outcomes and Research Surveillance (CanCORS) multicenter prospective study show that fatalistic beliefs among patients with colorectal cancer are associated with higher risk of advanced stage at diagnosis.[47]

Genetic differences and tumor biology are less likely important mediators of racial disparities in colorectal cancer outcomes; however, some studies have reported biological differences based on race. For example, more accelerated epigenetic aging has been observed in colorectal cancers of young-onset Black patients, and higher rates of KRAS mutations and lower rates of BRAF mutations have been observed in node-positive cancers.[48,49]

Providers and health care systems also play an important role in racial disparities in colorectal cancer through their impact on access and health promotion. Provider recommendation for colorectal cancer screening has been shown to be a barrier to achieving successful colorectal cancer screening, and the method of communication and cultural sensitivity in which these recommendations are delivered may influence whether patients adopt the recommendation.[16,43] Health care systems and providers are key drivers that may contribute to any structural racism that could influence racial disparities in colorectal cancer mortality. For example, physicians may exhibit an implicit bias for providing colonoscopy screening recommendations viewing some patients as less likely to adopt their recommendation.[17] An example of structural racism in a health system may be an endoscopy center that is strategically placed for reimbursement purposes as opposed to patient need. Evaluation of potential structural racism in medicine and how it contributes to colorectal cancer outcomes is necessary to eliminate disparities in colorectal cancer.

DISCUSSION
Potential interventions to Address Disparities in Colorectal Cancer

Given the various factors influencing racial disparities in colorectal cancer care, multi-level interventions will be necessary to address racial disparities in colorectal cancer incidence and mortality. An integrated approach with individual elements directed at the patient, provider, health care system, and policy-level will be necessary.[44] For example, to increase screening measures, specific efforts may be directed toward increasing demand and access from a community perspective and improving access and direction from the provider front.[44]

One example of an intervention that could impact disparities in multiple phases of colorectal cancer care is patient navigation. Patient navigation may be used to promote and guide patients to effective colorectal screening practices, steering patients from detection to high-quality care in a timely fashion, and providing information throughout the treatment process and posttreatment surveillance.[7,43,50,51] A randomized trial to promote colorectal cancer screening among patients not meeting recommendations in community health centers showed that the provision of patient navigation was associated with significantly higher rates of screening compared with usual care especially among patients of color: 40% of patients achieved successful screening at 1-year postintervention compared with 17% with usual care.[50]

Other innovative mechanisms to address racial disparities in colorectal cancer include addressing barriers in health literacy and cultural competency.[43,52] Health literacy, or a patient's ability to obtain, interpret, and act on health-related information, had been shown to be an important predictor of receipt of colonoscopy screening.[52] The development of health literacy sensitive interventions has shown to improve the success of colorectal screening programs.[53] Improvements in physician strategies to effectively communicate to patients with low health literacy may also help break racial barriers. Interventions to improve provider-based cultural competency can improve provider's ability to deal with various social cultures, psychosocial behaviors, and beliefs including fear, isolation, fatalism, trust, and respect.[43]

Public policy provides another important avenue to impact racial disparities in colorectal cancer mortality. Before the 2021 United States Preventive Task Force (USPTF) update for the recommended screening age for colorectal cancer to asymptomatic patients with ages greater than 45, there were several calls to reduce screening age to greater than 45 for Black patients given the historically increased incidence in younger Black adults.[43,54] Thus, this new USPTF policy may provide a new avenue for a physician to promote effective screening and decrease disparities in colorectal cancer incidence and mortality. Calls for other policy changes have been made centered around payments for screening efforts.[55] Specifically, recommendations have been made to congress to eliminate unexpected cost-sharing that patients become responsible for when polyps are identified during screening procedures requiring diagnostic/pathology review and procedure type changes.[55]

The Delaware Cancer Consortium provides an example of an effective multilevel intervention designed to address health care disparities in colorectal cancer with highly effective results.[56] In response to high cancer incidence and mortality, the Delaware legislature adopted recommendations that provided (1) coverage for uninsured patients to undergo colonoscopic screening for colorectal cancer, (2) establishment of a patient navigator system to facilitate screening efforts and subsequent cancer care, and (3) coverage for 2 years of cancer care for affected individuals. The Black patient population was specifically targeted through outreach in community programs. Overall screening rates increased from 57% in 2001% to 74% in 2009 and for Black patients screening numbers increased from 48% to 74%. The percentage of Black patients presenting with late-stage disease significantly decreased. The 3-year average Black/White mortality ratio for colorectal cancer decreased from 1.63 to 1.06. Thus, by addressing financial and social barriers, significant strides toward equity in colorectal cancer outcomes are possible.

SUMMARY

Health care disparities in colorectal cancer are avoidable, unnecessary, and unjust. Black patients represent a major population who suffer from these disparities, which manifests in many forms.[4] The mortality differences in colorectal cancer experienced by Black patients are driven by an accumulation of disparities in prevention/screening, detection, treatment, and posttreatment care. The underlying reasons for these differences may be attributable to patient, provider, health-system, and policy-level reasons. Future multilevel interventions to drive change in each of these levels provide the opportunity to make significant reductions in such health care disparities.

CLINICS CARE POINTS

- Racial disparities in colorectal cancer mortality exist—disparities in prevention, detection, treatment, and posttreatment care contribute to these differences.
- Physician recommendation for age-appropriate colorectal screening is an important mechanism to ensure colorectal cancer screening in minority populations.
- Patient navigators represent one effective mechanism to maximize effective colorectal cancer screening and subsequent treatment.

DISCLOSURE

The authors have nothing to disclose.

FUNDING

DIC is supported in part by the NIH [K23 MD013903 2019–2022].

REFERENCES

1. Siegel RL, Miller KD, Fuchs HE, et al. Cancer Statistics, 2021. CA Cancer J Clin 2021;71:7–33.
2. The Secretary's Advisory Committee on National Health Promotion and Disease Prevention Objectives for 2020. Phase 1 Report. Recommendations for the framework and format of healthy people 2020. Available at. http://www.healthypeople.gov/sites/default/files/PhaseI_0.pdf. August 26, 2021.
3. Ellis L, Canchola AJ, Spiegel D, et al. Racial and ethnic disparities in cancer survival: the contribution of tumor, sociodemographic, institutional, and neighborhood characteristics. J Clin Oncol 2018;36:25–33.
4. Jackson CS, Oman M, Patel AM, et al. Health disparities in colorectal cancer among racial and ethnic minorities in the United States. J Gastrointest Oncol 2016;7(Suppl 1):S32–43.
5. Siegel RL, Miller KD, Goding Sauer A, et al. Colorectal cancer statistics, 2020. CA Cancer J Clin 2020;70:145–64.
6. National Cancer Institute. Surveillance Epidemiology, and End Result Program; SEER*EXPLORER. Available at. https://seer.cancer.gov/explorer/. August 26, 2021.
7. Williams R, White P, Nieto J, et al. Colorectal Cancer in African Americans: an update: prepared by the committee on minority affairs and cultural diversity, American College of Gastroenterology. Clin Transl Gastroenterol 2016;7:e185.

8. Holowatyj AN, Ruterbusch JJ, Rozek LS, et al. Racial/Ethnic disparities in survival among patients with young-onset colorectal cancer. J Clin Oncol 2016;34: 2148–56.

9. Inadomi JM. Screening for colorectal neoplasia. N Engl J Med 2017;376:149–56.

10. Clinical Preventive Services|Healthy People. 2020. Available at: https://www. healthypeople.gov/2020/leading-health-indicators/2020-lhi-topics/Clinical-Preventive-Services/data. August 26, 2021.

11. Hall IJ, Tangka FKL, Sabatino SA, et al. Patterns and trends in cancer screening in the United States. Prev Chronic Dis 2018;15:E97.

12. Warren Andersen S, Blot WJ, Lipworth L, et al. Association of race and socioeconomic status with colorectal cancer screening, colorectal cancer risk, and mortality in Southern US Adults. JAMA Netw Open 2019;2:e1917995.

13. Murphy MM, Tevis SE, Kennedy GD. Independent risk factors for prolonged postoperative ileus development. J Surg Res 2016;201:279–85.

14. Fedewa SA, Flanders WD, Ward KC, et al. Racial and Ethnic disparities in interval colorectal cancer incidence: a Population-Based Cohort Study. Ann Intern Med 2017;166:857.

15. Dimou A, Syrigos KN, Saif MW. Disparities in colorectal cancer in African-Americans vs Whites: before and after diagnosis. World J Gastroenterol 2009; 15:3734–43.

16. Jernigan JC, Trauth JM, Neal-Ferguson D, et al. Factors that influence cancer screening in older African American men and women: focus group findings. Fam Community Health 2001;24:27–33.

17. May FP, Almario CV, Ponce N, et al. Racial minorities are more likely than whites to report lack of provider recommendation for colon cancer screening. Am J Gastroenterol 2015;110:1388–94.

18. Lansdorp-Vogelaar I, Kuntz KM, Knudsen AB, et al. Contribution of screening and survival differences to racial disparities in colorectal cancer rates. Cancer Epidemiol Biomarkers Prev 2012;21:728–36.

19. Laiyemo AO, Doubeni C, Pinsky PF, et al. Race and Colorectal cancer disparities: health-care utilization vs different cancer susceptibilities. JNCI J Natl Cancer Inst 2010;102:538–46.

20. Rolnick S, Hensley Alford S, Kucera GP, et al. Racial and age differences in colon examination surveillance following a diagnosis of colorectal cancer. J Natl Cancer Inst Monogr 2005;35:96–101.

21. Polite BN, Dignam JJ, Olopade OI. Colorectal cancer model of health disparities: understanding mortality differences in minority populations. J Clin Oncol 2006;24: 2179–87.

22. Howard J, Hankey BF, Greenberg RS, et al. A collaborative study of differences in the survival rates of black patients and white patients with cancer. Cancer 1992; 69:2349–60.

23. Mayberry RM, Coates RJ, Hill HA, et al. Determinants of black/white differences in colon cancer survival. J Natl Cancer Inst 1995;87:1686–93.

24. Robbins AS, Siegel RL, Jemal A. Racial disparities in stage-specific colorectal cancer mortality rates from 1985 to 2008. J Clin Oncol 2012;30:401–5.

25. Marcella S, Miller JE. Racial differences in colorectal cancer mortality. The importance of stage and socioeconomic status. J Clin Epidemiol 2001;54:359–66.

26. Morris AM. Racial disparities in rectal cancer treatment: a population-based analysis. Arch Surg 2004;139:151.

27. Le H, Ziogas A, Lipkin SM, et al. Effects of socioeconomic status and treatment disparities in colorectal cancer survival. Cancer Epidemiol Biomark Prev 2008;17: 1950–62.
28. Snyder RA, He J, Le-Rademacher J, et al. Racial differences in survival and response to therapy in patients with metastatic colorectal cancer: a secondary analysis of CALGB/SWOG 80405 (Alliance A151931), Cancer, 0. Cancer; 2021. p. 1–8, cncr.33649.
29. Dignam JJ, Colangelo L, Tian W, et al. Outcomes among African-Americans and Caucasians in colon cancer adjuvant therapy trials: findings from the National Surgical Adjuvant Breast and Bowel Project. J Natl Cancer Inst 1999;91:1933–40.
30. Yothers G, Sargent DJ, Wolmark N, et al. Outcomes among black patients with stage ii and iii colon cancer receiving chemotherapy: an analysis of ACCENT adjuvant trials. JNCI J Natl Cancer Inst 2011;103:1498–506.
31. Esnaola NF, Gebregziabher M, Finney C, et al. Underuse of surgical resection in black patients with nonmetastatic colorectal cancer: location, location, location. Ann Surg 2009;250:549–57.
32. Morris AM, Wei Y, Birkmeyer NJO, et al. Racial disparities in late survival after rectal cancer surgery. J Am Coll Surg 2006;203:787–94.
33. Sineshaw HM, Ng K, Flanders WD, et al. Factors that contribute to differences in survival of black vs white patients with colorectal cancer. Gastroenterology 2018; 154:906–15.e7.
34. Daly MC, Jung AD, Hanseman DJ, et al. Surviving rectal cancer: examination of racial disparities surrounding access to care. J Surg Res 2017;211:100–6.
35. Lu PW, Scully RE, Fields AC, et al. Racial disparities in treatment for rectal cancer at minority-serving hospitals. J Gastrointest Surg 2021;25:1847–56.
36. Snyder RA, Hu C-Y, Zafar SN, et al. Racial disparities in recurrence and overall survival in patients with locoregional colorectal cancer. J Natl Cancer Inst 2021; 113:770–7.
37. Lai Y, Wang C, Civan JM, et al. Effects of cancer stage and treatment differences on racial disparities in survival from colon cancer: A United States Population-Based Study. Gastroenterology 2016;150:1135–46.
38. Flanagin A, Frey T, Christiansen SL, et al. Updated guidance on the reporting of race and ethnicity in medical and science journals. JAMA 2021;326:621–7.
39. White AL, Vernon SW, Franzini L, et al. Racial disparities in colorectal cancer survival: to what extent are racial disparities explained by differences in treatment, tumor or hospital characteristics? Cancer 2010;116:4622–31.
40. Poulson M, Cornell E, Madiedo A, et al. The impact of racial residential segregation on colorectal cancer outcomes and treatment. Ann Surg 2021;273:1023–30.
41. Eaglehouse YL, Georg MW, Shriver CD, et al. Racial comparisons in timeliness of colon cancer treatment in an equal-access health system. JNCI J Natl Cancer Inst 2020;112:410–7.
42. Doubeni CA, Field TS, Buist DSM, et al. Racial differences in tumor stage and survival for colorectal cancer in an insured population. Cancer 2007;109:612–20.
43. Coughlin SS, Blumenthal DS, Seay SJ, et al. Toward the elimination of colorectal cancer disparities among African Americans. J Racial Ethn Health Disparities 2016;3:555–64.
44. Carethers JM, Doubeni CA. Causes of socioeconomic disparities in colorectal cancer and intervention framework and strategies. Gastroenterology 2020;158: 354–67.

45. Doubeni CA, Major JM, Laiyemo AO, et al. Contribution of behavioral risk factors and obesity to socioeconomic differences in colorectal cancer incidence. JNCI J Natl Cancer Inst 2012;104:1353–62.

46. Katz ML, Fisher JL, Fleming K, et al. Patient activation increases colorectal cancer screening rates: a randomized trial among low-income minority patients. Cancer Epidemiol Biomark Prev 2012;21:45–52.

47. Lyratzopoulos G, Liu MP-H, Abel GA, et al. The Association between fatalistic beliefs and late stage at diagnosis of lung and colorectal cancer. Cancer Epidemiol Biomarkers Prev 2015;24:720–6.

48. Devall M, Sun X, Yuan F, et al. Racial disparities in epigenetic aging of the right vs left colon. J Natl Cancer Inst 2020;113:1779–82.

49. Yoon HH, Shi Q, Alberts SR, et al. Racial Differences in *BRAF/KRAS* Mutation Rates and Survival in Stage III Colon Cancer Patients. J Natl Cancer Inst 2015; 107:djv186.

50. Lasser KE, Murillo J, Lisboa S, et al. Colorectal cancer screening among ethnically diverse, low-income patients: a randomized controlled trial. Arch Intern Med 2011;171:906–12.

51. Raich PC, Whitley EM, Thorland W, et al. Patient navigation improves cancer diagnostic resolution: an individually randomized clinical trial in an underserved population. Cancer Epidemiol Biomark Prev 2012;21:1629–38.

52. Davis TC, Dolan NC, Ferreira MR, et al. The role of inadequate health literacy skills in colorectal cancer screening. Cancer Invest 2001;19:193–200.

53. Davis TC, Hancock J, Morris J, et al. Impact of health literacy-directed colonoscopy bowel preparation instruction sheet. Am J Health Behav 2017;41:301–8.

54. US Preventive Services Task Force, Davidson KW, Barry MJ, et al. Screening for colorectal cancer: US preventive services task force recommendation statement. JAMA 2021;325:1965–77.

55. Doubeni CA, Corley DA, Zauber AG. Colorectal cancer health disparities and the Role of US Law and Health Policy. Gastroenterology 2016;150:1052–5.

56. Grubbs SS, Polite BN, Carney J, et al. Eliminating racial disparities in colorectal cancer in the real world: it took a village. J Clin Oncol 2013;31:1928–30.

Nonoperative Management of Rectal Cancer
The Watch and Wait Strategy

Bruna Borba Vailati, MD[a,b,c,1],
Guilherme Pagin São Julião, MD[a,b,c,1],
Angelita Habr-Gama, MD, PhD[a,b,d,1],
Rodrigo Oliva Perez, MD, PhD[a,b,c,*]

KEYWORDS

- Watch & wait • Organ preservation • Rectal cancer • Neoadjuvant therapy
- Clinical complete response

KEY POINTS

- The single necessary requirement to consider the Watch and Wait strategy in rectal cancer is the achievement of a complete clinical response (cCR) following neoadjuvant treatment.
- Strict criteria of a cCR, including clinical, endoscopic, and radiological findings, are usually achieved after 12 to 16 weeks and preferably within 6 months from radiation completion.
- Patients managed by the Watch and Wait strategy have very good functional and oncological outcomes.
- Patients who initially achieve a cCR followed by tumor regrowth may represent a distinct subgroup of patients in terms of risk for distant metastases development.

INTRODUCTION

Over the past few decades, rectal cancer management has become increasingly challenging for multiple reasons. Proper imaging using dedicated magnetic resonance (MR), standardization of total mesorectal excision (TME), and incorporation of neoadjuvant treatment regimens have contributed to a significant decrease in local recurrence rates while minimizing the need for definitive stomas (therefore allowing for sphincter-preservation alternatives).[1–3] However, the observation of complete tumor response to radiation (RT) or chemoradiation (CRT) led to the proposal of organ-preservation strategies with avoidance of immediate surgery and close surveillance (Watch and Wait strategy) in selected patients.[4] Initially considered for a very

[a] Angelita & Joaquim Gama Institute, Sao Paulo, Brazil; [b] Hospital Alemão Oswaldo Cruz, Sao Paulo, Brazil; [c] Hospital Beneficência Portuguesa, Sao Paulo, Brazil; [d] Colorectal Surgery Division, University of São Paulo School of Medicine, Sao Paulo, Brazil
[1] Praça Amadeu Amaral, 47/111, São Paulo, São Paulo 01327-010, Brazil.
* Corresponding author. Praça Amadeu Amaral, 47/111, São Paulo, São Paulo 01327-010, Brazil.
E-mail address: Rodrigo.operez@gmail.com

Surg Oncol Clin N Am 31 (2022) 171–182
https://doi.org/10.1016/j.soc.2021.11.003
1055-3207/22/© 2021 Elsevier Inc. All rights reserved.
surgonc.theclinics.com

restricted subgroup of patients, the use of more contemporary neoadjuvant treatment regimens has resulted in a higher proportion of patients achieving complete tumor regression.[5] The purpose of the present article is to review the current evidence related to the selection criteria and outcomes in patients enrolled in this Watch and Wait strategy.

RATIONALE

Since the beginning, with early reports on nonoperative management for rectal cancer following neoadjuvant chemoradiation (nCRT), the purpose of Watch and Wait was to avoid potentially unnecessary TME. Although many believe that this was a strategy exclusively used for elderly and frail patients, this is actually a misconception as the idea was to spare any given patient from the morbidity, mortality, and functional consequences of radical proctectomy.[6]

Even though proper TME with or without nCRT may result in excellent local disease control, postoperative morbidity, mortality, need for temporary or definitive stomas, and functional consequences (including urinary, sexual, and anorectal dysfunctions) are common and quite significant.

DEFINITIONS AND TERMS

As organ-preservation strategies became an interesting alternative for patients, several new terms and definitions were commonly used by multiple authors during the last decades.

Complete pathologic response (pCR) refers to the absence of residual cancer cells detected during pathologic examination of a resected TME specimen (ypT0N0). Although many authors still use pCR for local excision specimens with the absence of residual primary cancer, the preferred term for the latter clinical entity would be ypT0.

Clinical complete response (cCR) refers to the absence of clinical, endoscopic, and radiological evidence for residual rectal cancer following any kind of neoadjuvant treatment (nonsurgical). Although there is intrinsic subjectivity in the definition of a cCR, there are objective endoscopic and radiological findings to be used for the identification of these patients[7] (**Fig. 1**).

A common term used in contemporary literature and clinical practice has been "near" complete clinical response to neoadjuvant treatment. This is a much less

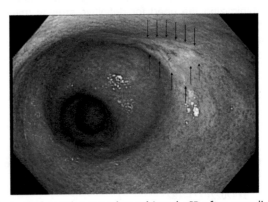

Fig. 1. Endoscopic view of rectal cancer that achieved cCR after neoadjuvant chemoradiation, showing whitening of the mucosa and teleangiectasia (*arrows*).

objective term, with no commonly agreed radiological or endoscopic features. The "near" complete clinical response usually refers to the presence of minimal residual disease and often relies on the individual authors' definitions of clinical, endoscopic, and/or radiological findings (**Fig. 2**).

nCRT usually refers to the use of long-course RT regimens with concomitant chemotherapy (5FU-based) as reported in the early randomized clinical trials.[8,9] Since the incorporation of total neoadjuvant treatment (TNT) regimens with either induction (delivered before RT) or consolidation (delivered after RT) chemotherapy, TNT regimens now typically need to provide the exact type of RT used (long or short-course) and chemotherapy type (induction or consolidation).[10]

In contrast to the term local recurrence, which is defined as the presence of recurrent cancer in the pelvis (including the anastomosis) following any type of surgical resection (TME or transanal local excision), the term used for recurrent disease after the achievement of a cCR managed nonoperatively is local regrowth[11] (**Fig. 3**). Local regrowth includes the presence of recurrent disease within the rectal wall, within the mesorectal compartment, or within lateral internal iliac/obturator lymph nodes following initial achievement of cCR and nonoperative management.

INDICATIONS AND SELECTION CRITERIA

The single necessary requirement to be considered eligible for the Watch and Wait strategy is the achievement of a cCR following any kind of neoadjuvant treatment. An important distinction needs to be clearly established here with patients undergoing exclusively nonoperative treatment due to medical comorbidities or who refuse surgical management. Although these patients may eventually achieve a cCR, the simple fact that they have avoided surgery (even in the absence of a cCR) does not mean they have been managed by Watch and Wait.

ASSESSMENT OF RESPONSE

As the prerequisite to be included in the Watch and Wait strategy is the achievement of a cCR, several aspects in the assessment of tumor response to neoadjuvant treatment should be taken into account.

Tumor response to RT or CRT is clearly time-dependent and multiple studies have suggested that higher rates of complete response (clinical or pathologic) are achieved

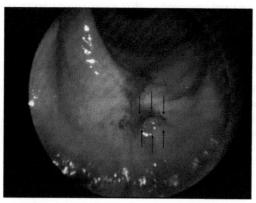

Fig. 2. Endoscopic assessment at 16 weeks from nCRT completion showing a small residual irregularity (*arrows*).

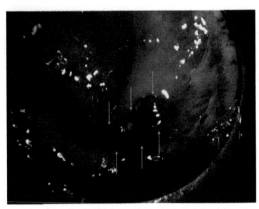

Fig. 3. Endoscopic assessment at 20 weeks from nCRT completion with a local regrowth (*arrows*) after initial achievement of cCR.

as longer intervals are used following completion of treatment.[12,13] However, not all patients will achieve a complete tumor response to treatment, regardless of the amount of time one allows for tumors to respond. Interesting studies using PET/CT assessment of tumor response have suggested that after nCRT, response (measured by a decrease in metabolic activity) is quite consistent between the end of treatment and 6 weeks.[14] However, only 50% of tumors kept on responding to treatment between 6 and 12 weeks from RT completion. The remaining 50% of tumors have somewhat regained metabolic activity between 6 and 12 weeks, suggesting that routine use of longer (>6 weeks) intervals would not necessarily benefit the entirety of patients with rectal cancer undergoing nCRT.[14] Similar findings from the prospective randomized controlled trial comparing 7 to 11 weeks after nCRT to achieve complete TRG found no statistically significant differences between groups.[15]

Using PET/CT imaging (metabolic tumor uptake) and MR (tumor volume estimates), it appears that most tumor response after nCRT occur within the first 6 weeks (or even less) after RT completion.[16,17] The achievement of ≥70% of tumor response (% of standard uptake value) at 6 weeks from RT completion was an independent feature associated with the achievement of a cCR.[16]

Although patients who ultimately achieve a cCR have excellent response at their first assessment, they rarely achieve all clinical, endoscopic, and radiological criteria at this time.[18] Most patients who underwent successful organ preservation through Watch and Wait (nearly 75%) only presented all 3 strict criteria for a cCR after 16 weeks from RT completion.[18] Finally, very few patients required more than 26 to 30 weeks (6 months) to achieve a cCR.[18]

Altogether, the current evidence suggests that patients undergoing neoadjuvant treatment interested in organ preservation with Watch and Wait should:

1. necessarily present excellent response in their first round of assessment
2. undergo successive reassessment of tumor response as most patients will only fulfill all 3 criteria after 16 weeks from RT completion.
3. Preferably achieve all 3 (clinical, endoscopic, and radiological) strict criteria of a cCR within 6 months from RT completion.

CRITERIA FOR cCR
Clinical Findings

The clinical findings consistent with the achievement of a cCR should preferably be obtained by digital rectal examination (DRE) from someone with clinical expertise in rectal cancer assessment. DRE findings commonly encountered among these patients include an entirely normal examination, slight induration of the area harboring the scar (area of the primary tumor), and definitely absence of any detectable ulceration, irregularity, stenosis, or mass.[7]

Endoscopic Findings

Usually, the ideal endoscopic finding of a cCR is a white flat scar with no ulceration covered by fibrin. Only teleangiectasias and slight hyperemia of the surroundings are accepted[7] (see **Fig. 1**). The presence of ulcers (even superficial/shallow ulcers) or significant areas of irregularity should be considered suspicious. An excellent tumor response may warrant additional subsequent assessments before defining ultimate management. However, "near-complete" or excellent response is not equal to cCR. Unless the excellent response becomes a cCR, these patients should not be kept under surveillance as in Watch and Wait.

Endoscopic Biopsies

Endoscopic biopsies should not be considered as part of the criteria for the identification of patients with cCR. The results of these biopsies should be interpreted with care.[19] In the setting of an incomplete clinical response, frequently observed negative biopsies may be misleading (suggesting the absence of residual cancer). In the setting of cCR, there is a minimal role for endoscopic biopsies as patients may exhibit a positive biopsy in the early stages following completion of therapy, despite the presence of an ongoing clinical response.

Excisional Biopsies

Excisional biopsies for the sole purpose of confirming a ypT0 in the setting of a cCR are not recommended.[20] One of the main reasons includes the high risk of wound breakdown and resulting morbidity following local excision in the setting of neoadjuvant RT.[21] These wound breakdowns are often very symptomatic even though not life-threatening.[22] The wound breakdown following local excision may have significant consequences in terms of subsequent clinical, endoscopic, and radiological surveillance (significant scarring and frequent presence of granulomas/distorted architecture).[23] In addition, functional outcomes after local excision are reportedly worse than observation alone.[24] Finally, in the event of a local recurrence and need for salvage resection, outcomes in the setting of previous transanal local excision are far worse than for salvage for local regrowths with an intact rectum/mesorectum.[25,26]

Radiological Findings

MR has become the preferred radiological tool to assess tumor response to neoadjuvant treatment. Ideally, patients with cCR should present with low signal intensity areas within the area harboring the initial tumor using T2-weighted sequences in a well-standardized dedicated MR protocol.[27] The amount of low-signal intensity areas within the area of the primary tumor has been used to estimate magnetic resonance tumor regression grade (mrTRG). Therefore, mrTRG grades 1 and 2 usually indicate complete or near-complete tumor regression grades [28] (**Fig. 4**). Diffusion-weighted sequences provide additional information to assist radiologists and clinicians to identify patients who are best candidates for organ-preserving strategies.[29–33]

PET/CT imaging may also assist in the identification of patients with complete response to treatment.[34] Although less available in clinical practice, multiple studies using different parameters provided by PET/CT have reported positive outcomes.[35,36]

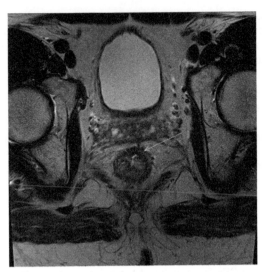

Fig. 4. Axial high-resolution T2WI magnetic resonance (MR) after neoadjuvant treatment showing complete radiological response, indicated by a low signal intensity area (*arrows*).

SURVEILLANCE STRATEGY

Surveillance after the achievement of a cCR can be divided into surveillance for detection of local regrowth and for distant metastases. Patients should follow currently available guidelines for systemic disease surveillance as for any colorectal cancer following primary surgical resection. Local regrowth surveillance may require a more detailed attention for a couple of reasons. First, most local regrowths develop during the first 3 years of follow-up.[37] This means that a more intensive follow-up should be recommended during these first 3 years.[38] Second, nearly 90% of local regrowths will have an endoluminal component of the disease rendering them detectable by simple DRE and/or flexible/rigid proctoscopy.[39] This highlights the importance of offering this organ-preserving strategy to patients with tumors at the reach of DRE. Finally, radiological imaging is also useful for the detection of regrowth, particularly among patients with exclusively mesorectal recurrent disease.[39]

In this setting, local surveillance should include routine DRE, flexible/rigid proctoscopy, and dedicated high-resolution MR. Our group has recommended close surveillance of these patients during the first 3 years (as the risk of local regrowth significantly decreases after cCR is sustained for 3 years).[38] Usually, follow-up visits with these studies are recommended every 8 to 12 weeks until 3 years of a sustained clinical response. The risk for subsequent local regrowth following a sustained cCR for 3 years is less than 5%. Therefore, less intensive surveillance may be considered between 3 and 5 years (every 6 months). Even though the risk of local regrowth beyond 5 years is infrequent, the potential risk remains. Therefore, these patients are usually followed for life (at least once a year).

OUTCOMES

Overall, the risk of local regrowth seems to be between 25% and 35% in 3 years after the achievement of a cCR managed by Watch and Wait.[37,40,41] The risk of local regrowth is significantly decreased after patients have sustained a cCR during this 3-year period. Conditional survival estimates suggest that the risk of subsequent local regrowth after this period is less than 5%.[38] Data from individual series and meta-analyses using individual patient data suggest that baseline T-status is a significant risk factor for local regrowth once patients have achieved a cCR.[41] The risk of local regrowth is nearly 20% for cT2, 30% for cT3, and almost 40% for cT4 disease. Radiological nodal status (cN) has not been associated with the risk of local regrowth or surgery-free survival.[42]

SALVAGE

Data from individual series as well as systematic reviews suggest that salvage surgery is feasible in the vast majority of patients (≥90%) with local regrowth.[39,43] In addition, salvage resection of the primary tumor is often associated with an R0 resection.[44,45] As a consequence, excellent local disease control is obtained (≥90% of the cases).[39] Usually, salvage surgery follows the same procedure originally considered. An exception to this are cases that have previously been managed by transanal local excision, which can significantly interfere with subsequent TME at salvage.

DISTANT METASTASES

Even patients with pCR are at risk for developing distant metastases. The risk of distant metastases among patients who achieve a cCR and are managed by Watch and Wait is low and similar when compared to those with pCR.[40] However, among patients with initial apparent cCR, 25% to 30% of patients will develop local regrowth. Local regrowth represents a microscopic residual disease that was clinically undetectable at the time of tumor response assessment. Therefore, it is not surprising that patients who experience local regrowth are also at significantly higher risk for the development of distant metastases (nearly 30%).[46]

SURVIVAL

Data from pooled analyses of patients managed by radical TME who exhibited a pCR showed 3-year overall survival rates of nearly 90%.[47] These patients were frequently treated by adjuvant chemotherapy. In contrast, meta-analysis data suggest that patients with cCR managed most frequently without adjuvant chemotherapy had 93.5% overall survival at 3 years.[40] The same interesting effect was observed in one study using propensity score matching of patients managed by radical surgery or Watch and Wait. The study was designed to show noninferiority of Watch and Wait in comparison to surgery but surprisingly overall survival was significantly superior for this former subgroup of patients.[48]

FUNCTIONAL OUTCOMES

The majority of data available suggest excellent post-treatment function after Watch and Wait. Outcomes seem to be particularly better when compared with both TME or even transanal local excision.[24,49,50] However, excellent outcomes are different from perfect outcomes. This needs to be explained to patients upfront as any type of radiation treatment will inevitably affect anorectal function.

PREDICTION OF TUMOR RESPONSE/MOLECULAR MARKERS

Ideally, we would be able to accurately predict tumor response before treatment, facilitating the selection of appropriate patients for the Watch and Wait approach. This would allow the selection of "winners" upfront, therefore minimizing the risk of local regrowth. In addition, one could avoid the use of unnecessary RT among patients where the sole purpose of using nCRT is to achieve a cCR and avoid surgery.

Unfortunately, however, accurate prediction of tumor response to neoadjuvant treatment has proven unsuccessful thus far. Although multiple specific individual genes or groups of genes have been associated with better or worse response to treatment, there is a series of problems associated with their use.[51,52] First, many of the genetic alterations (such as p53/Kras mutations or microsatellite instability) that commonly predict worse response to treatment are rarely present in most patients with rectal cancer.[53,54] Secondly, groups of genes that have been associated with favorable treatment responses are inconsistent across different studies.[51] Thirdly, intertumoral heterogeneity reflects distinct intrinsic tumor biology and explains why tumors within different patients may have completely different biological behavior despite sharing similar staging and clinical features. Finally, intratumoral heterogeneity (ITH) may have also contributed for the difficulties in predicting response based on pre-treatment samples. Ultimately, ITH may result in the fact that pre-treatment samples are not representative of the entirety of the cancer.[55]

The quality of patients' immune response to the primary cancer has been independently correlated with survival in colon cancer. Preliminary data in patients with rectal cancer suggest that it may be useful to predict response to nCRT.[56,57]

Another future concept is the use of cancer cell lines from particular patients to test the efficacy of multiple agents or regimens before initiation of treatment.[57] Finally, the use of circulating tumor DNA has been used to predict survival among patients with colorectal cancer and holds promise for monitoring response to treatment.[58]

CLINICS CARE POINTS

- Assessment of response to neoadjuvant treatment is critical to the consideration of patients for non-operative management of rectal cancer. Inherent subjectivity of such assessment remains a significant challenge in the Watch and Wait Strategy.

- Achievement of a cCR after neoadjuvant treatment for rectal cancer may allow avoidance of radical protectomy and all of its consequences in terms of morbidity/functional outcomes. However, a significant proportion of these patients will develop local regrowth requiring the need for salvage resection and determining a considerable risk for distant metastases.

DISCLOSURE

The authors have nothing to disclose.

REFERENCES

1. Burton S, Brown G, Daniels IR, et al. MRI directed multidisciplinary team preoperative treatment strategy: the way to eliminate positive circumferential margins? Br J Cancer 2006;94(3):351–7.
2. Heald RJ, Ryall RD. Recurrence and survival after total mesorectal excision for rectal cancer. Lancet 1986;1(8496):1479–82.
3. Heald RJ, Husband EM, Ryall RD. The mesorectum in rectal cancer surgery–the clue to pelvic recurrence? Br J Surg 1982;69(10):613–6.
4. Habr-Gama A, de Souza PM, Ribeiro U Jr, et al. Low rectal cancer: impact of radiation and chemotherapy on surgical treatment. Dis Colon Rectum 1998;41(9):1087–96.
5. Habr-Gama A, Sabbaga J, Gama-Rodrigues J, et al. Watch and wait approach following extended neoadjuvant chemoradiation for distal rectal cancer: are we

getting closer to anal cancer management? Dis Colon Rectum 2013;56(10): 1109–17.

6. Habr-Gama A, Perez RO, Nadalin W, et al. Operative versus nonoperative treatment for stage 0 distal rectal cancer following chemoradiation therapy: long-term results. Ann Surg 2004;240(4):711–7.

7. Habr-Gama A, Perez RO, Wynn G, et al. Complete clinical response after neoadjuvant chemoradiation therapy for distal rectal cancer: characterization of clinical and endoscopic findings for standardization. Dis Colon Rectum 2010;53(12): 1692–8.

8. Sauer R, Becker H, Hohenberger W, et al. Preoperative versus postoperative chemoradiotherapy for rectal cancer. N Engl J Med 2004;351(17):1731–40.

9. Sauer R, Liersch T, Merkel S, et al. Preoperative versus postoperative chemoradiotherapy for locally advanced rectal cancer: results of the German CAO/ARO/ AIO-94 randomized phase III trial after a median follow-up of 11 years. J Clin Oncol 2012;30(16):1926–33.

10. Cercek A, Roxburgh CSD, Strombom P, et al. Adoption of Total Neoadjuvant Therapy for Locally Advanced Rectal Cancer. JAMA Oncol 2018;4(6):e180071.

11. Heald RJ, Beets G, Carvalho C. Report from a consensus meeting: response to chemoradiotherapy in rectal cancer - predictor of cure and a crucial new choice for the patient: on behalf of the Champalimaud 2014 Faculty for 'Rectal cancer: when NOT to operate. Colorectal Dis 2014;16(5):334–7.

12. Kalady MF, de Campos-Lobato LF, Stocchi L, et al. Predictive factors of pathologic complete response after neoadjuvant chemoradiation for rectal cancer. Ann Surg 2009;250(4):582–9.

13. Sloothaak DA, Geijsen DE, van Leersum NJ, et al. Optimal time interval between neoadjuvant chemoradiotherapy and surgery for rectal cancer. Br J Surg 2013; 100(7):933–9.

14. Perez RO, Habr-Gama A, São Julião GP, et al. Optimal timing for assessment of tumor response to neoadjuvant chemoradiation in patients with rectal cancer: do all patients benefit from waiting longer than 6 weeks? Int J Radiat Oncol Biol Phys 2012;84(5):1159–65.

15. Lefevre JH, Mineur L, Kotti S, et al. Effect of Interval (7 or 11 weeks) Between Neoadjuvant Radiochemotherapy and Surgery on Complete Pathologic Response in Rectal Cancer: A Multicenter, Randomized, Controlled Trial (GREC-CAR-6). J Clin Oncol 2016;34(31):3773–80.

16. Perez RO, Habr-Gama A, Sao Juliao GP, et al. Predicting complete response to neoadjuvant CRT for distal rectal cancer using sequential PET/CT imaging. Tech Coloproctol 2014;18(8):699–708.

17. Van den Begin R, Kleijnen JP, Engels B, et al. Tumor volume regression during preoperative chemoradiotherapy for rectal cancer: a prospective observational study with weekly MRI. Acta Oncol 2018;57(6):723–7.

18. Habr-Gama A, Sao Juliao GP, Fernandez LM, et al. Achieving a Complete Clinical Response After Neoadjuvant Chemoradiation That Does Not Require Surgical Resection: It May Take Longer Than You Think! Dis Colon Rectum 2019;62(7): 802–8.

19. Perez RO, Habr-Gama A, Pereira GV, et al. Role of biopsies in patients with residual rectal cancer following neoadjuvant chemoradiation after downsizing: can they rule out persisting cancer? Colorectal Dis 2012;14(6):714–20.

20. Habr-Gama A, Sao Juliao GP, Perez RO. Pitfalls of transanal endoscopic microsurgery for rectal cancer following neoadjuvant chemoradiation therapy. Minim Invasive Ther Allied Technol 2014;23(2):63–9.

21. Marks JH, Valsdottir EB, DeNittis A, et al. Transanal endoscopic microsurgery for the treatment of rectal cancer: comparison of wound complication rates with and without neoadjuvant radiation therapy. Surg Endosc 2009;23(5):1081–7.
22. Perez RO, Habr-Gama A, Sao Juliao GP, et al. Transanal endoscopic microsurgery for residual rectal cancer after neoadjuvant chemoradiation therapy is associated with significant immediate pain and hospital readmission rates. Dis Colon Rectum 2011;54(5):545–51.
23. Sao Juliao GP, Ortega CD, Vailati BB, et al. Magnetic resonance imaging following neoadjuvant chemoradiation and transanal endoscopic microsurgery for rectal cancer. Colorectal Dis 2017;19(6):O196–203.
24. Habr-Gama A, Lynn PB, Jorge JM, et al. Impact of Organ-Preserving Strategies on Anorectal Function in Patients with Distal Rectal Cancer Following Neoadjuvant Chemoradiation. Dis Colon Rectum 2016;59(4):264–9.
25. Hompes R, McDonald R, Buskens C, et al. Completion surgery following transanal endoscopic microsurgery: assessment of quality and short- and long-term outcome. Colorectal Dis 2013;15(10):e576–81.
26. Morino M, Allaix ME, Arolfo S, et al. Previous transanal endoscopic microsurgery for rectal cancer represents a risk factor for an increased abdominoperineal resection rate. Surg Endosc 2013;27(9):3315–21.
27. Patel UB, Brown G, Rutten H, et al. Comparison of magnetic resonance imaging and histopathological response to chemoradiotherapy in locally advanced rectal cancer. Ann Surg Oncol 2012;19(9):2842–52.
28. Patel UB, Blomqvist LK, Taylor F, et al. MRI after treatment of locally advanced rectal cancer: how to report tumor response–the MERCURY experience. AJR Am J Roentgenol 2012;199(4):W486–95.
29. Lambregts DM, Maas M, Bakers FC, et al. Long-term follow-up features on rectal MRI during a wait-and-see approach after a clinical complete response in patients with rectal cancer treated with chemoradiotherapy. Dis Colon Rectum 2011;54(12):1521–8.
30. Lambregts DM, van Heeswijk MM, Delli Pizzi A, et al. Diffusion-weighted MRI to assess response to chemoradiotherapy in rectal cancer: main interpretation pitfalls and their use for teaching. Eur Radiol 2017;27(10):4445–54.
31. Lambregts DM, Lahaye MJ, Heijnen LA, et al. MRI and diffusion-weighted MRI to diagnose a local tumour regrowth during long-term follow-up of rectal cancer patients treated with organ preservation after chemoradiotherapy. Eur Radiol 2016;26(7):2118–25.
32. Maas M, Lambregts DM, Nelemans PJ, et al. Assessment of Clinical Complete Response After Chemoradiation for Rectal Cancer with Digital Rectal Examination, Endoscopy, and MRI: Selection for Organ-Saving Treatment. Ann Surg Oncol 2015;22(12):3873–80.
33. Lambregts DM, Rao SX, Sassen S, et al. MRI and Diffusion-weighted MRI Volumetry for Identification of Complete Tumor Responders After Preoperative Chemoradiotherapy in Patients With Rectal Cancer: A Bi-institutional Validation Study. Ann Surg 2015;262(6):1034–9.
34. Perez RO, Habr-Gama A, Gama-Rodrigues J, et al. Accuracy of positron emission tomography/computed tomography and clinical assessment in the detection of complete rectal tumor regression after neoadjuvant chemoradiation: long-term results of a prospective trial (National Clinical Trial 00254683). Cancer 2012;118(14):3501–11.

35. Rymer B, Curtis NJ, Siddiqui MR, et al. FDG PET/CT Can Assess the Response of Locally Advanced Rectal Cancer to Neoadjuvant Chemoradiotherapy: Evidence From Meta-analysis and Systematic Review. Clin Nucl Med 2016;41(5):371–5.

36. Dos Anjos DA, Perez RO, Habr-Gama A, et al. Semiquantitative Volumetry by Sequential PET/CT May Improve Prediction of Complete Response to Neoadjuvant Chemoradiation in Patients With Distal Rectal Cancer. Dis Colon Rectum 2016;59(9):805–12.

37. van der Valk MJM, Hilling DE, Bastiaannet E, et al. Long-term outcomes of clinical complete responders after neoadjuvant treatment for rectal cancer in the International Watch & Wait Database (IWWD): an international multicentre registry study. Lancet 2018;391(10139):2537–45.

38. Fernandez LM, Sao Juliao GP, Figueiredo NL, et al. Conditional recurrence-free survival of clinical complete responders managed by watch and wait after neoadjuvant chemoradiotherapy for rectal cancer in the International Watch & Wait Database: a retrospective, international, multicentre registry study. Lancet Oncol 2021;22(1):43–50.

39. Habr-Gama A, Gama-Rodrigues J, Sao Juliao GP, et al. Local recurrence after complete clinical response and watch and wait in rectal cancer after neoadjuvant chemoradiation: impact of salvage therapy on local disease control. Int J Radiat Oncol Biol Phys 2014;88(4):822–8.

40. Dattani M, Heald RJ, Goussous G, et al. Oncological and Survival Outcomes in Watch and Wait Patients With a Clinical Complete Response After Neoadjuvant Chemoradiotherapy for Rectal Cancer: A Systematic Review and Pooled Analysis. Ann Surg 2018;268(6):955–67.

41. Chadi SA, Malcomson L, Ensor J, et al. Factors affecting local regrowth after watch and wait for patients with a clinical complete response following chemoradiotherapy in rectal cancer (InterCoRe consortium): an individual participant data meta-analysis. Lancet Gastroenterol Hepatol 2018;3(12):825–36.

42. Habr-Gama A, Sao Juliao GP, Vailati BB, et al. Organ Preservation Among Patients With Clinically Node-Positive Rectal Cancer: Is It Really More Dangerous? Dis Colon Rectum 2019;62(6):675–83.

43. Kong JC, Guerra GR, Warrier SK, et al. Outcome and Salvage Surgery Following "Watch and Wait" for Rectal Cancer after Neoadjuvant Therapy: A Systematic Review. Dis Colon Rectum 2017;60(3):335–45.

44. Fernandez LM, Figueiredo NL, Habr-Gama A, et al. Salvage Surgery With Organ Preservation for Patients With Local Regrowth After Watch and Wait: Is It Still Possible? Dis Colon Rectum 2020;63(8):1053–62.

45. Nasir I, Fernandez L, Vieira P, et al. Salvage surgery for local regrowths in Watch & Wait - Are we harming our patients by deferring the surgery? Eur J Surg Oncol 2019;45(9):1559–66.

46. Smith JJ, Strombom P, Chow OS, et al. Assessment of a Watch-and-Wait Strategy for Rectal Cancer in Patients With a Complete Response After Neoadjuvant Therapy. JAMA Oncol 2019;e185896.

47. Maas M, Nelemans PJ, Valentini V, et al. Long-term outcome in patients with a pathological complete response after chemoradiation for rectal cancer: a pooled analysis of individual patient data. Lancet Oncol 2010;11(9):835–44.

48. Renehan AG, Malcomson L, Emsley R, et al. Watch-and-wait approach versus surgical resection after chemoradiotherapy for patients with rectal cancer (the OnCoRe project): a propensity-score matched cohort analysis. Lancet Oncol 2016;17(2):174–83.

49. Hupkens BJP, Martens MH, Stoot JH, et al. Quality of Life in Rectal Cancer Patients After Chemoradiation: Watch-and-Wait Policy Versus Standard Resection - A Matched-Controlled Study. Dis Colon Rectum 2017;60(10):1032–40.

50. Vailati BB, Habr-Gama A, Mattacheo AE, et al. Quality of Life in Patients With Rectal Cancer After Chemoradiation: Watch-and-Wait Policy Versus Standard Resection-Are We Comparing Apples to Oranges? Dis Colon Rectum 2018; 61(3):e21.

51. Lopes-Ramos C, Koyama FC, Habr-Gama A, et al. Comprehensive evaluation of the effectiveness of gene expression signatures to predict complete response to neoadjuvant chemoradiotherapy and guide surgical intervention in rectal cancer. Cancer Genet 2015;208(6):319–26.

52. Perez RO, Habr-Gama A, Sao Juliao GP, et al. Should We Give Up The Search for a Clinically Useful Gene Signature for the Prediction of Response of Rectal Cancer to Neoadjuvant Chemoradiation? Dis Colon Rectum 2016;59(9):895–7.

53. Chow OS, Kuk D, Keskin M, et al. KRAS and Combined KRAS/TP53 Mutations in Locally Advanced Rectal Cancer are Independently Associated with Decreased Response to Neoadjuvant Therapy. Ann Surg Oncol 2016;23(8):2548–55.

54. Hasan S, Renz P, Wegner RE, et al. Microsatellite Instability (MSI) as an Independent Predictor of Pathologic Complete Response (PCR) in Locally Advanced Rectal Cancer: A National Cancer Database (NCDB) Analysis. Ann Surg 2018; 271(4):716–23.

55. Bettoni F, Masotti C, Habr-Gama A, et al. Intratumoral Genetic Heterogeneity in Rectal Cancer: Are Single Biopsies representative of the entirety of the tumor? Ann Surg 2017;265(1):e4–6.

56. El Sissy C, Kirilovsky A, Van den Eynde M, et al. A Diagnostic Biopsy-Adapted Immunoscore Predicts Response to Neoadjuvant Treatment and Selects Patients with Rectal Cancer Eligible for a Watch-and-Wait Strategy. Clin Cancer Res 2020; 26(19):5198–207.

57. Ganesh K, Wu C, O'Rourke KP, et al. A rectal cancer organoid platform to study individual responses to chemoradiation. Nat Med 2019;25(10):1607–14.

58. Carpinetti P, Donnard E, Bettoni F, et al. The use of personalized biomarkers and liquid biopsies to monitor treatment response and disease recurrence in locally advanced rectal cancer after neoadjuvant chemoradiation. Oncotarget 2015; 6(35):38360–71.

Technological Advances in the Surgical Treatment of Colorectal Cancer

Sue J. Hahn, MD, Patricia Sylla, MD*

KEYWORDS

- Complete mesocolic excision (CME) • Transanal • Total mesorectal excision (TME)
- Colon and rectal cancer • Laparoscopy • Robotic • Minimally invasive surgery (MIS)
- Transanal TME (taTME)

KEY POINTS

- Adoption of minimally invasive surgery (MIS) for colorectal cancer resections has continued to increase, largely driven by improved short-term clinical outcomes and shorter time to recovery.
- Anastomotic and septic complications following colorectal cancer resections are equivalent across all MIS approaches.
- Published data support the short- and long-term oncologic safety of laparoscopic and robotic colon and rectal resection for cancer.
- The impact of total mesorectal excision (TME) on functional outcomes remains significant despite the increased adoption of MIS.
- Transanal TME is mostly used to facilitate sphincter salvage and reduce the risk of conversion in patients with low rectal cancer.

INTRODUCTION

The understanding of the oncologic principles of surgical resection for colorectal cancer has evolved greatly over the last few decades since the concept of total mesorectal excision (TME) was proposed by Heald and colleagues.[1] TME includes the removal of the rectum and mesorectum as one intact specimen by dissection along the mesorectal fascial plane. This concept has also been applied to surgical resection for colon cancer. Hohenberger and colleagues[2] first described complete mesocolic excision (CME) in 2009; namely, the dissection of the visceral fascia from the parietal fascia of the retroperitoneum and central ligation of the central colonic vessels for maximal lymph node harvest. Alongside this progress in oncologic surgical technique,

Division of Colon and Rectal Surgery, Department of Surgery, Icahn School of Medicine at Mount Sinai Hospital, 5 East 98th Street, Box 1259, New York, NY 10029, USA
* Corresponding author.
E-mail addresses: sue.hahn@mountsinai.org (S.J.H.); Patricia.sylla@mountsinai.org (P.S.)

Surg Oncol Clin N Am 31 (2022) 183–218
https://doi.org/10.1016/j.soc.2022.01.001
1055-3207/22/© 2022 Elsevier Inc. All rights reserved.

surgonc.theclinics.com

minimally invasive approaches, such as laparoscopy, robotic surgery, and transanal minimally invasive surgery (TAMIS), evolved with the aim to improve patient morbidity and mortality associated with traditional open approaches. These technological advances are addressed, as well as their short- and long-term outcomes in colorectal cancer.

EVOLUTION OF MINIMALLY INVASIVE COLORECTAL RESECTION

Surgical resection remains the mainstay treatment for patients with colorectal cancer. Open surgery has been the standard of care, but it is associated with significant morbidity and results in a large operation from which the patient must recover. The first laparoscopic colon resection was described in 1991.[3,4] This procedure, however, represented a technical challenge for surgeons and generated concerns about oncologic outcomes for patients with colon cancer. Overall, the minimally invasive technique was found to have improved short-term patient outcomes and noninferior oncologic outcomes.

The success of laparoscopic surgery led to further attempts to improve patient outcomes with the introduction of reduced port laparoscopy and robot-assisted laparoscopy. Single-incision laparoscopic surgery (SILS) uses a single entry point, typically the patient's umbilicus, resulting in a single scar and improved cosmesis.[5] Compared with standard multiport laparoscopy, SILS for colon cancer surgery has been shown to have comparable short-term outcomes.[6,7] Some studies have shown that SILS also results in shorter length of hospital stay than multiport laparoscopy.[8,9] Despite these benefits, widespread adoption has been limited because it is more technically difficult to perform owing to the proximity of the working instruments to each other, restricted freedom of movement, and fewer port availability.[10] Robotic-assisted colorectal surgery has increased significantly over the last decade.[11,12] However, the benefits of the robotic approach over standard laparoscopy have yet to be fully elucidated. Data from randomized controlled trials (RCTs) suggest lower conversion rates, longer operative times, and higher costs with a robotic compared with laparoscopic approach, whereas complication rates are similar.[11–15]

Natural orifice specimen extraction (NOSE) was introduced as a minimally invasive extraction method using a natural opening for specimen delivery. This is typically performed transvaginally or transrectally. NOSE for colon cancer has been associated with decreased pain and lower analgesia requirements when compared with conventional laparoscopic surgery.[16] Transanal specimen extraction after laparoscopic colorectal cancer surgery has been found to be safe, feasible, and oncologically comparable in highly selected cases.[17,18] RCTs are required to verify these findings and study long-term outcomes.

Natural orifice transluminal endoscopic surgery (NOTES) represents one of the most significant surgical innovations since the introduction of laparoscopy. In colorectal surgery, transanal endoscopic microsurgery (TEM; Richard Wolf Company, Tubingen, Germany) was introduced in 1983 and used a closed multiport proctoscope system to perform endoluminal local excision of rectal lesion using high-definition visualization, carbon dioxide (CO_2) insufflation, and adapted instrumentation.[19] When used to perform full-thickness excision of carefully selected low-risk early-stage rectal cancer, TEM demonstrates equivalent oncologic outcomes to radical resection.[20] The rigid TEM platform was subsequently adapted for use with conventional laparoscopic instruments, camera, and video tower in the form of a Transanal Endoscopic Operating System (TEO; Karl Storz, Tuttlingen, Germany).[21] Given the high costs of the TEM and TEO platforms and steep learning curve associated with their use, a novel approach using existing single-incision laparoscopic disposable ports, TAMIS, was developed.[22] Currently, this approach using transanal endoscopic platforms is referred to as transanal endoscopic surgery (TES) and is mostly used for local excision of benign and highly selected T1 malignant upper and middle rectal lesions with predicted low risk of lymph node metastasis. Local excision and endoscopic strategies for early colorectal tumors are further described in another article in this issue. For high-risk T1 lesions and more locally advanced tumors, TME remains the gold-standard surgical approach, in combination with neoadjuvant therapy for locally advanced stage II and III disease.

Transanal total mesorectal excision (taTME), whereby TME dissection is primarily performed using a transanal endoscopic approach with transabdominal assistance (open, laparoscopic, or robotic) represents the latest innovation in TME technique. taTME was developed as a convergence of multiple existing techniques in colorectal and minimally invasive surgery (MIS). First, from the experience gained from TES, inadvertent transcolonic or transrectal entry into the peritoneal cavity was shown to be safely managed endoscopically, which helped establish the feasibility and safety of purposeful transrectal access to the peritoneal entry, which is a core principle of taTME.[23] Second, taTME expands on the technique of the transanal transabdominal approach (TATA), whereby for very low rectal tumors, sphincter preservation can be achieved using intersphincteric resection.[24] During TATA, extending TME dissection beyond a few centimeters proximally is not possible because of poor exposure. However, this dissection can be effectively extended cephalad through the use of TES platforms, hence the concept of TME being performed using a bottom-up to complement a top-down approach (**Fig. 1**). Third, taTME was derived from the NOTES paradigm, whereby transanal access can be used for specimen extraction (NOSE), and as

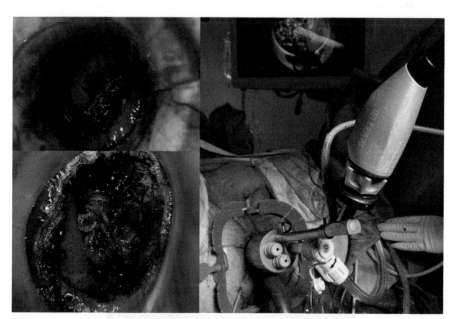

Fig. 1. For eligible low rectal tumors ≤5 cm from the anal verge, partial or complete intersphincteric resection is performed through an open transanal approach, followed by purse-string closure of the anorectal stump and insertion of a transanal platform to initiate taTME.

primary access to perform complex gastrointestinal procedures endoscopically, including colorectal resections.[25] It is the promise of incisionless surgery transluminal endoscopic surgery that propelled taTME forward.[25,26] Although "Pure" NOTES taTME is rarely feasible because of a limitation in instrumentation, this approach has been described in selected reports and case series.[27] taTME was cautiously transitioned from the experimental model to clinical application. Extensive preclinical work in porcine models and human cadavers demonstrated the feasibility of a transanal approach to rectosigmoid resection.[27–29] This preclinical work was instrumental to highlight that although a significant portion of the TME dissection could be performed by transanal dissection, abdominal assistance was required in order to perform safe ligation of the inferior mesenteric vessels, proximal mobilization of the colonic conduit, and splenic flexure takedown, and to reduce the risk of inadvertent organ injury.[30] For this reason, most taTME procedures are performed as a 2-team approach and include an abdominal and transanal team working simultaneously or sequentially (**Fig. 2**). This preclinical work set the stage for the first clinical case of taTME reported by Sylla and collegues[31] in 2010. After this report, the field rapidly expanded with publication of numerous case series that have since grown in sample size, alongside the international taTME registry whose first publication of the first 720 cases was published in 2016,[32] and the most recent publication of 1540 taTME cases performed for rectal cancer in 2021.[33] In addition to an enlarging body of evidence in support of the perioperative and early oncologic safety of this approach in carefully selected cases, several large taTME institutional and multicenter cohort series have recently published their mid-term 3- to 5-year oncologic outcomes, whereas several phase II and phase III clinical trials are currently ongoing.[34,35]

OUTCOMES
Short-Term Outcomes

Colon cancer
Since the COST trial was reported in 2004, laparoscopic colon resection for colon cancer has been widely performed in the United States. Various RCTs have found the

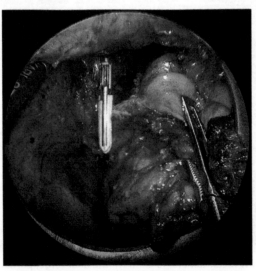

Fig. 2. Combined transanal and abdominal mobilization of residual rectal and mesorectal pelvic side attachments performed as a 2-team approach.

minimally invasive colectomy approach to be superior to the traditional open approach for colon cancer in regard to short-term outcomes (**Table 1**). The Barcelona trial, which was the first RCT that compared laparoscopic with open approaches, reported faster recovery and shorter hospital length of stay with the laparoscopic approach.[36] Although the COST trial found that the rates of intraoperative complications, 30-day postoperative mortality, complications at 60 days, hospital readmission, and reoperation were distributed similarly between the treatment groups, it also demonstrated faster perioperative recovery, shorter median hospital stay, and briefer use of parenteral and oral analgesics for the laparoscopic group.[37] The COST trial also found that recurrence rates in surgical wounds were less than 1% in both groups, addressing concerns for tumor seeding in port sites in laparoscopic colectomy. The COLOR trial similarly found that laparoscopic colectomy was associated with earlier return of bowel function, need for fewer analgesics, and a shorter hospital stay compared with open colectomy. It also reported that 28-day morbidity (including wound infection) and mortality did not differ between the groups.[38] The ALCCaS trial demonstrated the same advantages for the laparoscopic group and found no differences in the rates of wound infection, pneumonia, or other types of complications.[39] The Japan Clinical Oncology Group Study 0404 performed a noninferiority study to compare laparoscopic with open D3 dissection and resection of advanced T3 or T4 (without other organ involvement) colon cancers and likewise demonstrated that patients in the laparoscopic arm had shorter hospital stay, faster return of bowel function, decreased narcotic use, and fewer complications.[40]

A topic of ongoing discussion in colon cancer surgery focuses on the technical considerations of the ileocolic anastomosis following MIS right colectomy. The anastomosis can be performed either intracorporeally or extracorporeally depending on surgeon preference. The advantage with an intracorporeal anastomosis is that the specimen can be extracted through a Pfannenstiel or transverse incision off the midline. For an extracorporeal anastomosis, an incision is usually made in the midline, above the umbilicus, which traditionally carries a higher risk of hernia formation.

Although intracorporeal anastomosis is considered more challenging to perform as compared with extracorporeal anastomosis, particularly when done via laparoscopy, it has become more widely available with the increased adoption of the robotic platform owing to its robotic articulating instruments and ergonomic advantages. Studies comparing the 2 anastomotic techniques for laparoscopic and robotic right colectomy have demonstrated advantages for the intracorporeal approach, including earlier return to bowel function, shorter hospital length of stay, shorter extraction incisions, decreased incisional hernia rate, and reduced short-term morbidity (**Table 2**).

Rectal cancer
Just as with colon cancers cases, various RCTs demonstrated the improved short-term outcomes of the minimally invasive approach, as compared with the more traditional open approach, for rectal cancer surgery (**Table 3**). The COLOR II trial compared laparoscopic with open resection of rectal cancer within 15 cm from the anal verge and found that bowel function returned sooner and hospital stay was shorter in the laparoscopic group with no differences in morbidity and mortality within 28 days after surgery between the 2 groups.[41] The ALaCaRT trial included patients with T1–T3 tumors within 15 cm of the anal verge and found earlier return of bowel function in the laparoscopic group, with no differences in length of stay, analgesic requirement, or major complications between the 2 groups.[42] The conversion rate in this trial was 9%. The ACOSOG Z6051 trial included 486 patients undergoing laparoscopic and

Table 1
Trials comparing laparoscopic and open surgery for colon cancer: oncologic outcomes

Study	Study Period	No.	Mean Follow-Up Duration, mo	Postoperative Morbidity, %	Overall Recurrence, %	Disease-Free Survival, %	Overall Survival, %	Other
Barcelona, et al, 2002[36]	1993–1998	Lap: 106 Open: 102	95	11 29	18 28	– –	64 57	• 30 d mortality similar
COST, 2007[54]	1994–2001	Lap: 435 Open: 428	53	21 20	19.4 21.8	69.2 68.2	76.4 74.6	
COLOR, 2005[35,121]	1997–2003	Lap: 534 Open:542	84	21 20	19.6 16.9	76.2 74.2	84.2 81.8	• Conversion rate 17% • BMI >30 excluded
CLASICC, 2007[99,122]	1996–2002	Lap: 230 Open: 118	62.9	35 35	23.8 22.2	57.6 64.0	55.7 62.7	• Positive CRM: 5% open vs 7% lap ($P = .45$)
ALCCaS, 2012[55]	1998–2005	Lap: 290 Open: 297	62	37.8 45.3	13.7 14.8	72.3 71.7	77.7 76.0	• Conversion rate 14.6%

Abbreviation: lap, laparoscopic.

Table 2
Studies comparing intracorporeal and extracorporeal anastomosis in right colectomy

Authors	Year	Study Design	LRC	RRC	ICA	ECA	Results
Grams et al[123]	2010	Retrospective	X	X	14	15	ICA: Earlier ROBF, decreased postoperative narcotic use, decreased morbidity, decreased LOS
Cirocchi et al[124]	2012	Systematic review & meta-analysis	X		177	145	No significant differences between groups
Park et al[68]	2012	RCT	X	X	30 RRC 7 LRC	5 RRC 28 LRC	No significant differences between groups
Lee et al[125]	2013	Retrospective	X		51	35	Comparable short- and long-term outcomes in LRC in colon cancer
Stein et al[126]	2013	Review	X		164	195	No significant differences between groups
Feroci et al[127]	2013	Systematic review & meta-analysis	X		202	223	ICA: Earlier ROBF, earlier po intake, decreased analgesic use and LOS
Morpurgo et al[128]	2013	Case control	X		48 RRC ICA	48 LRC ECA	RRC ICA: Earlier ROBF, shorter LOS, lower anastomotic complication rate
Milone et al[129]	2015	Multicenter case-control	X		286	226	ECA: Higher complication rate and higher severity of morbidity (per Clavien-Dindo classification), higher rate of wound infections ICA: Earlier ROBF
Trastulli et al[130]	2015	Retrospective multicenter	X	X	102 RRC 40 LRC	94 LRC ECA	RRC ICA vs LRC ECA: longer OR time, earlier ROBF and shorter LOS RRC ICA vs LRC ICA: earlier ROBF, no difference in LOS
Vignali et al[131]	2016	RCT	X		64	64	ICA: Earlier ROBF, lower incisional hernia rate

(continued on next page)

Table 2
(continued)

Authors	Year	Study Design	LRC	RRC	ICA	ECA	Results
van Oostendorp et al[132]	2017	Systematic review & meta-analysis	X		763	729	ICA: Shorter LOS, reduced short-term morbidity
Cleary et al[133]	2018	Multicenter case control	X	X	335 RRC 44 LRC	253 RRC 397 LRC	ICA: Longer OR times, lower conversion rate, shorter LOS, lower complication rate
Mari et al[134]	2018	RCT	X		30	30	ICA: Earlier ROBF, earlier po intake No significant difference in LOS
Allaix et al[135]	2019	RCT	X		70	70	ICA: Earlier ROBF No significant difference in LOS
Emile et al[136]	2019	Systematic review & meta-analysis	X	X	2123	2327	ICA: Shorter extraction site incisions, earlier ROBF, fewer complications, lower rates of conversion, leak, SSI, and incisional hernia
Bollo et al[137]	2020	RCT	X		69	70	ICA: Longer OR times, shorter extraction site incision, earlier ROBF, less postoperative analgesia, less LGIB, lower CD grade I and grade II complications, lower LOS
Creavin et al[138]	2021	Systematic review & meta-analysis	X		199	200	ICA: Earlier ROBF, less ileus, improved pain scores No significant difference in LOS or overall morbidity

Abbreviations: CD, Clavien-Dindo; ECA, extracorporeal anastomosis; ICA, intracorporeal anastomosis; LGIB, lower gastrointestinal bleeding; LOS, length of stay; LRC, laparoscopic right colectomy; ROBF, return of bowel function; RRC, robotic right colectomy; OR, operating room; po, per oral; SSI, surgical site infection.

Table 3
Trials comparing laparoscopic and open surgery for rectal cancer: oncologic outcomes

Trial	Inclusion Criteria	Primary Endpoint	Results				
			Negative CRM	Clear Distal Margin	Complete or Near-Complete TME	Other	
Kang et al,[49] (COREAN) 2010	Stage II-III tumors within 9 cm of AV 340 patients	3-y DFS	97.1% lap vs 95.9% open (P = .77)	100% lap vs 100% open (P = .54)	91.8% lap vs 88% open (P = .41)	• 3-y LR, DFS, OS: similar • EBL: 200 mL lap vs 217 mL open • OR time: 245 min lap vs 197 min open • ROBF: 38 h lap vs 60 h open • LOS: 8 d lap vs 9 d open • Conversion rate: 1.5%	
Van der Pas et al,[41] (COLOR II) 2013	T1-T3 tumors within 15 cm of AV 1044 patients	3-y LR	90% lap vs 90% open (P = .85)	100% lap vs 100% open (P = .67)	97% lap vs 98% open (P = .25)	• 3-y LR, DFS, OS: similar • EBL: 200 mL lap vs 400 mL open • OR time: 240 min lap vs 188 min open • ROBF: 2 d lap vs 3 d open • LOS: 8 d lap vs 9 d open • Conversion rate: 17%	

(continued on next page)

Table 3
(continued)

Trial	Inclusion Criteria	Primary Endpoint	Results			Other
			Negative CRM	Clear Distal Margin	Complete or Near-Complete TME	
Stevenson et al,[42,119] (ALaCaRT) 2015	T1-T3 tumors within 15 cm of AV 475 patients	Meeting all of the following: Complete TME, CRM ≥ 1 mm, distal margin ≥ 1 mm	93% lap vs 97% open ($P = .06$)	98% lap vs 98% open ($P = .91$)	97% lap vs 99% open ($P = .06$)	• Successful resection: 82% lap vs 89% open • Conversion rate: 9% • 2-y LRR: 5.4% lap vs 3.1% open (HR, 1.7; 95% CI, −9.2% to 5.4%) • 2-y DFS, OS: similar • OR time: 266 min lap vs 220 min open • LOS: similar
Fleshman et al,[43,120] (ACOSOG Z6051) 2015	Stage II-III tumors within 12 cm of AV 248 patients	Composite of following: CRM >1 mm, negative distal margin, completeness of TME	87.9% lap vs 92% open ($P = .11$)	99% lap vs 99% open ($P = .67$)	92% lap vs 95% open ($P = .20$)	• Successful resection: 81.7% lap vs 86.9% open • Conversion rate: 11.3% • 2-y DFS, OS: similar

Abbreviation: AV, anal verge.

open resection of stage II or III rectal cancer within 12 cm of the anal verge and found no differences in length of stay, readmission, or severe complications.[43] The conversion rate in this trial was 11.3%. Compared with laparoscopic surgery, robotic surgery in recent systematic reviews has been associated with earlier time to oral diet or return to bowel function, shorter hospital stays, and lower conversion rate at the cost of longer operative times.[44–47] The ROLARR trial, however, found that robotic surgery results in comparable short-term outcomes and does not significantly reduce the risk of conversion to open laparotomy. The trial concluded thereby that robotic surgery does not confer a significant enough benefit clinically in the short term, as compared with conventional laparoscopic surgery, to justify its higher cost.[48]

Overall, laparoscopic TME has shown some advantages, including decreased pain and wound infection rates, reduced length of hospital stay, but impact on anastomotic complications and functional outcomes has been limited.[41,49,50] In addition, laparoscopic TME has been plagued with high rates of conversion to an open approach, ranging from 9% to 30% in large trials, although centers with experienced laparoscopic surgeons demonstrate conversion rates of 10% or less.[42,43,49,50] Conversion to open surgery has been associated with worse patient outcomes.[41,51–53] Converted patients are more likely to have higher body mass index (BMI), prolonged length of stay, and increased overall postoperative complication rates, such as increased anastomotic leak rate. The COST and CLASICC trials also found that conversion was associated with worse overall survival (OS).[54,55] However, these outcomes may also be partially attributable to the stage of the patients' disease, with more advanced disease necessitating conversion.

Robotic TME offers the advantages of 3-dimensional visualization and articulated instrumentation. In nonrandomized studies, robotic TME has had lower rates of conversion compared with laparoscopic TME (odds ratio, 0.26; 95% confidence interval [CI], 0.12–0.57).[56,57] However, a large randomized study, ROLARR, showed no advantage of robotic TME in terms of margin positivity, mortality, morbidity, or conversions as compared with laparoscopic TME.[48] Furthermore, in high-risk groups (men, obesity, distal tumors), rates of conversion were very high in both the robotic (7.2%–18.9%) and the laparoscopic (13.3%–27.8%) arms of the trial. Finally, there are ongoing concerns about the high overall costs of robotic TME when compared with laparoscopic TME.[58]

Transanal Total Mesorectal Excision

Rates of abdominal conversion in taTME appear to be relatively low, ranging from 0% to 5.6% in the taTME registry that included 720 patients (**Table 4**). A propensity-matched analysis of taTME compared with laparoscopic TME found a significantly lower rate of conversion in the taTME group (1.5% vs 8.6%; P<.001).[59] Thus, it appears that taTME is associated with similar, if not improved, outcomes with regards to intraoperative conversion, particularly in the hands of experienced operators. With respect to postoperative morbidity with taTME, there are no significant differences in the rate of major or minor complications (see **Table 4**). Transanal specimen extraction, when possible, eliminates the need for an abdominal extraction site, which could help lower the risk of wound infection. However, most taTME procedures performed still use an abdominal extraction site in order to decrease the risk of specimen fragmentation and disruption that can occur when extraction is attempt through a narrow pelvis.[32]

Transabdominal TME requires firing of a stapler low in the pelvis, frequently resulting in multiple staple firings to achieve transection at the distal margin. Multiple firings of the stapling device have been associated with higher rates of anastomotic leak; thus,

Table 4
Patient characteristics and outcomes reported in published transanal total mesorectal excision series with ≥80 patients

	Veltcamp Helbach, 2016[139]	de Lacy, 2018[140]	Perdawood, 2021[141]	Detering, 2019[59]	Kang, 2019
Study period	6/2012 - 9/2014	11/2011–6/2016	12/2013–7/2019	1/2015–12/2017	5/2010–4/2016
Study location	Amsterdam, The Netherlands	Barcelona, Spain	Slagelse, Denmark	The Netherlands	China
Number of institutions	2	1	1	44	10
Transanal device used	GelPOINT or SILS	GelPOINT	GelPOINT	—	—
Total number of patients	80	186	200	416	211
Patient & tumor characteristics					
Male sex, n (%)	48 (60.0)	118 (63.4)	147 (73.5)	301 (72.4)	124 (58.8)
Age, mean ± standard deviation (SD) or median (interquartile range [IQR]), y	65.3 ± 2.7	65 (56–75)	67 ± 10	—	58.6 ± 13.6
BMI, mean ± SD or median (IQR), kg/m^2	28.6 ± 1.8	25.1 ± 3.9	26.7 ± 4.3	—	22.9 ± 3.1
Tumor height from anal verge, mean ± SD or median (IQR), cm[a]	5.3 (1–10)[b]	7.9 ± 1.5 (mid) 3.5 ± 1.3 (low)	8 ± 2	—	5.9 ± 2.0
Preoperative stage, n (%)					
T1–2	All T2–T3	44 (23.6)	86 (43.0)	121 (29.0)	67 (31.7)
T3		126 (67.7)	105 (52.5)	266 (63.9)	106 (50.2)
T4		14 (7.5)	9 (4.5)	21 (5.0)	29 (13.7)
Neoadjuvant therapy, n (%)	65 (81.3)	116 (62.4)	44 (22.0)	151 (36.3)	58 (27.5)
Clinical outcomes					
Total operative time, mean ± SD or median (IQR), minutes	204 (91–447)	147.8 ± 51.2	286 ± 63	—	280.0 ± 110
Conversions, n (%)	—	—	1 (0.5)	6 (1.4)	2 (0.9)
Overall morbidity at 28 d, n (%)	31 (28.3)	—	49 (24.5)	176 (42.3)	59 (27.9)
Minor	21 (26.3)	—	22 (11.0)	—	—
Major	10 (12.0)	—	27 (13.5)	—	—
Overall mortality at 28 d, n (%)	1 (1.3)	—	—	1 (0.2)	—

	Hol, 2019[86]	Zeng, 2020[78]	Wasmuth, 2020[84]	Oostendorp, 2020[85]	Roodbeen, 2021[87]
Anastomotic leak, n (%)	—	13 (9.3)	—	53 (16)	17 (8.1)
Unplanned reoperation, n (%)	9 (11.3)	—	—	—	7 (3.3)
Length of hospital stay, mean ± SD or median (IQR), d	8 (3–41)	—	—	—	13 (3–65)
Pathologic outcomes					
Positive CRM, n (%)	2 (2.5)[c]	15 (8.1)	11 (5.5)	18 (4.4)	5 (2.3)
Positive DRM, n (%)	0	6 (3.2)	1 (0.5)	—	—
TME quality, n (%)					
Complete	71 (88.8)	178 (95.7)	133 (66.5)	—	175 (82.9)
Moderate/near complete	7 (8.8)	3 (1.6)	45 (22.5)	—	33 (15.6)
Incomplete	2 (2.5)	2 (1.1)	22 (11.0)	—	3 (1.4)
Number of lymph nodes, mean ± SD or median (IQR)	16 ± 2	14 (11–18)	—	—	14.2 ± 7.3
Median follow-up, mo	21	—	29[c]	—	35
Recurrence rate,[a] n (%)					
Local	2 (2.5)	—	7 (3.5)	—	13 (6.2)
Distant	—	—	24 (12.0)	—	27 (12.8)
Both local and distant	—	—	6 (3.0)	—	—
Study period	1/2012–5/2016	4/2016–11/2018	10/2014–10/2018	3/2015–10/2018	8/2011–12/2018
Study location	Amsterdam, The Netherlands	Guangzhou, China	Norway	The Netherlands	The Netherlands; Italy; France; Belgium; United States
Number of institutions	2	1	7	12	6
Transanal device used	GelPOINT	SILS or Starr Port	GelPOINT	GelPOINT	GelPOINT
Total number of patients	159	128	157	120	767

(continued on next page)

Table 4
(continued)

	Hol, 2019[86]	Zeng, 2020[78]	Wasmuth, 2020[84]	Oostendorp, 2020[85]	Roodbeen, 2021[87]
Patient & tumor characteristics					
Male sex, n (%)	106 (67)	83 (64.8)	109 (69.4)	109 (91)	552 (72.0)
Age, mean ± SD or median (IQR), years	66.9 ± 10.2	56.1 ± 11.2	66 ± 11	65 ± 10	64 (55–70)
BMI, mean ± SD or median (IQR), kg/m²	26.4 ± 4.3	22.5 ± 3.1	—	27 ± 4	25.8 (23.2–28.8)
Tumor height from anal verge, mean ± SD or median (IQR), cm^d	5.7 ± 3.5	5.0 ± 1.7	8 (range, 2–13)	7 ± 3	3.0 (1.0–5.0)
Preoperative stage, n (%)					
T1–2	41 (25.8)	22 (17.1)	—	103 (85.9)	219 (31.5)
T3	103 (64.8)	100 (78.1)	—	17 (14.2)	421 (60.7)
T4	11 (6.9)	1 (0.8)	—	—	52 (7.5)
Neoadjuvant therapy, n (%)	112 (70.4)	(46.1)	33 (21.0)	77 (64.2)	527 (68.7)
Clinical outcomes					
Total operative time, mean ± SD or median (IQR), min	—	213.2 ± 58.9	274 ± 74	—	240 (200–300)
Conversions, n (%)	—	0	2 (1.3)	0	22 (2.9)
Overall morbidity at 28 d, n (%)	83 (52.2)	—	—	54 (45.0)	306 (39.9)
Minor	44 (27.7)	—	—	31 (25.8)	210 (27.4)
Major	39 (24.5)	13 (10.2)	—	23 (19.2)	96 (12.5)
Overall mortality at 28 d, n (%)	—	0	4 (2.5)	0	1 (0.1)
Anastomotic leak, n (%)	10 (6.3)	7 (5.4)	11 (8.4)	17 (17)	—
Unplanned reoperation, n (%)	36 (22.6)	2 (1.6)	—	—	—
Length of hospital stay, mean ± SD or median (IQR), d	—	10.8 ± 6.6	—	—	6 (4–10)
Pathologic outcomes					
Positive CRM, n (%)	1 (0.6)		20 (12.7)	6 (5.0)	56 (7.3)

	Simo, 2021[88]	Klein, 2021[142]	Caceydo, 2021[143]	Alhanafy, 2020[144]
Positive DRM, n (%)	0	—	0	14 (1.7)
TME quality, n (%)				
Complete	139 (87)		107 (89.2)	607 (80.6)
Moderate/near complete	16 (10)		13 (10.8)	94 (12.5)
Incomplete	4 (3)		0	52 (6.9)
Number of lymph nodes, mean ± SD or median (IQR)	—	—	—	16 (11–22)
Median follow-up, mo	52	19.5	21.9	25.5
Recurrence rate, n (%)				
Local	6 (3.8)	12 (7.9)	12 (10.0)	24 (3.1)
Distant	22 (13.8)	—	23 (19.2)	—
Both local and distant	2 (1.3)	3 (2.6)	9 (7.5)	11 (1.4)
Study period	5/2013–2/2019	8/2016–4/2019	1/2014–12/2018	1/2014–12/2017
Study location	Madrid, Spain	Denmark	Canada	Seoul, South Korea
Number of institutions	4	4	8	1
Transanal device used	GelPOINT	—	GelPOINT or Richard Wolf	—
Total number of patients	173	115	608	208
Patient & tumor characteristics				
Male sex, n (%)	121 (70)	85 (74)	423 (69.6)	132 (63.5)
Age, mean ± SD or median (IQR), y	69 (56–77)	69 (61–73)	63 (54–70)	62.5 ± 10.1
BMI, mean ± SD or median (IQR), kg/m²	27 (24–29)	25.2 (23.1–28.4)	27 24.1–31.3)	24 ± 3.1
Tumor height from anal verge, mean ± SD or median (IQR), cm[e]	5 (4–7)	8 (0–5 cm), 88 (6–10 cm), 11 (11–15 cm)	6 (4–8)	88 (<5 cm), 112 (<10 cm), 8 (≥10 cm)
Preoperative stage, n (%)				
T1–2	58 (33.6)	47 (40)	—	52 (25)
T3	44 (25.4)	58 (50)	—	139 (66.8)

(continued on next page)

Table 4
(continued)

	Simo, 2021[88]	Klein, 2021[142]	Caceydo, 2021[143]	Alhanafy, 2020[144]
T4	11 (6.4)	5 (4.3)	—	17 (8.2)
Neoadjuvant therapy, n (%)	118 (68.2)	19 (17%)	425 (69.9)	135 (64.9)
Clinical outcomes				
Total operative time, mean ± SD or median (IQR), min	240 ± 42	253 (210–300)	276 (234–338)	215 (range, 90–705)
Conversions, n (%)	—	0	26 (4.3)	5 (2.5)
Overall morbidity at 28 d, n (%)	—	37 (32.1)	339 (55.8)	75 (37.1)
Minor	—	33 (28.7)	243 (40.2)	—
Major	17 (10)	9 (7.8)	93 (15.4)	11 (5.5)
Overall mortality at 28 d, n (%)	—	0	3 (0.5)	—
Anastomotic leak, n (%)	—	6 (9.1)	46 (7.6)	18 (8.9)
Unplanned reoperation, n (%)	—	—	64 (10.5)	—
Length of hospital stay, mean ± SD or median (IQR), d	6 (5–10)	6 (5–13)	—	9 (range, 6–49)
Pathologic outcomes				
Positive CRM, n (%)	2 (1.4)	2 (1.7)[f]	43 (7.1)	26 (12.9)
Positive DRM, n (%)	2 (1.1)	7 (6)	15 (2.5)	6 (3)
TME quality, n (%)				
Complete	126 (72.8)[e]	67 (60)	565 (92.9)	134 (66.3)
Moderate/near complete	24 (13.9)[e]	32 (28)	-	61 (30.2)
Incomplete	6 (3.5)[e]	13 (12)	27 (4.4)	7 (3.5)
Number of lymph nodes, mean ± SD or median (IQR)	13 (9–17)	32 (23–46)	—	—
Median follow-up, mo	23	23	27	34
Recurrence rate, n (%)				

		taTME Registry, 2017[32]	taTME Registry, 2019[33]	taTME Registry, 2021[145]
Local	5 (2.9)	4 (3.5)	22 (3.6)	(1.7)
Distant	14 (8.1)	11 (9.6)	57 (9.4)	(3.6)
Both local and distant				
Study period		7/2014–12/2015	7/2014–12/2016	2/2010–12/2018
Study location		International	International	International
Number of institutions		66	107	203
Transanal device used		—	Rigid and flexible	—
Total number of patients		720	1594	2803
Patient & tumor characteristics				
Male sex, n (%)		489 (67.9)	1080 (67.8)	1991 (71)
Age, mean ± SD or median (IQR), y		62.4 ± 13	63.7 ± 12.4	65 (57–73)
BMI, mean ± SD or median (IQR), kg/m^2		26.5 ± 4.3	26.3 ± 4.4	25.8 (23.3–28.9)
Tumor height from anal verge, mean ± SD or median (IQR), cm[9]		6 (range, 0–13)	6 (range, 0–17)	4 (2–6)[h]
Pre-operative stage, n (%)				
T1–2		—	—	695 (28.5)
T3		≥T3, 374 (66.9)	≥T3, 930 (69)	1544 (63.2)
T4				176 (7.2)
Neoadjuvant therapy, n (%)		355 (57.1)	895 (56.1)	1710 (60.9)
Clinical outcomes				

(continued on next page)

Table 4
(continued)

	taTME Registry, 2017[32]	taTME Registry, 2019[33]	taTME Registry, 2021[145]
Total operative time, mean ± SD or median (IQR), min	—	252 ± 102	—
Conversions, n (%)	60 (9.1)	90 (5.6)	—
Overall morbidity at 28 d, n (%)	213 (32.6)	564 (35.4)	—
Minor	142 (21.7)	354 (22.2)	
Major	8 (1.3)	201 (25.8)	
Overall mortality at 28 d, n (%)	3 (0.5)	9 (0.6)	—
Anastomotic leak, n (%)	40 (6.7)	250 (15.7)	—
Unplanned reoperation, n (%)	44 (6.1)	128 (8)	—
Length of hospital stay, mean ± SD or median (IQR), d	—	8 (range, 2–94)	—
Pathologic outcomes			
Positive CRM, n (%)	14 (2.4)	—	125 (5.1)
Positive DRM, n (%)	2 (0.3)	—	25 (1)
TME quality, n (%)			
Complete	503 (85)	—	2280 (86.2)
Moderate/near complete	65 (11)	—	285 (10.8)
Incomplete	24 (4.1)	—	79 (3)
Number of lymph nodes, mean ± SD or median (IQR)	—	—	—
Median follow-up, mo	—	—	24 (12–38)

Recurrence rate, n (%)		
Local	—	(4.8)
Distant	—	(23.4)
Both local and distant	—	—

Less than 2 mm.
[a] Among patients with nonmetastatic disease.
[b] From anorectal junction.
[c] Less than 2 mm.
[d] Pathologic T stage.
[e] Pathologic T stages.
[f] CRM status missing in 60 (9.9%).
[g] TME specimen quality missing in 9.8% of patients.
[h] From anorectal junction, +Mean follow-up time.

there was hope that taTME, by virtue of eliminating the need for rectal stapling, would reduce the risk of this complication.[60] Generally, anastomotic leak rates reported in the largest series from experienced centers have ranged from 5.4% to 17% (see **Table 4**), which are not significantly different from rates following laparoscopic TME. An analysis of 1594 patients in the taTME registry found that early anastomotic leak (within 30 days of the operation) occurred in 7.8% of patients.[33] Overall, 15.7% of patients experienced some form of anastomotic complication, including early leak, delayed leak (2.0%), pelvic abscess (4.7%), fistula (0.8%), chronic sinus (0.9%), and stricture (3.6%). For patients that experienced early leak, a majority could be managed nonoperatively (82%).

PROCEDURE-SPECIFIC ADVERSE EVENTS

Surgical advancement does not come without new concerns. Pathologic oncologic markers regarding the quality of the rectal specimen after TME are especially relevant when comparing a newer surgical technique (laparoscopy) with the conventional approach (open).[43] Quirke and colleagues[61] correlated completeness of the TME specimen with oncologic survival and recurrence. Several studies have demonstrated that the open approach produces better pathologic specimens, although long-term outcomes were found to be similar.[42,43,46]

Transanal Total Mesorectal Excision

Urethral injury and visceral injury

Urethral injury predominately in male patients has been identified as an intraoperative complication of particular concern in taTME. During the anterior dissection from below, the prostate can be inadvertently mobilized, exposing the prostatic urethra. Incidence of urethral injury has varied in case series, ranging from 0% all the way up to 6.7% in a small series of 30 male patients by Rouanet and colleagues.[62] In reports from the international registry, the incidence of urethral injury has been reported around 0.8%.[33] An examination of 34 patients with urethral injury during taTME found that most of these injuries occurred early in the surgeon's experience (during the first 8 cases performed).[63] This indicates potential to reduce the incidence of urethral injury with explicit training on anatomic landmarks and pitfalls. Most injuries were identified intraoperatively, and many were repaired via a transperineal approach and without conversion to an open or laparoscopic approach.

In female patients undergoing taTME, vaginal perforation is also of concern during the anterior resection and can be associated with later rectovaginal fistula development. The international registry reported a 0.3% rate of vaginal perforation during taTME.[33] The injury can be repaired using a simple suture approach.[64] In addition to the concern of vaginal perforation, incorporation of the vaginal wall in a coloanal anastomosis can lead to formation of a neo-recto-vaginal fistula, and care must be taken to avoid this complication. Other visceral injuries that have been reported include ureteric injuries, bladder perforation, enterotomy, hypogastric nerve division, and splenic injury.[33,63]

Carbon dioxide embolism

Because of the high flow of CO_2 in a small space, risk of venous injury, and low pressure in the pelvic veins owing to Trendelenburg positioning, there is an increased risk of CO_2 embolism during taTME.[65] Harnsberger and colleagues[66] examined 80 cases of taTME and found that 3 patients had an abrupt decrease in end-tidal CO_2, drop in blood pressure, and poor oxygenation consistent with development of CO_2 embolus during the transanal portion of the operation. Analysis of the international registry demonstrated that approximately 0.4% of patients (25/6375 cases) had concern for CO_2 embolism.[67] There was no mortality, although 2 patients required cardiopulmonary resuscitation. Although the incidence is low, surgeons should be prepared to recognize and treat CO_2 embolism during taTME.

Oncologic Outcomes

Laparoscopic and robotic total mesorectal excision

The oncologic outcomes of minimally invasive and open surgeries for colon cancer have been shown to be similar (see **Table 1**). The COST, CLASICC, and COLOR trials reported that overall recurrence, disease-free survival (DFS), and OS rates were comparable in the 2 groups.[41,50,54,55] The COST trial found that patients who underwent conversion had worse 5-year OS rates compared with those that were completed open or laparoscopically. However, there was no significant difference in 5-year DFS or recurrence associated with conversion. The CLASICC trial reported that conversion to open approach for patients with colon cancer was associated with worse OS and DFS regardless of the experience of the surgeon.[50,55] This difference was attributed to advanced cancer pathology. RCTs studying long-term outcomes after robotic colectomy for colon cancer, albeit scant, appear to also report similar oncologic outcomes when compared with laparoscopic colectomy.[68]

Like trials in colon cancer, COREAN, CLASICC, and COLOR II trials found little to no difference in the oncologic outcomes (eg, local recurrence, OS, or DFS rates) between laparoscopic and open surgery for rectal cancer (see **Table 3**).[38,55,69] However, a debate arose over the safety of laparoscopic rectal cancer surgery. The controversy began when the ALaCaRT trial in Australia and New Zealand and the ACOSOG Z6051 trial in the United States failed to demonstrate the advantages of laparoscopic surgery when applying a new composite assessment score of successful resections. The rubric for this score considered distal resection margin (DRM), circumferential radial margin (CRM), and the completeness of the TME specimen. Successful TME is essential to reduce local recurrence and improve DFS, and CRM is the most important factor among pathologic quality indicators.[61,70] The AlaCaRT study indicated positive circumferential resection margins in 7% of the laparoscopic group versus 3% in the open group.[42] ACOSOG Z6051 reported a negative CRM involvement in 87.9% of the laparoscopic specimens and in 92.3% of open resections.[71] Both studies also found similar 2-year DFS and OS rates. Furthermore, recent systematic analyses reported that the pathologic results of laparoscopic surgery are comparable to that of open surgery, but do not guarantee better pathologic specimens.[46,72,73] As for robotic TME, RTCs and meta-analyses describing long-term oncologic outcomes are scarce. Current evidence suggests that pathologic outcomes after robotic TME are similar to laparoscopic TME but may have longer distal resection margins.[74–76]

The CLASICC and COLOR II trials demonstrated equivalent long-term oncologic outcomes for laparoscopic versus open TME.[41,77] However, concerns have been raised about oncologic safety of laparoscopic TME after 2 large randomized trials, ACOSOG Z6051 and AlaCaRT, were unable to demonstrate noninferiority compared with an open approach for morbidity and short-term oncologic outcomes.[37,38] Concerns have been raised regarding high rates of positive margins in very low tumors.[41]

Thus, even in expert hands, both laparoscopic and robotic TME have been shown to have significant limitations, particularly with regards to dissection and exposure deep in the narrow pelvis. These ongoing challenges provided the impetus for the development of a transanal approach to TME.

Transanal Total Mesorectal Excision

Total mesorectal excision grade and margin positivity

Overall, the rates of margin positivity in the largest series of taTME have been low, ranging from 0.6% to 12.9% for positive CRM ($\geq$1 mm) and 0% to 3.2% for positive DRM ($\geq$1 mm). Similarly, rates of complete and near-complete TME specimens according to Quirke's classification have generally ranged from 96% to 100% (see **Table 4**).

In a propensity-matched analysis, Detering and colleagues[59] found no differences in the rate of positive CRM between taTME and laparoscopic TME (4.3% vs 4%, P = 1.00). In an ongoing randomized study, Zeng and colleagues[78] found a 1.5% CRM-positive rate in both laparoscopic and taTME groups. A 2016 systematic review found lower rates of CRM positivity (4.5 vs 10.3%) and higher rates of complete or near-complete TME specimens (95.3% vs 88.2%) for taTME versus laparoscopic TME.[79]

In an analysis of results from the international taTME registry, Roodbeen and colleagues[80] found that positive CRM occurred in 4% of cases. Risk factors for positive CRM included tumors that were low in the rectum (<1 cm from the anorectal junction (ARJ)), tumors that were anterior, and T4 tumors. Extramural venous invasion and threatened or involved CRM on MRI were also risk factors for positive CRM. In addition, they noted a DRM positivity rate of 1% and found that 91.2% of specimens were graded as complete or near complete. This was only slightly lower than prior analysis of the registry finding that 96.6% of TME specimens were complete or near complete.[32]

D'Andrea and colleagues[81] reported a 3.7% positive CRM rate, with 83% complete and 94.4% complete/near-complete TME specimens in a cohort of 54 patients with relatively complex tumor characteristics, including prior pelvic surgery, local recurrence, and T3 and T4 tumors with threatened CRM. All cases were selected carefully when curative resection was deemed possible based on multidisciplinary team review.

Lymph nodes

Numerous case series have reported adequate rates of lymph node harvest with taTME, with mean number of nodes harvested generally between 16 and 32 nodes (see **Table 4**). The number of harvested lymph nodes in taTME seems comparable to laparoscopic TME. In its matched analysis, Detering and colleagues[59] found a similar proportion of patients had greater than 10 lymph nodes harvested between taTME and laparoscopic TME (84.3% vs 80.8%; P = .23). Another propensity-matched analysis by Roodbeen and colleagues[82] found a median of 18 versus 14 nodes in the taTME and laparoscopic groups, respectively (P = .10). In a randomized study, Zeng and colleagues[78] found no difference in median number of resected nodes: 15 versus 16 in the taTME and laparoscopic TME groups, respectively (P = .07).

Local and distant recurrence

Early case series of taTME reported favorable rates of local and distant recurrence, ranging from 1.7% to 7.9% and 12%–23.4%, respectively (see **Table 4**). However, there is recent alarm about several studies that presented high rates of local recurrence following taTME. A Norwegian report has questioned the oncologic safety of the transanal approach by reporting a 9.5% local relapse rate, characterized as rapid and multifocal along the pelvic side wall.[83] The Norwegian authorities temporarily halted the use of taTME and performed an audit that confirmed an estimated local recurrence rate (LR) of 11.6% with taTME compared with 2.4% for patients undergoing laparoscopic or open TME in the Norwegian Colorectal Cancer Registry at 2.5 years following surgery.[84] This raised concern that air flow during dissection from below could result in tumor seeding and adverse outcomes.

van Oostendorp and colleagues[85] also reported a higher rate of local recurrence at 10% following taTME performed in 12 centers undergoing a structured training pathway for implementation of taTME. They reported on a cohort of 120 patients early in the learning curve (first 10 cases at each center) with 21.9 months of follow-up. Of the 12 patients with local recurrence, 8 patients experienced multifocal pelvic recurrence similar to what was found in the Norwegian study. Although the rate of positive CRMs was similar to earlier studies (5.0%), the investigators found that there was a high rate of early complications, including anastomotic leak (17%). They found that in addition to positive CRM and pT3 tumors, intraoperative complications and postoperative pelvic sepsis were significant predictors of local recurrence, indicating that the technical execution of taTME, as opposed to the technique itself, may be the issue. In examining a larger cohort from 4 centers that had performed more than 41 cases, they found that the rate of local recurrence decreased with institutional experience, with 15% of the initial 10 cases at each center experiencing LR, as compared with 4.2% in the next 30 cases, and 3.8% from there onward.[85] Hol and colleagues found similar risk factors for local recurrence in a single-center study.[86] Deijen and colleagues[34] in a systemic review also noted the role that experience plays in LRs following taTME, finding that low-volume centers experienced a recurrence rate of 8.9% as compared with a recurrence rate of 2.8% in high-volume centers.

A recent multicenter study by Roodbeen and colleagues[87] estimated a 2-year actuarial LR of 3.3% and a 3-year actuarial LR of 4.4%, with a median time to local recurrence of 13.5 months. None of these patients had a multifocal pattern of pelvic recurrence. Of 24 patients with local recurrence, 13 had isolated recurrence, and nearly all of these patients (n = 10) were able to undergo salvage surgery, with 8 patients free of disease at the end of follow-up. Several ongoing studies hope to better address the question of local recurrence, including the COLOR III, GRECCAR, and North American taTME trial (clinicaltrials.gov).[34,35]

Overall and disease-free survival

Several studies have estimated DFS at 2 years to be between 82% and 89%.[87–89] Similarly, at 3 years, DFS was between 78% and 80% for these same studies, although Hol and colleagues[86] found a higher rate of 92% at 3 years and 81% at 5 years. In terms of OS, this was estimated between 95% and 96% at 2 years and 93% at 3 years, although Hol and colleagues found lower rates of 84% at 3 years and 77% at 5 years.[86–89]

CURRENT CHALLENGES AND CONTROVERSIES
Learning Curve for Laparoscopic and Robotic Resections

Despite its postoperative benefits, laparoscopic colectomy and proctectomy have not been as quickly accepted as laparoscopic cholecystectomy. Indeed, approximately 55% colon resections use the laparoscopic approach in the United States.[90] This is primarily due to its steep learning curve, with large urban teaching hospitals having greater utilization of laparoscopy. Studies have reported that a range of approximately 30 to 70 completed laparoscopic colectomies are needed to achieve proficiency.[91,92] Compared with the open approach, laparoscopy is technically more difficult because it requires operating with a 2-dimensional vision, decreased tactile feedback, and limited degrees of instrument maneuverability. Robotic surgery has thereby emerged as a potential tool to overcome such disadvantages. The robotic system provides better ergonomics, ambidextrous capability, elimination of tremor, motion scaling, articulating instruments that provide greater degrees of freedom, and an assistant-independent 3-dimensional viewing capability. Indeed, competency in robotic-assisted colorectal surgery is reportedly attained after 13 to 15 cases, possibly shortening the learning curve for MIS.[93,94] However, literature evaluating robotic technology for colorectal cancer surgery, including risks, outcomes, and costs, remains limited.

Learning Curve for Transanal Total Mesorectal Excision

taTME is a complex and challenging technique, even for surgeons already skilled in MIS. The initial analysis from the first 720 patients in the international taTME registry found that the procedure was safe and effective with acceptable short-term patient outcomes. However, incorrect plane dissection was reported in 7.8% of patients, as well as technical problems in almost 40% of cases. Although the most frequently reported intraoperative problems during the transanal phase were unstable pneumopelvis and poor smoke evacuation, there were also cases of pelvic bleeding and severe complications, including prostate and urethral injuries. It is important for the surgeon to master the anatomy as viewed during this "bottoms up" approach to avoid pitfalls, such as urethral injury or injury to the lateral neurovascular bundles.[95] In addition, performing the perineal or transanal phase through a single-port platform adds difficulty to the procedure because of the lack of triangulation and collision of instruments.

Several studies have focused on this steep learning curve, finding that improved outcomes occur with increased experience with the procedure. Koedam and colleagues[96] noted that surgeons had a significant reduction in postoperative complications (17.5% vs 47.5%) as well as anastomotic leak rate (5.0% vs 27.5%) after the first 40 cases. Lee and colleagues[97] determined that providers reached proficiency, defined by acceptable rates of high-quality TME similar to laparoscopic or open approaches, at around 45 to 50 cases. Deijen and colleagues have noted lower rates of conversion, higher rates of complete TME, and lower rates of local recurrence for high-volume taTME centers (more than 30 cases) versus low-volume centers.[34] Similarly, it has been noted that many of the reported urethral injuries occurred early in the surgeon's learning curve during the first 8 cases performed.[63]

In light of this difficult learning curve, several societies and expert centers from Europe and the United States have started providing training courses and guidelines for taTME beginners. However, a defined pathway is yet to be accepted by the colorectal surgical community. The International taTME Educational Collaborative Group proposed a framework for a structured taTME training curriculum via a consensus of experts in 2017.[98] Structured training generally includes practice of skills on cadavers and other simulated models, mentorship, and precepted cases with a taTME expert, and mandatory participation in submission of early cases to a national or international registry.[98] Prior experience and accreditation in laparoscopic colorectal surgery are required, and experience with transanal surgery is highly recommended. Training should take place in centers with a high volume of rectal cancer, and ideally 2 surgeons per unit should undergo training together; indeed, some national societies have recommended that new adopters of taTME should be trained exclusively at centers with expertise in taTME with a high volume of patients with rectal cancer.[99] Mentors should have at least 5 years in the surgical specialty, and they should have performed at least 30 taTME cases independently and should also provide training courses for this operation. Experts have also recommended that centers perform at least 20 to 30 cases per year to maintain skills in this challenging procedure.[96,100]

This structured training model has been shown to be feasible at a national level, and trainees have demonstrated acceptable rates of complications, conversions, and short-term oncologic results.[98,101,102] However, as previously noted, a group in the Netherlands recently published the oncologic results of the first 10 patients treated with taTME in 12 adopting centers that followed a structured training pathway.[85] Histopathologic outcomes, including CRM positivity, were good. However, the locoregional recurrence rate was 10%, and more than half of the pelvic relapses presented with multifocal characteristics. Thus, it is unclear whether these structured training pathways, as currently implemented, are adequate to overcome the steep learning curve associated with taTME, particularly by centers that have no prior experience with the technique.

Further guidelines have recently been proposed by the taTME Guidance Group, comprising representatives from numerous international societies.[100] The optimal training pathway, similar to the pathway defined by the taTME Educational Collaborative Group, was further clarified. Furthermore, the group recommended that challenging cases, such as T4 tumors, and cases of prior pelvic irradiation, prostate resection, or other complex pelvic surgery should be reserved for experienced providers at expert centers.[100] Expert centers were defined as those with an experienced taTME surgeon beyond the learning curve, multidisciplinary support, excellent clinical and pathologic outcomes as compared with registry data, and annual case volume of at least 25 taTME resections for rectal cancer annually, and preferably more than 40 annual taTME cases for any indication. The group also issued guidelines defining surgical quality and recommended prospective measurement of these outcomes with benchmarking against historical standards. Overall, standardization of the taTME technique and structured training is an ongoing discussion among the international surgical societies with the goal of facilitating safe and appropriate implementation into clinical practice.

FUNCTIONAL OUTCOMES

Low anterior resection syndrome (LARS) describes the constellation of symptoms, including diarrhea, incomplete emptying, fecal urgency and frequency, and incontinence, that occurs following rectal resection. Data regarding anorectal function after robotic TME compared with that after laparoscopic surgery are lacking and conflicting. Kim and colleagues[103] demonstrated that there was no difference in incidence of LARS in patients undergoing robotic or laparoscopic TME. Grass and colleagues[104] demonstrated improved anorectal function after robotic TME when compared with laparoscopic, open, or taTME, with the robotic group experiencing no LARS in 60.5%. The ROLARR trial found no difference in major LARS between the robotic group and laparoscopic group, with an 82.6% incidence rate of LARS in patients undergoing robotic TME, which consisted of minor symptoms in 19.7% and major symptoms in 62.9%. The most common symptoms were incontinence to flatus (65.2%) and clustering of bowel movements (66.7%).[105]

Data regarding functional outcomes after robotic TME are limited but largely demonstrate better urogenital function in patients undergoing robotic TME when compared with laparoscopic TME. A controlled study by Kim and colleagues[106] reported robotic TME for rectal cancer is associated with earlier recovery of normal voiding and sexual function compared with laparoscopic TME. D'Annibale and colleagues[107] compared functional outcomes between laparoscopic and robotic TME. The International Prostate Symptom Score (IPSS) scores normalized at 1 year after surgery in both groups. Patients undergoing robotic TME retained better erectile function at 1 year after surgery compared with those undergoing laparoscopic TME (6% vs 57%). A phase II RCT reported better sexual function 1 year after surgery in the robotic group than in the laparoscopic group.[103] A systematic review demonstrated favorable urologic and sexual function in patients undergoing robotic TME when compared with laparoscopic TME. Specifically, IPSS scores 3 months after robotic surgery were better than that of laparoscopic surgery, and International Index of Erectile Function (IIEF) scores changed from baseline to 6 months after a robotic approach were better than that of the laparoscopic approach. The ROLARR trial demonstrated no significant difference between the robotic and laparoscopic arms in regard to IPSS and IIEF scores.

Transanal Total Mesorectal Excision versus Laparoscopic Total Mesorectal Excision

A meta-analysis of functional outcomes after taTME as compared with laparoscopic TME found that there was no difference in incidence of LARS (relative risk, 1.13; 95% CI, 0.94–1.35), but that there was significant heterogeneity between studies.[108] The incidence of LARS was relatively high in both groups; however, few patients underwent colostomy for management of symptoms.

Despite concerns of higher rates of urologic injury and dysfunction after taTME, several small comparative studies have found no differences in urologic function between taTME and laparoscopic TME in men as measured by the IPSS.[109–111] Foo and colleagues[112] noted in a small study (n = 23) that men complained of worsened erectile function immediately following surgery ($P = .002$), but that function returned to normal after 6 months. They found no differences in scores measuring urologic function at 3 and 6 months following surgery. Few studies have examined outcomes in women, with Pontallier and colleagues[111] reporting 2 out of 5 women reporting sexual dysfunction after taTME, similar to rates after laparoscopic TME.

Effects of taTME on quality-of-life (QOL) scores have been mixed, with most studies showing an initial decrease following taTME followed by recovery to baseline by 6 to 12 months.[96,113] Keller and colleagues[114] actually found an increase in emotional function of patients at 1 year following surgery ($P<.01$). However, Koedam and colleagues[96] found that although other decreases in QOL measures had resolved to baseline at 6 months following taTME, social function remained significantly worse than baseline ($P = .01$).

In comparison to laparoscopic TME, some studies have found that scores favor laparoscopic taTME in certain areas, such as role functioning, fatigue, fecal incontinence, and buttock pain.[109,110] However, a systematic review and meta-analysis found no differences across comparative studies.[108]

FUTURE DIRECTIONS

New technological advancements for colorectal surgery are on the horizon. Augmented reality technology, such as head-mounted display, seeks to offer free head motion, instrument tracking, information overlay, and improved ergonomics for the surgeon.[115] Telementoring technology has also been introduced as a surgical training aid and aims to improve remote connectivity and education for surgeons within and between hospitals. However, there are limitations to widespread implementation, including technical limitations, such as minimum resolution requirements, Internet bandwidth limitations, and cybersecurity concerns, given the transmission of highly sensitive patient information.[116] Robotic transanal surgery has naturally evolved since TAMIS, using current abdominal robotic systems through flexible transanal platforms. However, these bulky multiarm systems with inflexible instruments are limited in their ability to access the proximal rectum and beyond. To overcome these issues, flexible endoluminal robotic systems were introduced with flexible cameras and instruments. Current iterations of this system are limited, however, because the instruments inherently lack the stability otherwise existing in robot-assisted technology and because they have a steep learning curve for utilization of advanced maneuvers, such as endoluminal suturing.[117] Most recently, the single-port robotic system was introduced that provides multiple wristed, elbowed instruments, as well as a wristed endoscope, and improves triangulation of instruments in tight spaces. Although this device is currently limited to urologic procedures, early evidence demonstrates satisfactory intraoperative performance when compared with conventional multiarm robotic systems.[118]

SUMMARY

MIS for colorectal cancer has been shown to improve short-term patient outcomes with earlier return of bowel function, decreased length of hospital stay, and reduced analgesic use, while providing similar long-term oncologic outcomes when compared with the open approach. More recent advancements, such as robotic surgery and TaTME, do not come without new risks and require sufficient surgical experience and skill. Further research is needed to evaluate the safety and feasibility of these newer approaches. As advancements continue, surgical innovations have the potential to improve surgeon capability, surgical education, and patient outcomes, which are otherwise not possible with conventional methods.

CLINICS CARE POINTS

- Laparoscopic colectomy for colorectal cancer is safe and has better short-term and similar long-term oncologic outcomes compared with an open approach.
- Higher-level evidence is needed for assessment of safety and patient outcomes in regard to robotic surgery and transanal total mesorectal excision.

DISCLOSURE

Dr P. Sylla serves as consultant to Ethicon, Medtronic, Karl Storz, Stryker. Dr S. Hahn has nothing to disclose.

REFERENCES

1. Heald RJ, Husband EM, Ryall RD. The mesorectum in rectal cancer surgery—the clue to pelvic recurrence? Br J Surg 1982;69(10):613–6.
2. Hohenberger W, Weber K, Matzel K, et al. Standardized surgery for colonic cancer: complete mesocolic excision and central ligation—technical notes and outcome. Colorectal Dis 2009;11(4):354–64.
3. Jacobs M, Verdeja JC, Goldstein HS. Minimally invasive colon resection (laparoscopic colectomy). Surg Laparosc Endosc 1991;1(3):144–50.
4. Fowler DL, White SA. Laparoscopy-assisted sigmoid resection. Surg Laparosc Endosc 1991;1(3):183–8.
5. Evans L, Manley K. Is there a cosmetic advantage to single-incision laparoscopic surgical techniques over standard laparoscopic surgery? A systematic review and meta-analysis. Surg Laparosc Endosc Percutan Tech 2016;26(3):177–82.
6. Athanasiou C, Pitt J, Malik A, et al. A systematic review and meta-analysis of single-incision versus multiport laparoscopic complete mesocolic excision colectomy for colon cancer. Surg Innov 2020;27(2):235–43.

7. Song Z, Li Y, Liu K, et al. Clinical and oncologic outcomes of single-incision laparoscopic surgery for right colon cancer: a propensity score matching analysis. Surg Endosc 2019;33(4):1117–23.

8. Liu X, Yang WH, Jiao ZG, et al. Systematic review of comparing single-incision versus conventional laparoscopic right hemicolectomy for right colon cancer. World J Surg Oncol 2019;17(1):179.

9. Hoyuela C, Juvany M, Carvajal F. Single-incision laparoscopy versus standard laparoscopy for colorectal surgery: a systematic review and meta-analysis. Am J Surg 2017;214(1):127–40.

10. Poon JT, Cheung CW, Fan JK, et al. Single-incision versus conventional laparoscopic colectomy for colonic neoplasm: a randomized, controlled trial. Surg Endosc 2012;26(10):2729–34.

11. Sheetz KH, Norton EC, Dimick JB, et al. Perioperative outcomes and trends in the use of robotic colectomy for Medicare beneficiaries from 2010 through 2016. JAMA Surg 2020;155(1):41–9.

12. Solaini L, Bazzocchi F, Cavaliere D, et al. Robotic versus laparoscopic right colectomy: an updated systematic review and meta-analysis. Surg Endosc 2018; 32(3):1104–10.

13. Roh HF, Nam SH, Kim JM. Robot-assisted laparoscopic surgery versus conventional laparoscopic surgery in randomized controlled trials: a systematic review and meta-analysis. PloS One 2018;13(1):e0191628.

14. Huang YJ, Kang YN, Huang YM, et al. Effects of laparoscopic vs robotic-assisted mesorectal excision for rectal cancer: an update systematic review and meta-analysis of randomized controlled trials. Asian J Surg/Asian Surg Assoc 2019;42(6):657–66.

15. Giuliani G, Guerra F, Coletta D, et al. Robotic versus conventional laparoscopic technique for the treatment of left-sided colonic diverticular disease: a systematic review with meta-analysis. Int J Colorectal Dis 2021;37(1):101–9.

16. Wolthuis AM, Fieuws S, Van Den Bosch A, et al. Randomized clinical trial of laparoscopic colectomy with or without natural-orifice specimen extraction. Br J Surg 2015;102(6):630–7.

17. Franklin ME Jr, Liang S, Russek K. Integration of transanal specimen extraction into laparoscopic anterior resection with total mesorectal excision for rectal cancer: a consecutive series of 179 patients. Surg Endosc 2013;27(1):127–32.

18. Nishimura A, Kawahara M, Suda K, et al. Totally laparoscopic sigmoid colectomy with transanal specimen extraction. Surg Endosc 2011;25(10):3459–63.

19. Buess G, Theiss R, Hutterer F, et al. [Transanal endoscopic surgery of the rectum - testing a new method in animal experiments]. Leber Magen Darm 1983;13(2):73–7.

20. Winde G, Nottberg H, Keller R, et al. Surgical cure for early rectal carcinomas (T1). Transanal endoscopic microsurgery vs. anterior resection. Dis Colon Rectum 1996;39(9):969–76.

21. Nieuwenhuis DH, Draaisma WA, Verberne GH, et al. Transanal endoscopic operation for rectal lesions using two-dimensional visualization and standard endoscopic instruments: a prospective cohort study and comparison with the literature. Surg Endosc 2009;23(1):80–6.

22. Atallah S, Albert M, Larach S. Transanal minimally invasive surgery: a giant leap forward. Surg Endosc 2010;24(9):2200–5.

23. Gavagan JA, Whiteford MH, Swanstrom LL. Full-thickness intraperitoneal excision by transanal endoscopic microsurgery does not increase short-term complications. Am J Surg 2004;187(5):630–4.

24. Marks J, Mizrahi B, Dalane S, et al. Laparoscopic transanal abdominal transanal resection with sphincter preservation for rectal cancer in the distal 3 cm of the rectum after neoadjuvant therapy. Surg Endosc 2010;24(11):2700–7.

25. Rattner D, Kalloo A, Group ASW. ASGE/SAGES Working Group on Natural Orifice Translumenal Endoscopic Surgery. 2005. Surg Endosc 2006;20(2): 329–33.

26. Sylla P, Willingham FF, Sohn DK, et al. NOTES rectosigmoid resection using transanal endoscopic microsurgery (TEM) with transgastric endoscopic assistance: a pilot study in swine. J Gastrointest Surg 2008;12(10):1717–23.

27. Leroy J, Barry BD, Melani A, et al. No-scar transanal total mesorectal excision: the last step to pure NOTES for colorectal surgery. JAMA Surg 2013;148(3): 226–30.

28. Sylla P, Sohn DK, Cizginer S, et al. Survival study of natural orifice translumenal endoscopic surgery for rectosigmoid resection using transanal endoscopic microsurgery with or without transgastric endoscopic assistance in a swine model. Surg Endosc 2010;24(8):2022–30.

29. Whiteford MH, Denk PM, Swanstrom LL. Feasibility of radical sigmoid colectomy performed as natural orifice translumenal endoscopic surgery (NOTES) using transanal endoscopic microsurgery. Surg Endosc 2007;21(10):1870–4.

30. Telem DA, Han KS, Kim MC, et al. Transanal rectosigmoid resection via natural orifice translumenal endoscopic surgery (NOTES) with total mesorectal excision in a large human cadaver series. Surg Endosc 2013;27(1):74–80.

31. Sylla P, Rattner DW, Delgado S, et al. NOTES transanal rectal cancer resection using transanal endoscopic microsurgery and laparoscopic assistance. Surg Endosc 2010;24(5):1205–10.

32. Penna M, Hompes R, Arnold S, et al. Transanal total mesorectal excision: international registry results of the first 720 cases. Ann Surg 2017;266(1):111–7.

33. Penna M, Hompes R, Arnold S, et al. Incidence and risk factors for anastomotic failure in 1594 patients treated by transanal total mesorectal excision: results from the International TaTME Registry. Ann Surg 2019;269(4):700–11.

34. Deijen CL, Velthuis S, Tsai A, et al. COLOR III: a multicentre randomised clinical trial comparing transanal TME versus laparoscopic TME for mid and low rectal cancer. Surg Endosc 2016;30(8):3210–5.

35. Lelong B, Meillat H, Zemmour C, et al. Short- and mid-term outcomes after endoscopic transanal or laparoscopic transabdominal total mesorectal excision for low rectal cancer: a single institutional case-control study. J Am Coll Surg 2017;224(5):917–25.

36. Lacy AM, Garcia-Valdecasas JC, Delgado S, et al. Laparoscopy-assisted colectomy versus open colectomy for treatment of non-metastatic colon cancer: a randomised trial. Lancet 2002;359(9325):2224–9.

37. Clinical Outcomes of Surgical Therapy Study Group, Nelson H, Sargent DJ, et al. A comparison of laparoscopically assisted and open colectomy for colon cancer. N Engl J Med 2004;350(20):2050–9.

38. Veldkamp R, Kuhry E, Hop WC, et al. Laparoscopic surgery versus open surgery for colon cancer: short-term outcomes of a randomised trial. Lancet Oncol 2005;6(7):477–84.

39. Hewett PJ, Allardyce RA, Bagshaw PF, et al. Short-term outcomes of the Australasian randomized clinical study comparing laparoscopic and conventional open surgical treatments for colon cancer: the ALCCaS trial. Ann Surg 2008;248(5): 728–38.

40. Yamamoto S, Inomata M, Katayama H, et al. Short-term surgical outcomes from a randomized controlled trial to evaluate laparoscopic and open D3 dissection for stage II/III colon cancer: Japan Clinical Oncology Group Study JCOG 0404. Ann Surg 2014;260(1):23–30.

41. van der Pas MH, Haglind E, Cuesta MA, et al. Laparoscopic versus open surgery for rectal cancer (COLOR II): short-term outcomes of a randomised, phase 3 trial. Lancet Oncol 2013;14(3):210–8.

42. Stevenson AR, Solomon MJ, Lumley JW, et al. Effect of laparoscopic-assisted resection vs open resection on pathological outcomes in rectal cancer: the AlaCaRT randomized clinical trial. JAMA 2015;314(13):1356–63.

43. Fleshman J, Branda M, Sargent DJ, et al. Effect of laparoscopic-assisted resection vs open resection of stage II or III rectal cancer on pathologic outcomes: the ACOSOG Z6051 randomized clinical trial. JAMA 2015;314(13):1346–55.

44. Ng KT, Tsia AKV, Chong VYL. Robotic versus conventional laparoscopic surgery for colorectal cancer: a systematic review and meta-analysis with trial sequential analysis. World J Surg 2019;43(4):1146–61.

45. Lim S, Kim JH, Baek SJ, et al. Comparison of perioperative and short-term outcomes between robotic and conventional laparoscopic surgery for colonic cancer: a systematic review and meta-analysis. Ann Surg Treat Res 2016;90(6):328–39.

46. Simillis C, Lal N, Thoukididou SN, et al. Open versus laparoscopic versus robotic versus transanal mesorectal excision for rectal cancer: a systematic review and network meta-analysis. Ann Surg 2019;270(1):59–68.

47. Jones K, Qassem MG, Sains P, et al. Robotic total meso-rectal excision for rectal cancer: a systematic review following the publication of the ROLARR trial. World J Gastrointest Oncol 2018;10(11):449–64.

48. Jayne D, Pigazzi A, Marshall H, et al. Effect of robotic-assisted vs conventional laparoscopic surgery on risk of conversion to open laparotomy among patients undergoing resection for rectal cancer: the ROLARR randomized clinical trial. JAMA 2017;318(16):1569–80.

49. Kang SB, Park JW, Jeong SY, et al. Open versus laparoscopic surgery for mid or low rectal cancer after neoadjuvant chemoradiotherapy (COREAN trial): short-term outcomes of an open-label randomised controlled trial. Lancet Oncol 2010;11(7):637–45.

50. Guillou PJ, Quirke P, Thorpe H, et al. Short-term endpoints of conventional versus laparoscopic-assisted surgery in patients with colorectal cancer (MRC CLASICC trial): multicentre, randomised controlled trial. Lancet 2005;365(9472):1718–26.

51. Palanivelu C, Sendhilkumar K, Jani K, et al. Laparoscopic anterior resection and total mesorectal excision for rectal cancer: a prospective nonrandomized study. Int J Colorectal Dis 2007;22(4):367–72.

52. Tjandra JJ, Chan MK, Yeh CH. Laparoscopic- vs. hand-assisted ultralow anterior resection: a prospective study. Dis Colon Rectum 2008;51(1):26–31.

53. Selvindos PB, Ho YH. Multimedia article. Laparoscopic ultralow anterior resection with colonic J-pouch-anal anastomosis. Dis Colon Rectum 2008;51(11):1710–1.

54. Fleshman J, Sargent DJ, Green E, et al. Laparoscopic colectomy for cancer is not inferior to open surgery based on 5-year data from the COST Study Group trial. Ann Surg 2007;246(4):655–62.

55. Jayne DG, Thorpe HC, Copeland J, et al. Five-year follow-up of the Medical Research Council CLASICC trial of laparoscopically assisted versus open surgery for colorectal cancer. Br J Surg 2010;97(11):1638–45.
56. Liao G, Zhao Z, Lin S, et al. Robotic-assisted versus laparoscopic colorectal surgery: a meta-analysis of four randomized controlled trials. World J Surg Oncol 2014;12:122.
57. Zhang X, Wei Z, Bie M, et al. Robot-assisted versus laparoscopic-assisted surgery for colorectal cancer: a meta-analysis. Surg Endosc 2016;30(12):5601–14.
58. Tyler JA, Fox JP, Desai MM, et al. Outcomes and costs associated with robotic colectomy in the minimally invasive era. Dis Colon Rectum 2013;56(4):458–66.
59. Detering R, Roodbeen SX, van Oostendorp SE, et al. Three-year nationwide experience with transanal total mesorectal excision for rectal cancer in the Netherlands: a propensity score-matched comparison with conventional laparoscopic total mesorectal excision. J Am Coll Surg 2019;228(3):235–244 e231.
60. Braunschmid T, Hartig N, Baumann L, et al. Influence of multiple stapler firings used for rectal division on colorectal anastomotic leak rate. Surg Endosc 2017; 31(12):5318–26.
61. Quirke P, Steele R, Monson J, et al. Effect of the plane of surgery achieved on local recurrence in patients with operable rectal cancer: a prospective study using data from the MRC CR07 and NCIC-CTG CO16 randomised clinical trial. Lancet 2009;373(9666):821–8.
62. Rouanet P, Mourregot A, Azar CC, et al. Transanal endoscopic proctectomy: an innovative procedure for difficult resection of rectal tumors in men with narrow pelvis. Dis Colon Rectum 2013;56(4):408–15.
63. Sylla P, Knol JJ, D'Andrea AP, et al. Urethral injury and other urologic injuries during transanal total mesorectal excision: an international collaborative study. Ann Surg 2021;274(2):e115–25.
64. Adamina M, Buchs NC, Penna M, et al. Gallen Colorectal Consensus Expert G. St. Gallen consensus on safe implementation of transanal total mesorectal excision. Surg Endosc 2018;32(3):1091–103.
65. Ratcliffe F, Hogan AM, Hompes R. CO2 embolus: an important complication of TaTME surgery. Tech Coloproctol 2017;21(1):61–2.
66. Harnsberger CR, Alavi K, Davids JS, et al. CO2 embolism can complicate transanal total mesorectal excision. Tech Coloproctol 2018;22(11):881–5.
67. Dickson EA, Penna M, Cunningham C, et al. Carbon dioxide embolism associated with transanal total mesorectal excision surgery: a report from the international registries. Dis Colon Rectum 2019;62(7):794–801.
68. Park JS, Kang H, Park SY, et al. Long-term oncologic after robotic versus laparoscopic right colectomy: a prospective randomized study. Surg Endosc 2019; 33(9):2975–81.
69. Jeong SY, Park JW, Nam BH, et al. Open versus laparoscopic surgery for midrectal or low-rectal cancer after neoadjuvant chemoradiotherapy (COREAN trial): survival outcomes of an open-label, non-inferiority, randomisedandomized controlled trial. Lancet Oncol 2014;15(7):767–74.
70. Massarweh NN, Hu CY, You YN, et al. Risk-adjusted pathologic margin positivity rate as a quality indicator in rectal cancer surgery. J Clin Oncol 2014;32(27): 2967–74.
71. Fleshman J, Branda ME, Sargent DJ, et al. Disease-free survival and local recurrence for laparoscopic resection compared with open resection of stage II to III rectal cancer: follow-up results of the ACOSOG Z6051 randomized controlled trial. Ann Surg 2019;269(4):589–95.

72. Conticchio M, Papagni V, Notarnicola M, et al. Laparoscopic vs. open mesorectal excision for rectal cancer: are these approaches still comparable? A systematic review and meta-analysis. PloS One 2020;15(7):e0235887.
73. Knol JJ, D'Hondt M, Souverijns G, et al. Transanal endoscopic total mesorectal excision: technical aspects of approaching the mesorectal plane from below–a preliminary report. Tech Coloproctol 2015;19(4):221–9.
74. Han C, Yan P, Jing W, et al. Clinical, pathological, and oncologic outcomes of robotic-assisted versus laparoscopic proctectomy for rectal cancer: a meta-analysis of randomized controlled studies. Asian J Surg 2020;43(9):880–90.
75. Debakey Y, Zaghloul A, Farag A, et al. Robotic-assisted versus conventional laparoscopic approach for rectal cancer surgery, first Egyptian academic center experience, RCT. Minim Invasive Surg 2018;2018:5836562.
76. Baik SH, Ko YT, Kang CM, et al. Robotic tumor-specific mesorectal excision of rectal cancer: short-term outcome of a pilot randomized trial. Surg Endosc 2008;22(7):1601–8.
77. Green BL, Marshall HC, Collinson F, et al. Long-term follow-up of the Medical Research Council CLASICC trial of conventional versus laparoscopically assisted resection in colorectal cancer. Br J Surg 2013;100(1):75–82.
78. Zeng Z, Luo S, Chen J, et al. Comparison of pathological outcomes after transanal versus laparoscopic total mesorectal excision: a prospective study using data from randomized control trial. Surg Endosc 2020;34(9):3956–62.
79. Ma B, Gao P, Song Y, et al. Transanal total mesorectal excision (taTME) for rectal cancer: a systematic review and meta-analysis of oncological and perioperative outcomes compared with laparoscopic total mesorectal excision. BMC Cancer 2016;16:380.
80. Roodbeen SX, de Lacy FB, van Dieren S, et al. Predictive factors and risk model for positive circumferential resection margin rate after transanal total mesorectal excision in 2653 patients with rectal cancer. Ann Surg 2019;270(5):884–91.
81. D'Andrea AP, McLemore EC, Bonaccorso A, et al. Transanal total mesorectal excision (taTME) for rectal cancer: beyond the learning curve. Surg Endosc 2020;34(9):4101–9.
82. Roodbeen SX, Penna M, Mackenzie H, et al. Transanal total mesorectal excision (TaTME) versus laparoscopic TME for MRI-defined low rectal cancer: a propensity score-matched analysis of oncological outcomes. Surg Endosc 2019;33(8):2459–67.
83. Larsen SG, Pfeffer F, Korner H, et al. Norwegian moratorium on transanal total mesorectal excision. Br J Surg 2019;106(9):1120–1.
84. Wasmuth HH, Faerden AE, Myklebust TA, et al. Transanal total mesorectal excision for rectal cancer has been suspended in Norway. Br J Surg 2020;107(1):121–30.
85. van Oostendorp SE, Belgers HJ, Bootsma BT, et al. Locoregional recurrences after transanal total mesorectal excision of rectal cancer during implementation. Br J Surg 2020;107(9):1211–20.
86. Hol JC, van Oostendorp SE, Tuynman JB, et al. Long-term oncological results after transanal total mesorectal excision for rectal carcinoma. Tech Coloproctol 2019;23(9):903–11.
87. Roodbeen SX, Spinelli A, Bemelman WA, et al. Local recurrence after transanal total mesorectal excision for rectal cancer: a multicenter cohort study. Ann Surg 2021;274(2):359–66.

88. Simo V, Tejedor P, Jimenez LM, et al. Oncological safety of transanal total mesorectal excision (TaTME) for rectal cancer: mid-term results of a prospective multicentre study. Surg Endosc 2021;35(4):1808–19.
89. Kang DW, Kwak HD, Sung NS, et al. Oncologic outcomes in rectal cancer patients with a ≤1-cm distal resection margin. Int J Colorectal Dis 2017;32(3): 325–32.
90. Moghadamyeghaneh Z, Carmichael JC, Mills S, et al. Variations in laparoscopic colectomy utilization in the United States. Dis Colon Rectum 2015;58(10):950–6.
91. Simons AJ, Anthone GJ, Ortega AE, et al. Laparoscopic-assisted colectomy learning curve. Dis Colon Rectum 1995;38(6):600–3.
92. Schlachta CM, Mamazza J, Seshadri PA, et al. Defining a learning curve for laparoscopic colorectal resections. Dis Colon Rectum 2001;44(2):217–22.
93. Nasseri Y, Stettler I, Shen W, et al. Learning curve in robotic colorectal surgery. J Robot Surg 2021;15(3):489–95.
94. Shaw DD, Wright M, Taylor L, et al. Robotic colorectal surgery learning curve and case complexity. J Laparoendosc Adv Surg Tech A 2018;28(10):1163–8.
95. Atallah S, Albert M. The neurovascular bundle of Walsh and other anatomic considerations crucial in preventing urethral injury in males undergoing transanal total mesorectal excision. Tech Coloproctol 2016;20(6):411–2.
96. Koedam TWA, Veltcamp Helbach M, van de Ven PM, et al. Transanal total mesorectal excision for rectal cancer: evaluation of the learning curve. Tech Coloproctol 2018;22(4):279–87.
97. Lee L, Kelly J, Nassif GJ, et al. Defining the learning curve for transanal total mesorectal excision for rectal adenocarcinoma. Surg Endosc 2020;34(4): 1534–42.
98. Francis N, Penna M, Carter F, et al. Development and early outcomes of the national training initiative for transanal total mesorectal excision in the UK. Colorectal Dis 2020;22(7):756–67.
99. Fearnhead NS, Acheson AG, Brown SR, et al. The ACPGBI recommends pause for reflection on transanal total mesorectal excision. Colorectal Dis 2020;22(7): 745–8.
100. TaTme Guidance Group representing the Escp icwtAAEEECCCCJSSSS-MIS. International expert consensus guidance on indications, implementation and quality measures for transanal total mesorectal excision. Colorectal Dis 2020; 22(7):749–55.
101. Veltcamp Helbach M, van Oostendorp SE, Koedam TWA, et al. Structured training pathway and proctoring; multicenter results of the implementation of transanal total mesorectal excision (TaTME) in the Netherlands. Surg Endosc 2020;34(1):192–201.
102. Francis N, Penna M, Mackenzie H, et al. Consensus on structured training curriculum for transanal total mesorectal excision (TaTME). Surg Endosc 2017; 31(7):2711–9.
103. Kim MJ, Park SC, Park JW, et al. Robot-assisted versus laparoscopic surgery for rectal cancer: a phase II open label prospective randomized controlled trial. Ann Surg 2018;267(2):243–51.
104. Grass JK, Chen CC, Melling N, et al. Robotic rectal resection preserves anorectal function: systematic review and meta-analysis. Int J Med Robot 2021;17(6): e2329.
105. Bolton WS, Chapman SJ, Corrigan N, et al. The incidence of low anterior resection syndrome as assessed in an international randomized controlled trial (MRC/NIHR ROLARR). Ann Surg 2021;274(6):e1223–9.

106. Kim JY, Kim NK, Lee KY, et al. A comparative study of voiding and sexual function after total mesorectal excision with autonomic nerve preservation for rectal cancer: laparoscopic versus robotic surgery. Ann Surg Oncol 2012;19(8):2485–93.

107. D'Annibale A, Pernazza G, Monsellato I, et al. Total mesorectal excision: a comparison of oncological and functional outcomes between robotic and laparoscopic surgery for rectal cancer. Surg Endosc 2013;27(6):1887–95.

108. van der Heijden JAG, Koeter T, Smits LJH, et al. Functional complaints and quality of life after transanal total mesorectal excision: a meta-analysis. Br J Surg 2020;107(5):489–98.

109. Veltcamp Helbach M, Koedam TWA, Knol JJ, et al. Quality of life after rectal cancer surgery: differences between laparoscopic and transanal total mesorectal excision. Surg Endosc 2019;33(1):79–87.

110. Bjoern MX, Nielsen S, Perdawood SK. Quality of life after surgery for rectal cancer: a comparison of functional outcomes after transanal and laparoscopic approaches. J Gastrointest Surg 2019;23(8):1623–30.

111. Pontallier A, Denost Q, Van Geluwe B, et al. Potential sexual function improvement by using transanal mesorectal approach for laparoscopic low rectal cancer excision. Surg Endosc 2016;30(11):4924–33.

112. Foo CC, Kin Ng K, Tsang JS, et al. Low anterior resection syndrome after transanal total mesorectal excision: a comparison with the conventional top-to-bottom approach. Dis Colon Rectum 2020;63(4):497–503.

113. Leao P, Santos C, Goulart A, et al. TaTME: analysis of the evacuatory outcomes and EUS anal sphincter. Minim Invasive Ther Allied Technol 2019;28(6):332–7.

114. Keller DS, Reali C, Spinelli A, et al. Patient-reported functional and quality-of-life outcomes after transanal total mesorectal excision. Br J Surg 2019;106(4):364–6.

115. Rahman R, Wood ME, Qian L, et al. Head-mounted display use in surgery: a systematic review. Surg Innov 2020;27(1):88–100.

116. Erridge S, Yeung DKT, Patel HRH, et al. Telementoring of surgeons: a systematic review. Surg Innov 2019;26(1):95–111.

117. Atallah S. Assessment of a flexible robotic system for endoluminal applications and transanal total mesorectal excision (taTME): could this be the solution we have been searching for? Tech Coloproctol 2017;21(10):809–14.

118. Moschovas MC, Bhat S, Sandri M, et al. Comparing the approach to radical prostatectomy using the multiport da Vinci Xi and da Vinci SP robots: a propensity score analysis of perioperative outcomes. Eur Urol 2021;79(3):393–404.

119. Stevenson ARL, Solomon MJ, Brown CSB, et al. Disease-free Survival and Local Recurrence After Laparoscopic-assisted Resection or Open Resection for Rectal Cancer: The Australasian Laparoscopic Cancer of the Rectum Randomized Clinical Trial. Ann Surg. 2019;269(4):596–602.

120. Fleshman J, Branda ME, Sargent DJ, et al. Disease-free Survival and Local Recurrence for Laparoscopic Resection Compared With Open Resection of Stage II to III Rectal Cancer: Follow-up Results of the ACOSOG Z6051 Randomized Controlled Trial. Ann Surg. 2019;269(4):589–95.

121. Colon Cancer Laparoscopic or Open Resection Study Group, Buunen M, Veldkamp R, et al. Survival after laparoscopic surgery versus open surgery for colon cancer: long-term outcome of a randomised clinical trial. Lancet Oncol 2009;10(1):44–52, x.

122. Jayne DG, Guillou PJ, Thorpe H, et al. Randomized trial of laparoscopic-assisted resection of colorectal carcinoma: 3-year results of the UK MRC CLASICC Trial Group. J Clin Oncol 2007;25(21):3061–8.
123. Grams J, Tong W, Greenstein AJ, et al. Comparison of intracorporeal versus extracorporeal anastomosis in laparoscopic-assisted hemicolectomy. Surg Endosc 2010;24(8):1886–91.
124. Cirocchi R, Trastulli S, Farinella E, et al. Intracorporeal versus extracorporeal anastomosis during laparoscopic right hemicolectomy - systematic review and meta-analysis. Surg Oncol 2013;22(1):1–13.
125. Lee KH, Lee MR, Pigazzi A. Robotic-assisted laparoscopic segmental resection with rectoanal anastomosis: a new approach for the management of complicated rectourethral fistula. Tech Coloproctol 2013;17(5):585–7.
126. Stein SA, Bergamaschi R. Extracorporeal versus intracorporeal ileocolic anastomosis. Tech Coloproctol 2013;17(Suppl 1):S35–9.
127. Feroci F, Lenzi E, Garzi A, et al. Intracorporeal versus extracorporeal anastomosis after laparoscopic right hemicolectomy for cancer: a systematic review and meta-analysis. Int J Colorectal Dis 2013;28(9):1177–86.
128. Morpurgo E, Contardo T, Molaro R, et al. Robotic-assisted intracorporeal anastomosis versus extracorporeal anastomosis in laparoscopic right hemicolectomy for cancer: a case control study. J Laparoendosc Adv Surg Tech A 2013;23(5):414–7.
129. Milone M, Elmore U, Di Salvo E, et al. Intracorporeal versus extracorporeal anastomosis. Results from a multicentre comparative study on 512 right-sided colorectal cancers. Surg Endosc 2015;29(8):2314–20.
130. Trastulli S, Coratti A, Guarino S, et al. Robotic right colectomy with intracorporeal anastomosis compared with laparoscopic right colectomy with extracorporeal and intracorporeal anastomosis: a retrospective multicentre study. Surg Endosc 2015;29(6):1512–21.
131. Vignali A, Bissolati M, De Nardi P, et al. Extracorporeal vs. Intracorporeal Ileocolic Stapled Anastomoses in Laparoscopic Right Colectomy: An Interim Analysis of a Randomized Clinical Trial. J Laparoendosc Adv Surg Tech A 2016; 26(5):343–8.
132. van Oostendorp S, Elfrink A, Borstlap W, et al. Intracorporeal versus extracorporeal anastomosis in right hemicolectomy: a systematic review and meta-analysis. Surg Endosc 2017;31(1):64–77.
133. Cleary RK, Kassir A, Johnson CS, et al. Intracorporeal versus extracorporeal anastomosis for minimally invasive right colectomy: A multi-center propensity score-matched comparison of outcomes. PLoS One 2018;13(10):e0206277.
134. Mari GM, Crippa J, Costanzi ATM, et al. Intracorporeal Anastomosis Reduces Surgical Stress Response in Laparoscopic Right Hemicolectomy: A Prospective Randomized Trial. Surg Laparosc Endosc Percutan Tech 2018;28(2):77–81.
135. Allaix ME, Degiuli M, Bonino MA, et al. Intracorporeal or Extracorporeal Ileocolic Anastomosis After Laparoscopic Right Colectomy: A Double-blinded Randomized Controlled Trial. Ann Surg 2019;270(5):762–7.
136. Emile SH, Elfeki H, Shalaby M, et al. Intracorporeal versus extracorporeal anastomosis in minimally invasive right colectomy: an updated systematic review and meta-analysis. Tech Coloproctol 2019;23(11):1023–35.
137. Bollo J, Turrado V, Rabal A, et al. Randomized clinical trial of intracorporeal versus extracorporeal anastomosis in laparoscopic right colectomy (IEA trial). Br J Surg 2020;107(4):364–72.

138. Creavin B, Balasubramanian I, Common M, et al. Intracorporeal vs extracorporeal anastomosis following neoplastic right hemicolectomy resection: a systematic review and meta-analysis of randomized control trials. Int J Colorectal Dis 2021;36(4):645–56.

139. Veltcamp Helbach M, Deijen CL, Velthuis S, et al. Transanal total mesorectal excision for rectal carcinoma: short-term outcomes and experience after 80 cases. Surg Endosc 2016;30(2):464–70.

140. de Lacy FB, van Laarhoven JJEM, Pena R, et al. Transanal total mesorectal excision: pathological results of 186 patients with mid and low rectal cancer. Surg Endosc 2018;32(5):2442–7.

141. Perdawood SK, Kroeigaard J, Eriksen M, et al. Transanal total mesorectal excision: the Slagelse experience 2013–2019. Surg Endosc 2021;35(2):826–36.

142. Klein MF, Seiersen M, Buut O, et al. Short-term outcomes after transanal total mesorectal excision for rectal cancer in Denmark – a prospective multicentre study. Colorectal Dis 2021;23:834–42.

143. Caycedo-Marulanda A, Lee L, Chadi SA, et al. Association of transanal total mesorectal excision with local recurrence of rectal cancer. JAMA Netw Open 2021;4(2):e2036330.

144. Alhanafy M, Park SS, Park SC, et al. Early experience with transanal total mesorectal excision compared wi2th laparoscopic total mesorectal excision for rectal cancer: a propensity score-matched analysis. Dis Colon Rectum 2020; 63:1500–10.

145. Roodbeen SX, Penna M, van Dieren S, et al. Local recurrence and disease-free survival after transanal total mesorectal excision: Results from an international taTME registry. J Natl Compr Canc Netw 2021;19(11):1232–40.

Local Excision and Endoscopic Strategies for the Treatment of Colorectal Cancer

Ilker Ozgur, MD, Emre Gorgun, MD, FACS, FASCRS*

KEYWORDS

- Endoluminal surgery • Advanced endoscopic treatment • ESD • Organ preservation
- Colorectal cancer

KEY POINTS

- Endoluminal surgery consists of local excision, transanal endoscopic microsurgery, transanal minimal invasive surgery, single port transanal robotic surgery, and advanced endoscopic surgery.
- Endoluminal surgery should become a tool in surgeons' armamentarium as a standard of care in the treatment of colorectal cancer and precancerous lesions.
- Patient selection for endoluminal surgery depends on strict criteria primarily based on the prediction of lymph node metastasis.
- Precancerous lesions should be considered for endoluminal surgery.
- Patients with rectal cancer may significantly benefit from total neoadjuvant treatment (TNT).
- Proper evaluation of tumor response after TNT is crucial in managing patients with rectal cancer for organ preservation.
- Surgery remains the best option for patients without complete pathologic response.

INTRODUCTION

Colorectal cancer (CRC) is the fourth most commonly diagnosed cancer and the second most common cause of cancer death in both men and women in the United States. The American Cancer Society's estimate for annual CRC incidence in 2021 is approximately 150,000 new cases. The death rate and incidence in patients older than 50 years have been decreasing for several decades as a result of endoscopic

Department of Colorectal Surgery, Digestive Disease and Surgery Institute, Cleveland Clinic, Cleveland, OH, USA
* Corresponding author.
E-mail address: gorgune@ccf.org

Surg Oncol Clin N Am 31 (2022) 219–237
https://doi.org/10.1016/j.soc.2021.11.004
1055-3207/22/© 2021 Elsevier Inc. All rights reserved.
surgonc.theclinics.com

screening programs.[1] Meanwhile, the incidence is increasing among patients younger than 50 years, and most of these patients are reported as early-stage CRC.[2]

Furthermore, the incidence of polyp detection during colonoscopies is also increasing with screening programs.[3] Most polyps encountered during routine colonoscopy are suitable for simple polypectomy and are treated during these procedures. Polyps that are large in size and/or have advanced morphologic features and are not amenable to conventional endoscopic removal are referred for surgery. Nearly 30,000 patients in the United States annually undergo colectomy or proctectomy for benign disease.[4] We previously reported a similar finding that 92% of these surgical resections do not have cancer in the final pathology.[5] Accordingly, there appears to be an opportunity for organ preservation for these patients presenting with polyps.

Endoluminal surgery (ELS) may also offer additional treatment options in locally advanced rectal cancer patients with paradigm change toward total neoadjuvant treatment (TNT) of the disease. New chemoradiation treatment protocols provided the advantage of organ preservation in locally advanced patients with rectal cancer. The neoadjuvant chemoradiation treatment (NCRT) and TNT may result in the downstaging of locally advanced rectal cancer to mucosal disease, down to and superficial residual tumor restricted to the mucosa or complete pathologic response (pCR) after treatment. Patients with such suspicious lesions, which are limited to the mucosa, after completion of NCRT or TNT protocols may benefit from ELS and have organ preservation.

Finally, patients with advanced disease who are not appropriate for major resection due to comorbidities and require a palliative intervention may be candidates for ELS. Some patients may demonstrate a relentless desire not to have a permanent stoma and thus, may also benefit from endoluminal surgery if palliation is needed.

Briefly, patients diagnosed with precancerous lesions (polyps) or early-stage cancer with a low probability of lymph node metastasis should be considered for ELS. Patients with advanced rectal cancer who either have a suspicious mucosal lesion after oncologic chemoradiation treatment or are in need of palliative intervention may also be candidates for ELS.

When local treatment modalities for colorectal surgery are considered, they should be separated into 2 headings according to lesion location: rectum and colon. This division is due to differences in anatomy, physiology, accessibility, available treatment options, as well as easier description. Currently, there are a variety of treatment options available for rectal lesions, as they have easier access when compared with colonic lesions. Also, the concept of local treatment modalities after neoadjuvant treatment for colonic cancer has not yet developed. Thus, the following surgical interventions are mainly preferred for rectal tumors, whereas endoscopic interventions are preferred for colonic lesions.

ENDOLUMINAL SURGERY
Key Points—Indications for Local Excision

- All precancerous lesions.
- To verify any lesion in case of pathologic and clinical discordance.
- Treatment of early colorectal lesions (cT1-2N0).
- Palliation of advanced colorectal lesions.
- Reassessment after TNT for regrowth/recurrence of rectal cancer.

Need for Oncological Resection Versus Local Excision

The standard surgery for CRC is mesocolic or mesorectal excision (TME), depending on tumor location. The optimal surgical treatment for CRC should provide curative surgery with low morbidity, ideal postoperative functions, and organ preservation, which is not always the case. CRC surgery is associated with several postoperative complications, including surgical site infections, anastomotic leaks, anastomotic strictures, postoperative functional problems, permanent ostomies, and even rarely death. Therefore, surgeons would prefer to provide less invasive methods with similar/comparable oncological outcomes when possible.

Although the rectal cancer treatment approach has become more complex due to medical developments and new technological implementations, surgery remains the primary treatment modality. When comparing the surgical approach, open surgery was compared to laparoscopic surgery and demonstrated equivalent oncologic outcomes.[6,7] Laparoscopic surgery is technically demanding for several aspects, especially in patients with low rectal cancer. Robotic surgery and transanal total mesorectal excision were explored to overcome this problem, especially in patients with distal rectal cancer or narrow pelvis.[8] Recently, robotic surgery was compared to laparoscopic surgery for safety in patients with rectal cancer, and authors reported nonsuperiority for robotic surgery.[9] It is inherent for CRC surgery to shift toward more minimally invasive procedures, aiming for superior oncological and functional outcomes as compared with standard surgery.

The aforementioned techniques are primarily preferred for lesions with possible lymph node metastasis, whereas local excision (LE) is suitable for precancerous or low-risk T1 lesions and provides more favorable outcomes. Any patient with clinical evidence of lymph node metastasis should not be considered for LE. The procedure can be defined as a full-thickness resection of the wall, including the tumor with clear margins, and without intentional lymph node dissection. The dissection is continued until the perirectal fatty tissue and is not extended beyond. Conventional transanal local excision (TLE) has some visual limitations for proximal rectal lesions. Transanal endoscopic microsurgery (TEM) and transanal minimal invasive surgery (TAMIS) were developed to overcome these challenges of TLE. As previously reported from our center, a similar strategy may be used for colonic lesions, and physicians may prefer combined endoscopic laparoscopic surgery (CELS) to treat colonic lesions.[5] Lately, endoscopic mucosal resection (EMR)[10] and endoscopic submucosal dissection (ESD)[11] have been introduced as advanced endoscopic techniques to treat mucosal and superficial submucosal lesions while maintaining organ preservation.

Patient Selection and Evaluation

All patients with the possibility of CRC should be assessed via routine staging procedures including digital rectal examination, endoscopy, serum carcinoembryonic antigen level, and cross-sectional imaging, especially if there are any concerns for malignancy (**Figs. 1** and **2**). The imaging should include computed tomography (CT) of the chest, abdomen, and pelvis for systemic scanning and MRI) of rectum or possibly endorectal ultrasound (US) for local evaluation of the lesion. Routine imaging for every patient is not recommended. In particular, MRI may overestimate early rectal mucosal lesions that are limited to the mucosa and submucosa.[12,13] Clinical evaluation and assessment followed by LE may be preferred.

Thorough evaluation of the lesion is crucial. Physical examination, clinical characteristics, and surgeon experience play a major role in surgical decision-making. Previous colonoscopy reports with colored images of the lesion should be obtained before the procedure and individually evaluated. Lesion properties such as the surface morphology, size, and the previous pathology report are essential, and pathology slides could be obtained for a second pathology review. Certain pathologic criteria are important to safely proceed with ELS. The lesions reported as adenocarcinoma

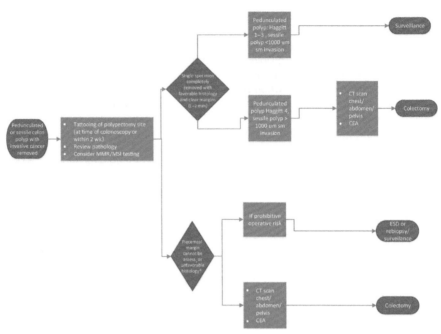

Fig. 1. Cancer in colon polyp care pathway performed at Cleveland Clinic. ªUnfavorable histology defined by: • Poorly differentiated • Angiolymphatic invasion • High tumor bidding

should meet the following criteria to avoid oncological organ resection: no vascular/neural invasion, tumor budding grade 1 (low grade), well/moderately differentiated, and negative vertical tumor margin. All criteria must be met otherwise endoscopic intervention is not recommended (see **Fig. 2**).

The potential for underlying malignancy can be assessed by endoscopic characterization of the lesion appearance. This step is critical and can be evaluated with one of the several available classification systems, including Paris,[14] Kudo pit pattern,[15] and Narrow-band imaging International Colorectal Endoscopic (NICE)[16] classification. The Paris classification describes the gross morphology of the lesion as polypoid or non-polypoid lesions. There is a clear inverse relationship between superficial lesion protrusion into the lumen and the risk of submucosal invasion, thus depressed lesions have an increased rate of malignancy.

The pit patterns are based on the specific arrangement of glands in different lesions and can help differentiate hyperplastic versus adenomatous versus malignant lesions. Narrow-band imaging (NBI) is a commonly available technology to evaluate the mucosal structure. NBI can be used to classify the polyp as hyperplastic, adenomatous, or malignant based on lesion color, vascular pattern, and surface pattern. Accurate endoscopic assessment allows appropriate selection of lesions for ELS and subsequent avoidance of resection due to concern for underlying malignancy.

Techniques
A 2-dose enema (one the night before and one in the morning before the surgery) is sufficient for most patients with rectal lesions. However, some patients may benefit from a full dose of mechanical preparation, especially if complaining of constipation. Preoperative antibiotics (ampicillin-sulbactam/cefuroxime acetate + metronidazole/

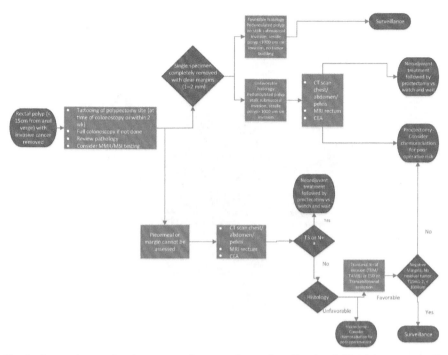

Fig. 2. Cancer in rectal polyp care pathway performed at Cleveland Clinic. [a]MRI generally unreliable to differentiate T1 versus T2. In that case, recommend local excision for pathological diagnosis. Unfavorable histology defined by: • Poorly differentiated • Angiolymphatic invasion • High tumor bidding

ciprofloxacin + metronidazole) are administered to minimize surgical site infections for ELS patients performed in the operating room. Deep venous thrombosis prophylaxis is done with either subcutaneous unfractionated heparin or low-molecular-weight heparin. Patients are placed in modified lithotomy, lateral decubitus, or prone jack-knife position depending on the anatomic orientation of lesion (anterior vs posterior vs lateral rectal wall), use of gravity, and surgeon preference. Administering local anesthesia before or after the procedure with pudendal nerve and perianal block helps to reduce postoperative pain. Either general anesthesia or sedation combined with local anesthesia under monitored ventilation is appropriate for surgery.

Transanal local excision
This surgery is confined to distal rectal lesions as mid-rectal or proximal-rectal lesions are technically not easily accessible. After attaining the desired position to start the surgery, the procedure begins with a digital examination and rectal irrigation. After verification of lesion location, the anal canal is dilated, and suture retraction (**Fig. 3**) or appropriate rectoscopes (**Fig. 4**) may be applied for adequate exposure. Physicians may prefer to use any of the retractors, including Hill-Ferguson, Sawyer, Parks, or Lone Star Retractor System (Cooper Surgical, Inc., Trumbull, CT, US) (**Fig. 5**), depending on personal expertise. The submucosal injection is performed for mucosal lesions. Peritumoral marking with electrocautery before the submucosal injection should not be performed, as this can lead to loss of injectate trough and create mucosal defects. Additional dye (indigo carmine, methylene blue, acetic acid) may be used for clear

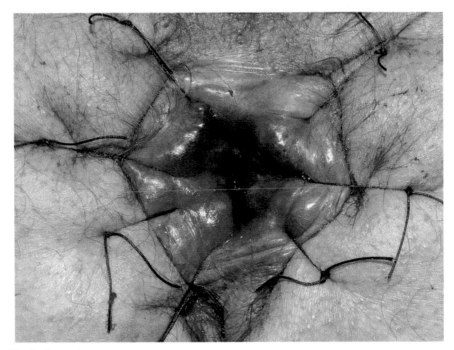

Fig. 3. Retraction sutures.

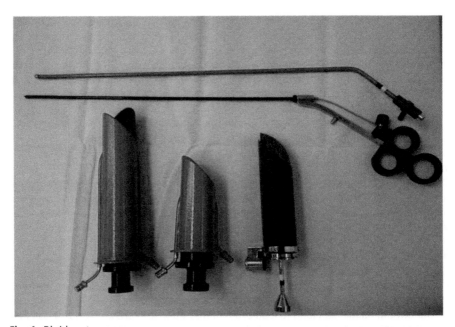

Fig. 4. Rigid rectoscopes.

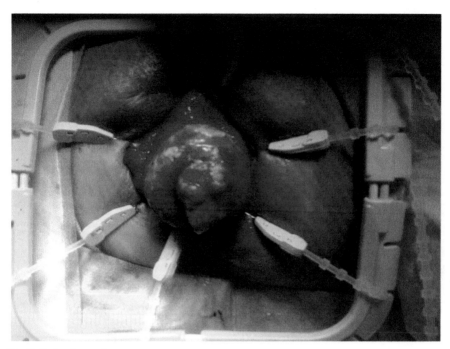

Fig. 5. Retractor system.

margin assessment. The tumor is then resected with at least 0.5 cm clear margin. The specimen is pinned on a corkboard with appropriate orientation marks (**Fig. 6**). The created full-thickness defect is closed transversely after proper hemostasis with polyglactin sutures. Although dissection with no violation to muscular layer of rectum is achievable with conventional TLE, due to lack of magnified scope views tendency is to create large full-thickness defects. The full-thickness repair is generally recommended unless there is only a minor defect on the muscular layer. The surgeon assesses the rectum with a proper endoscope if available. There is no need for the continuation of antibiotics after the procedure. After recovery, patients are discharged with a postoperative follow-up visit in 4 to 6 weeks and pathology discussion.

Transanal endoscopic microsurgery
The procedure requires specific unique rigid equipment developed for this surgery in the mid-1980s. It uses a special rectoscope 4 cm in diameter and special rectal tubing. The rectoscope diameter may cause procedural unsuitability for some patients. Patients are positioned prone for anterior lesions, lithotomy for posterior lesions, and lateral decubitus for lateral lesions to expose the lesion at 6 o'clock. After rectal administration of the rigid rectoscope, it is attached and secured to the operating table. After attaining pneumorectum with CO_2 insufflation, the procedure is performed with 4 laparoscopic instruments designed for TEM. Laparoscope fogging and smoke in the rectum is the major obstacle of the procedure. The dissection principles are the same as a conventional technique. Special attention is a must for proximal, full-thickness lesions due to probable peritoneal contamination. Therefore, patients should have full dose mechanical bowel preparation. Also, anterior lesions need specific attention in women as postoperative rectovaginal fistula is a potential

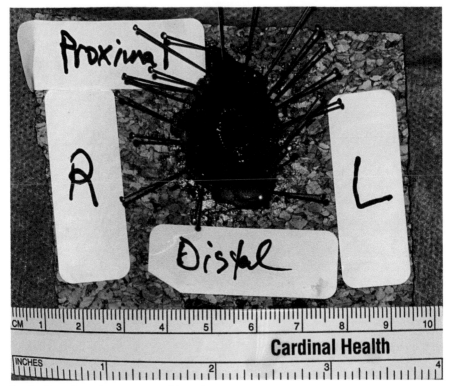

Fig. 6. Pinned specimens on a corkboard.

complication. The created defect is closed with laparoscopic needle drivers. TEM requires insufflation and thus may be difficult for lesions involving the distal anal canal. However, the beveled TEM proctoscope allows insufflation with visualization of the vast majority of the distal rectum. That is the main advantage of the Wolf system for TEM over TAMIS where the single access port completely covers the distal rectum/anal canal. If the lesion does involve the very distal anal canal, proximal dissection can be performed with the TEM equipment in place and then the last remaining distal dissection with the pratt retractor.

Transanal minimally invasive surgery
The surgery is very similar to TEM and does not require an expensive and specifically developed rigid rectoscope. The anal canal is intubated with a single-use laparoscopic entry device, and the desired number of trocars are placed through this device (**Fig. 7**). The surgeon introduces laparoscopic instruments through the trocars. The advantage of TAMIS to TEM is the four-quadrant possible surgery. The TAMIS access port covers more of the distal rectum than the TEM beveled proctoscope and thus may be less applicable than TEM for distal rectal lesions.

Transanal single-port robotic ELS
Robotic technology can be adapted for rectal lesions "within reach" as endoluminal robotic surgery. It is very similar to TAMIS and uses the same administration device. The single-port robot, Da Vinci SP (Intuitive Surgical, Inc. Sunnyvale, CA, USA), is a

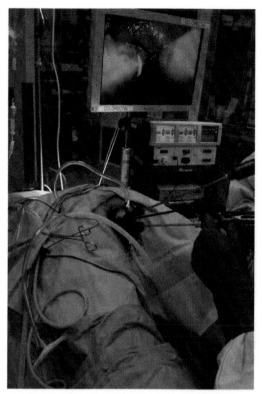

Fig. 7. Patient in prone position during TAMIS and introduced laparoscopic devices.

semiflexible endo robot that can reach up to 24 cm from the anal verge. It is docked under general anesthesia in a modified lithotomy position via GelPOINT Path Transanal Access Platform (Applied Medical Corporation, LA, CA, USA) (**Fig. 8**). The platform provides better visualization and controlled with semiflexible robotic arms. Mucosal resections just confined to the mucosal layer without unintentional full-thickness injury are feasible and achievable. The pneumorectum is attained with continuous CO_2 insufflation. Depending on the decided resection technique (mucosa or full-thickness), the procedure begins with either submucosal injection of lifting agent Orise Gel (Boston Scientific Corporation, Marlborough, MA, USA) or marking the lesion circumferentially. After achieving an adequate lift for mucosal lesions, the procedure is continued with either a hook or a spatula creating the dissection at the submucosal level. The smoke is evacuated from the rectum with an aspirator introduced from the gel port or continuous CO_2 insufflation systems. The injecting needle and aspiration device are directed with the help of a silk knot at the tip of the tubing to create a handle for robot arms. Thinner than the hook, the spatula tip delivers less energy to the dissection field and creates a more precise cut. The full-thickness defects are repaired in a similar fashion with other laparoscopic transanal procedures. There is no need for repair in case of pure mucosal resection.

Significant progress is expected in the near future with the development of fully flexible robotic-assisted surgical systems. These platforms might enable surgeons to perform incisionless surgeries with similar oncologic outcomes. Fully flexible endorobotic systems is an area for further research and future directions.

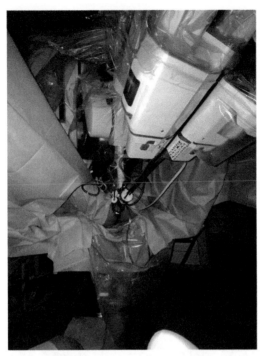

Fig. 8. SP robot docked.

Advanced endoscopy (EMR/ESD/hybrid ESD)

Although advanced polypectomy techniques initially became popular in Asia and were designed for the upper gastrointestinal system, they recently became more prevalent in the United States.[5] The challenging anatomy of the lower gastrointestinal system limits the popularity for application in the colon and rectum, as the colon has a thinner wall when compared with the stomach. Also, the colon has folds, corners, and flexures that provide extra difficulties in maintaining a stable scope position. Despite these technical demands and long learning curve, there is increased interest in ESD due to advantages over surgery. Advanced endoscopy offers multiple benefits to patients and could be the next big step for minimally invasive surgery. Conventional TLE or even TAMIS typically leads to full-thickness[17] defects with nonfavorable postoperative outcomes, especially after neoadjuvant treatment,[18] which is not the case with ELS. Salvage surgery may lead to abdominal perineal resection with end colostomy for patients who undergo LE even for early rectal cancer (pT1-2).[19] Also, patients with such salvage surgery have a much lower overall survival rate when compared with the standard surgery group.[20] On the other hand, advanced endoscopic techniques may avoid full-thickness defect or injury that will interfere with future surgery, according to our experience in more than 500 cases.[5] In this context, ELS is rapidly progressing while providing minimally invasive surgery in outpatient settings. Endoscopists face the challenge of operating through a flexible, unstable scope within a confined space that is frequently in motion.

Deciding on the type of advanced endoscopy procedure

The procedure consists of injection, dissection, resection, and removal of the lesion. The lesion is elevated from the underlying muscular layer with the proper injectate, creating a submucosal cushion enabling safe dissection. The primary aim is to achieve complete en bloc resection. Guidelines encourage performing EMR for lesions smaller than 20 mm and ESD to be reserved for larger lesions.[3] ESD is reported to have a higher en bloc resection and lower recurrence rates with similar complication rates compared to EMR.[21] A systematic review reported a 96% en bloc resection rate for ESD in colonic lesions.[22]

Consequently, preoperative lesion evaluation is essential. Previous colonoscopy reports should be obtained before the procedure, and colored images of the colonoscopies should be assessed by the physician. This provides the opportunity to evaluate the lesion in detail and decide if additional equipment might be needed during the procedure. The physicians use advanced endoscopic imaging techniques such as NBI and focal interrogation to predict the risk of invasion from the appearance of surface morphology, including pit patterns.[10,15–17] Therefore, a standard care pathway and decision-making tree for patients should be maintained (**Fig. 9**). Perioperative evaluation of patients is critical for successful results.

Careful selection of patients for attempted EMR, ESD, or hybrid ESD is critical. Procedural selection is based on the size of the tumor and the risk of underlying carcinoma. When lesion size is considered, it will be acceptable to perform EMR if the lesion is <2 cm. ESD is often reserved for lesions >2 cm without features of malignancy. For patients where the diagnosis is unclear, ESD is of preference. When there is potential for underlying malignancy, the lesion can be assessed by endoscopic characterization of surface appearance and the ability of the lesion to lift with submucosal injection properly. As previously described, the appearance of the lesion is critical and can be evaluated with one of several available classification systems.

Key points—preinterventional evaluation

- Attain detailed medical history and updated medication list. Anticoagulant use and dosage are crucial. The typical hold time for anticoagulants is 2 to 7 days before the procedure depending on the half-life of the specific medication.
- Physicians may perform ELS procedures both in endoscopy suites or operating room settings. Operating room settings may be reserved for patients with comorbidities or high-risk lesions as well as planned combined endolaparoscopy.
- Full dose mechanical bowel preparation is a standard of care, a day before the procedure, 4 L polyethylene glycol is preferred.
- Patients are prescribed peroral neomycin and metronidazole.

Injection Techniques and Type of Injectates

Creating a submucosal cushion is essential to proceed with ELS. Common submucosal lifting agents currently available include saline, hyaluronic acid, glycerol, dilute albumin, and proprietary gels. The submucosal saline injection will suffice and provides a lift that lasts approximately 3 minutes; however, ELS typically takes longer. There are also readily available, FDA-approved injectates on the market; ORISE Gel Submucosal Lifting Agent (Boston Scientific) and Eleview. They are preprepared and ready to use, which may help to decrease the procedure time. A self-prepared solution composed of diluted adrenalin (1 mL of 0.1% adrenalin) and hydroxyethyl starch solution mixed with methylene blue or any other dye can also be used.[23] Saline is not preferred as an injectate for ELS as its stay in tissue is limited, and it disperses quickly.[24]

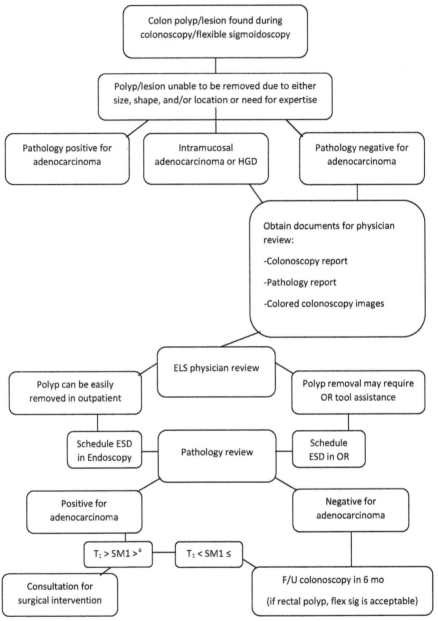

Fig. 9. ESD care pathway. [a]No vascular invasion, tumor budging grade 1 (low grade), and negative vertical tumor margin. (all criteria must meet).

Key points—injection technique

- The goal of the injection is to achieve a balanced and adequate lift for the mucosal lesion. The injection needle should be advanced tangentially along the mucosa (**Fig. 10**). The endoscopist positions and inserts the needle, and

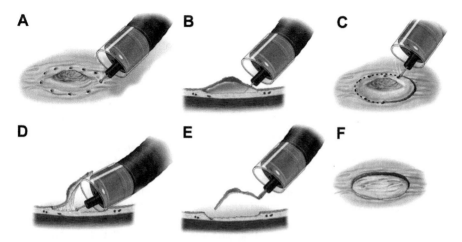

Fig. 10. Steps of ESD: marking (*A*), injection (*B*), mucosal incision (*C*), dissection in submucosal plane (*D*), resection (*E*), and muscular layer after completion (*F*).

the assistant starts the injection. If tissue elevation is not observed after starting the injection, this could be due to entry into an incorrect plane, typically into the muscular layer or abdominal cavity. The injection needle should be adjusted slightly and realigned before continuing.

- For lesions located on a fold, the injection should begin along the far aspect (oral side) of the lesion to lift the lesion toward the operative field of view. The lesion may fall away from the view if the injection is started from the distal side (anal side).
- If the correct plane is ensured, but the adequate lift cannot be achieved (nonlifting sign), this could be a sign of either deep invasion into the submucosa, or fibrosis due to previous resection/biopsy. When the deep invasion is suspected, the procedure should be stopped; however, we recently reported our institution's results that nonlifting may be due to previous attempts of tissue resection.[25] In those cases, the procedure can still safely proceed from an oncological perspective.

Endoscopic Mucosal Resection

EMR consists of snaring the lesion subsequent to the injection step. The goal is en bloc lesion removal sized less than 20 mm. There are many sizes and shapes for snares to perform EMR in the market. The selection of the appropriate one for the procedure is essential. Snaring is done with a 2 to 3 mm clear mucosal margin, and the lesion should fit entirely in the snare. Repeated snaring is not encouraged due to piecemeal resection, which will decrease specimen quality. Edges of resection site may be coagulated with snare tip to decrease recurrence rate.

Endoscopic Submucosal Dissection

ESD has surgical principles during endoscopic lesion removal. Endoscopic knives are crucial instruments for ESD, and different knives are available on the market, including the FlexKnife Electrosurgical Knife (Olympus, Tokyo, Japan), HookKnife (Olympus America Inc, Center Valley, PA), the DualKnife (Olympus America Inc, Center Valley, PA), the HybridKnife (ERBE, Tübingen, Germany) and more recently the ORISE Pro-Knife (Boston Scientific, Marlborough, MA). The combined electrosurgical knives aim to decrease the instrument change time by integrating the injection needle and knife functions into one instrument. Instrument referrals depend on the availability and the endoscopist's comfort level with the instrument.

The procedure begins after adequate tissue elevation with injection and lesion borders are marked. This step is sometimes omitted, especially if the lesion is in clear vision, depending on physician preference, as it may lead to injectate leak and loss of cushion created. The injection should extend outside of the mucosal lesion as there will be a clear mucosal margin. Once the lift is started, future injections should be directed at the edge of the last lift to stay in the same plane. The dissection is started from the distal (anal) border of the mucosa around the lesion and is incised in a semi-circular fashion with an endoscopic knife. The complete circumferential incision will result in an increased leak of submucosal fluid with more incredible difficulty of subsequent lift. However, the advantage of a complete circumferential mucosal incision at the start of the procedure is to avoid over dissection pass the lesion in the submucosal plane during ESD. After partial incision, further dissection proceeds tangential (parallel) to the submucosa to prevent digging into the colon wall and creating a full-thickness injury (Fig. 10). Visualization is aided with a clear cap distal attachment to allow the endoscope to elevate the overlying mucosa. Vessels are easily seen with a blue dye added to the injectate and are coagulated for hemostasis. As the dissection continues, repeat submucosal injection can be periodically used to expand the submucosa in front of the dissection.

Hybrid ESD

Occasionally, a hybrid method with ESD and EMR can be helpful and time-efficient. The technique is started after injection with adequate lift. The resection borders are marked with a snare tip, and dissection starts in a similar technique with ESD, and the lesion is liberated peripherally. Afterward, the remaining central dissection can be done with a large snare like in EMR. These steps should be continued until complete resection is achieved. En bloc resection should be the primary goal.

Key points—ELS

- Clear and visualize the resection area and inspect for any full-thickness defects.
- Use coagulation forceps for hemostasis if needed.
- Avoid excessive thermal energy.
- Close full-thickness defects with endoscopic hemoclip.
- Use over-the-scope clips for larger defects

Novel Endoluminal Platforms

Although ESD offers a way to avoid unnecessary surgery and provides better results comparing piecemeal resections, it is not widely applicable and adapted because of technical challenges like poor stabilization and visualization. In addition, the required technical skills are very hard to acquire with a steep learning curve. New endoluminal devices are being developed to facilitate the process and increase procedural success rates. They aim to help the endoscopist to stabilize the procedure field and incorporate surgical principles such as traction-counter traction.

ORISE Tissue Retractor System (ORISE TRS; Boston Scientific Corp, Marlborough, Mass, USA) consists of a cage-like structure that has 2 instrument channels and can be inserted over a standard colonoscope. This platform helps stabilization during resection, and endoscopic instruments can be introduced through the channels (Fig. 11).[26]

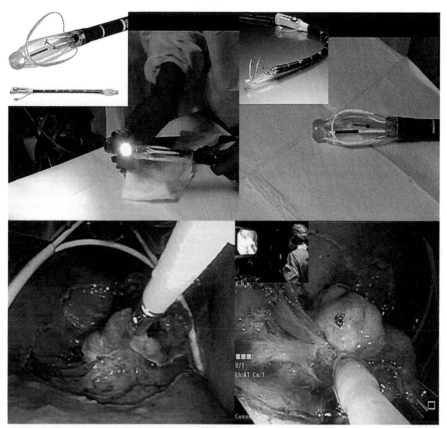

Fig. 11. ORISE Tissue Retractor System: This platform with a cage-like structure that has 2 instrument channels and is inserted over a standard colonoscope.

DiLumen C^2 is a novel endoscopic stabilization device facilitating traction and en bloc removal of complex colorectal lesions (**Fig. 12**A). DiLumen C^2 is introduced over endoscopes. The device uses 2 balloons, and when both balloons are deployed and inflated, the area in between is stabilized. In addition, DiLumen C^2 uses 2 working

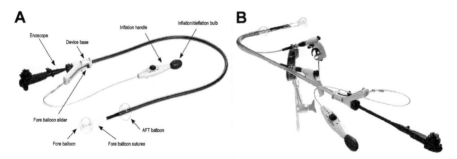

Fig. 12. Dilumen Endolumenal Interventional Platform: (*A*) Device introduced over the scope. (*B*) Device with introduced grasper and scissors.

channels at the 3 and 9 o'clock position to introduce DiLumen I_g Grasper and Scissors I_s (**Fig. 12**B). Standard ESD is started, and a solution is injected into the submucosal space to create the desired cushion. Dissection begins with an appropriate knife. Subsequently, the scope is withdrawn, and the Dilumen C^2 platform is introduced around the scope into the lumen. The platform is positioned at the level of the lesion, and both balloons are inflated for stabilization of the system and lumen. Once the platform is stabilized, the tissue grasper is introduced through the instrument guide. It is used to retract the tissue to create adequate traction and counter-traction, which facilitates dissection.

Complications of Advanced Polypectomy

Complications can occur during or after the procedure. The most commonly observed ones are perforation and bleeding. Bleeding occurs in approximately 2% to 7% of patients. Minimal bleeding may occur during the procedure and should not be alarming. Endoscopic clips and snare coagulation can be used to control bleeding. Delayed bleeding rates have been reported to be 2%, and these may require operative exploration and resections if they cannot be controlled.[5] When patients present with bleeding, our workup includes serial CBC checks and close monitoring. PRBC transfusion is given only when indicated, and patients are scoped in the endo unit if bleeding is continuous. In our experience, most bleedings are self-limiting and are more common in patients with chronic anticoagulation use. Delayed bleeding rates and perforation rates were 3.6% and 2.7% in our early experience with 110 patients.[5]

Perforation is reported between 5% and 20% of patients. The risk of perforation is associated with increased tumor size and the presence of fibrosis. Perforation is diagnosed based on the clinical presentation of the patient with abdominal pain and fever. Immediate perforation rates were reported to be higher than delayed perforation rates, with the latter being less than 0.5%.[5] Immediate perforations may warrant surgical intervention if the defect cannot be managed with clipping. Perforation during ESD of malignant lesions can result in potential tumor seeding, as evidenced from the more robust gastric cancer literature. However, in our series, no peritoneal seeding was seen due to perforation during the procedure.[5] Post-ESD electrocoagulation syndrome is similar to postpolypectomy syndrome and can be seen in up to 40% of patients. Lastly, endoscopic methods at the resection site carry the potential for recurrence. Local recurrence after ESD is approximately 1%.[27,28]

Surveillance after Mucosal Resections

The aim of the follow-up colonoscopy and surveillance after ESD or EMR is early detection of local recurrence and/or metachronous lesions. Currently, there is no consensus on surveillance after mucosal resection. The pathologic characteristics and quality of the resected specimen determine the proposed surveillance and individual risk factors, including more than one lesion, previous carcinoma history, and accompanying comorbidities. Although Eastern and Western guidelines offer different periods depending on these features, the follow-up endoscopy may be recommended at the sixth month after the index procedure and then at the first and third year.[3,29–31]

Early detection of a recurrent lesion is crucial, and every patient, after an advanced endoscopic procedure, should undergo surveillance. Belberdos and colleagues reported 20% recurrence after piecemeal resection, whereas it was 3% for the en bloc resection technique following EMR.[32]

SUMMARY

Local excision and ELS are promising organ preservation techniques and are becoming more widely accepted and practiced in CRC management. The main obstacle of the procedures is the careful selection and workup of patients. Proper selection of patients affects the outcomes, previously reported to be inferior with LE compared with radical surgery. Although ELS is considered challenging, it will continue to progress and gain more popularity over time. Increased education, research, and availability of the tools to perform these procedures will help more endoscopists be adept over time. Owing to the ability to avoid intraabdominal surgery, ELS can be the next big step for minimally invasive surgery. Through research and development, fully flexible endorobotic platforms with stable camera positioning and precision will become a reality and push the field of ELS forward.

DISCLOSURE

I. Ozgur has nothing to disclose. E. Gorgun has financial disclosures with Boston Scientific and DiLumen as a consultant.

REFERENCES

1. Zauber AG, Winawer SJ, O'Brien MJ, et al. Colonoscopic polypectomy and long-term prevention of colorectal-cancer deaths. N Engl J Med 2012;366(8):687–96. https://doi.org/10.1056/NEJMoa1100370.

2. Patel SG, Boland CR. Colorectal cancer in persons under age 50: seeking causes and solutions. Gastrointest Endosc Clin N Am 2020;30(3):441–55. https://doi.org/10.1016/j.giec.2020.03.001.

3. Kaltenbach T, Anderson JC, Burke CA, et al. Endoscopic removal of colorectal lesions-recommendations by the US multi-society task force on colorectal cancer. Gastroenterology 2020;158(4):1095–129. https://doi.org/10.1053/j.gastro.2019.12.018.

4. Peery AF, Cools KS, Strassle PD, et al. Increasing rates of surgery for patients with nonmalignant colorectal polyps in the United States. Gastroenterology 2018;154(5):1352–60.e3. https://doi.org/10.1053/j.gastro.2018.01.003.

5. Gorgun E, Benlice C, Abbas MA, et al. Experience in colon sparing surgery in North America: advanced endoscopic approaches for complex colorectal lesions. Surg Endosc 2018;32(7):3114–21. https://doi.org/10.1007/s00464-018-6026-2.

6. Stevenson ARL, Solomon MJ, Brown CSB, et al. Disease-free survival and local recurrence after laparoscopic-assisted resection or open resection for rectal cancer: the Australasian Laparoscopic Cancer of the rectum randomized clinical trial. Ann Surg 2019;269(4):596–602.

7. Fleshman J, Branda ME, Sargent DJ, et al. Disease-free survival and local recurrence for laparoscopic resection compared with open resection of stage II to III rectal cancer: follow-up results of the ACOSOG Z6051 randomized controlled trial. Ann Surg 2019;269(4):589–95.

8. Lacy AM, Tasende MM, Delgado S, et al. Transanal total mesorectal excision for rectal cancer: outcomes after 140 patients. J Am Coll Surg 2015;221(2):415–23. https://doi.org/10.1016/j.jamcollsurg.2015.03.046.

9. Robotic-assisted vs conventional laparoscopic surgery on risk of conversion to open laparotomy among patients undergoing resection for rectal cancer: the

ROLARR randomized clinical trial. JAMA 2017;318(16):1569–80. https://doi.org/10.1001/jama.2017.7219.

10. Moss A, Bourke MJ, Williams SJ, et al. Endoscopic mucosal resection outcomes and prediction of submucosal cancer from advanced colonic mucosal neoplasia. Gastroenterology 2011;140(7):1909–18. https://doi.org/10.1053/j.gastro.2011.02.062.

11. Saito Y, Uraoka T, Yamaguchi Y, et al. A prospective, multicenter study of 1111 colorectal endoscopic submucosal dissections (with video). Gastrointest Endosc 2010. https://doi.org/10.1016/j.gie.2010.08.004.

12. Scheele J, Schmidt SA, Tenzer S, et al. Overstaging: a challenge in rectal cancer treatment. Visc Med 2018;34(4):301–6. https://doi.org/10.1159/000488652.

13. Salinas HM, Dursun A, Klos CL, et al. Determining the need for radical surgery in patients with T1 rectal cancer. Arch Surg 2011;146(5):540–3. https://doi.org/10.1001/archsurg.2011.76.

14. The Paris endoscopic classification of superficial neoplastic lesions: esophagus, stomach, and colon: November 30 to December 1, 2002. Gastrointest Endosc 2003;58(6 Suppl):S3–43.

15. Kudo S, Tamura S, Nakajima T, et al. Diagnosis of colorectal tumorous lesions by magnifying endoscopy. Gastrointest Endosc 1996;44:8–14.

16. Hayashi N, Tanaka S, Hewett DG, et al. Endoscopic prediction of deep submucosal invasive carcinoma: validation of the Narrow-Band Imaging International Colorectal Endoscopic (NICE) classification. Gastrointest Endosc 2013. https://doi.org/10.1016/j.gie.2013.04.185.

17. Habr-Gama A, Perez RO, Nadalin W, et al. Operative versus nonoperative treatment for stage 0 distal rectal cancer following chemoradiation therapy: long-term results. Ann Surg 2004;240(4):711–8. https://doi.org/10.1097/01.sla.0000141194.27992.32.

18. Perez RO, Habr-Gama A, Sao Juliao GP, et al. Transanal endoscopic microsurgery for residual rectal cancer after neoadjuvant chemoradiation therapy is associated with significant immediate pain and hospital readmission rates. Dis Colon Rectum 2011;54:545–51.

19. Garcia-Aguilar J, Mellgren A, Sirivongs P, et al. Local excision of rectal cancer without adjuvant therapy: a word of caution. Ann Surg 2000;231(3):345–51. https://doi.org/10.1097/00000658-200003000-00007.

20. Madbouly KM, Remzi FH, Erkek BA, et al. Recurrence after transanal excision of T1 rectal cancer: should we be concerned? Dis Colon Rectum 2005;48(4):711–21. https://doi.org/10.1007/s10350-004-0666-0.

21. Wang J, Zhang XH, Ge J, et al. Endoscopic submucosal dissection vs endoscopic mucosal resection for colorectal tumors: a meta-analysis. World J Gastroenterol 2014. https://doi.org/10.3748/wjg.v20.i25.8282.

22. Repici A, Hassan C, De Paula Pessoa D, et al. Efficacy and safety of endoscopic submucosal dissection for colorectal neoplasia: a systematic review. Endoscopy 2012. https://doi.org/10.1055/s-0031-1291448.

23. Sapci I, Gorgun E. Endoscopic submucosal dissection. In: Bardakcioglu O, editor. Advanced techniques in minimally invasive and robotic colorectal surgery. Cham: Springer; 2019. p. 9–16.

24. Sanchez-Yague A, Kaltenbach T, Raju G, et al. Advanced endoscopic resection of colorectal lesions. Gastroenterol Clin North Am 2013. https://doi.org/10.1016/j.gtc.2013.05.012.

25. Nugent E, Sapci I, Steele SR, et al. Pushing the envelope in endoscopic submu-cosal dissection: is it feasible and safe in scarred lesions? Dis Colon Rectum 2021;64(3):343–8. https://doi.org/10.1097/DCR.0000000000001870.
26. Sapci I, Gorgun E. Removal of a large rectal lesion with endoscopic submucosal dissection using a new endolumenal platform. Dis Colon Rectum 2020;63(5):710. https://doi.org/10.1097/DCR.0000000000001661.
27. De Ceglie A, Hassan C, Mangiavillano B, et al. Endoscopic mucosal resection and endoscopic submucosal dissection for colorectal lesions: a systematic re-view. Crit Rev Oncol Hematol 2016;104:138–55. https://doi.org/10.1016/j.critrevonc.2016.06.008.
28. Akintoye E, Kumar N, Aihara H, et al. Colorectal endoscopic submucosal dissec-tion: a systematic review and meta-analysis. Endosc Int Open 2016;4(10): E1030–44. https://doi.org/10.1055/s-0042-114774.
29. Gupta S, Lieberman D, Anderson JC, et al. Recommendations for follow-up after colonoscopy and polypectomy: a consensus update by the US multi-society task force on colorectal cancer. Am J Gastroenterol 2020;115(3):415–34. https://doi.org/10.14309/ajg.0000000000000544.
30. Pimentel-Nunes P, Dinis-Ribeiro M, Ponchon T, et al. Endoscopic submucosal dissection: European Society of Gastrointestinal Endoscopy (ESGE) guideline. Endoscopy 2015;47(9):829–54. https://doi.org/10.1055/s-0034-1392882.
31. Tanaka S, Kashida H, Saito Y, et al. Japan Gastroenterological Endoscopy Soci-ety guidelines for colorectal endoscopic submucosal dissection/endoscopic mucosal resection. Dig Endosc 2020;32(2):219–39. https://doi.org/10.1111/den.13545.
32. Belderbos TD, Leenders M, Moons LM, et al. Local recurrence after endoscopic mucosal resection of nonpedunculated colorectal lesions: systematic review and meta-analysis. Endoscopy 2014;46(5):388–402. https://doi.org/10.1055/s-0034-1364970.

Surgical Principles of Rectal Cancer

Ebram Salama, MD, MBA[a], Jessica Holland, MD, FRCS(C)[a],
Marylise Boutros, MD, FRCS(C)[a,b],*

KEYWORDS

- Rectal cancer • Low anterior resection • Abdominal perineal resection
- Surgical quality improvement

INTRODUCTION

Although the management of rectal cancer has become increasingly dependent on multimodality and multidisciplinary approaches, surgery remains the mainstay of care. Understanding the anatomy of the rectum and pelvis is pivotal to ensuring the best oncological and functional outcomes for patients. Surgical management of rectal cancer continues to evolve, from the advent of total mesorectal excision (TME) in the 1980s to aggressive sphincter-sparing procedures in recent years. This article reviews some of the key anatomic and surgical principles in rectal cancer care.

RECTAL AND PELVIC ANATOMY

The rectum represents the distal-most aspect of the hindgut, connecting the sigmoid colon to the anal canal. Its proximal extent, the rectosigmoid junction, is marked by the splaying of the taeniae coli and absence of epiploic appendages, which corresponds to approximately the level of the third sacral vertebrae. Distally, the anorectal ring marks the surgical transition from the rectum to the anal canal. The rectum is divided into 3 segments: the lower rectum spans approximately 0-7 cm from the anal verge, the mid rectum 7 to 12 cm, and the upper rectum 12 to 15 cm.[1] Although the rectum is primarily an extraperitoneal structure, its upper third is covered by the visceral peritoneum. Despite considerable individual variation, this peritoneal reflection sits at about 9 cm from the anal verge anteriorly and 12 cm laterally.[2] The peritoneal reflection is a clinically important landmark that can be readily identified on preoperative MRI.[3]

The rectum derives its main blood supply from the superior rectal artery (SRA), a terminal branch of the inferior mesenteric artery (IMA). Additional blood supply comes from the paired middle rectal and inferior rectal arteries, supplying the distal rectum.

[a] Department of Surgery, McGill University, 1650 Cedar Avenue, L9.424, Montreal, Quebec H3G 1A4, Canada; [b] Division of Colon and Rectal Surgery, Jewish General Hospital, 3755 Côte-Sainte-Catherine G-317, Montreal, Quebec H3T 1E2, Canada
* Corresponding author.
E-mail address: marylise.boutros@mcgill.ca

Surg Oncol Clin N Am 31 (2022) 239–253
https://doi.org/10.1016/j.soc.2021.11.005
1055-3207/22/Crown Copyright © 2021 Published by Elsevier Inc. All rights reserved.

The presence of the middle rectal artery is highly variable, identified in only 28% to 57% of cases, and frequently encountered as a single unilateral vessel.[4–6] The distal venous return mirrors the arterial supply, with predominate drainage of the rectum occurring through the portal circulation via the superior rectal and inferior mesenteric vein (IMV). The IMV runs along the left lateral side of the IMA and travels superiorly in the descending colon mesentery. The middle and inferior rectal veins drain to the internal iliac vein and enter the systemic circulation. Lymphatic circulation of the proximal two-thirds of the rectum drains into nodal basins along the SRA toward the inferior mesenteric nodes and the para-aortic chain. The lymphatics of the distal third of the rectum likewise drain into the superior rectal nodes, and laterally toward the internal iliac chain.

The mesorectum is a cone-shaped collection of perirectal adipose tissue, blood vessels, nerves, and lymphatics. The sacrum, coccyx, and muscles of the pelvic sidewall are draped by the parietal endopelvic fascia. The mesorectal fascia (**Fig. 1**) is an upward visceral extension of this parietal endopelvic fascia, maintaining the integrity of the mesorectum and its contents. Posteriorly, the thickened parietal pelvic fascia courses over the presacral venous plexus, hypogastric nerves, and sacral vertebrae and is referred to as the presacral fascia. At the level of the third and fourth sacral vertebrae, the presacral fascia gives rise to the retrosacral fascia (Waldeyer fascia), which then fuses with the visceral fascia propria approximately 3 to 5 cm from the anorectal junction. Anteriorly, Denonvilliers fascia extends from the perineal body to the inferior-most aspect of the peritoneal reflection. In men, it overlies the seminal vesicles and prostate, and in women, it forms part of the rectovaginal septum. The cavernous nerves that regulate erectile function run along the anterolateral aspect of Denonvilliers fascia (**Fig. 2**).

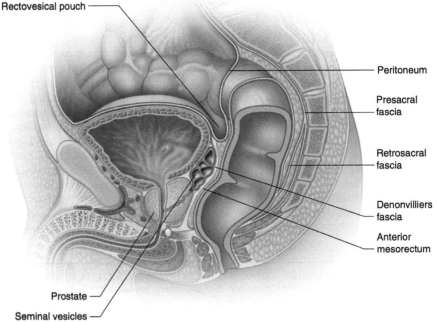

Fig. 1. Fascial relationships of the rectum. (*Permission granted from*: Carmichael J.C., Mills S. (2016) Anatomy and Embryology of the Colon, Rectum, and Anus. In: Steele S., Hull T., Read T., Saclarides T., Senagore A., Whitlow C. (eds) The ASCRS Textbook of Colon and Rectal Surgery. Springer, Cham.)

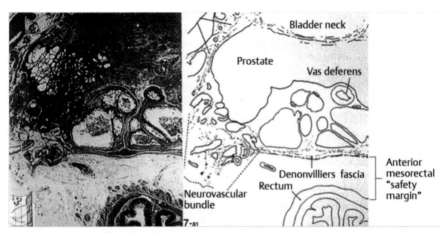

Fig. 2. Relationship of autonomic nerves to Denonvilliers fascia and mesorectum. (*Permission granted from:* Gordon PH, Nivatvongs S. Principles and Practice of Surgery for the Colon, Rectum, and Anus. CRC Press; 2007.)

Anterolaterally, the rectum is attached to the pelvic sidewall by the lateral stalks which are thickened folds of the mesorectal fascia. These structures can contain the middle rectal vessels (when present) and mixed automatic nerve branches of the inferior hypogastric plexus, which penetrate the mesorectal fascia to supply the rectum.

Understanding the autonomic nervous supply to the rectum is essential in minimizing the genitourinary consequences of rectal surgery. The lumbar splanchnic nerves are extensions of the sympathetic trunk, originating from the L1-L3 nerve roots, and provide sympathetic innervation to the rectum and pelvic organs. They contribute to the inferior mesenteric plexus, which courses along the IMA and innervates the left colon and upper rectum. More caudally, they form the superior hypogastric plexus, which subsequently divides into paired hypogastric nerves, coursing over the sacral promontory approximately 1 cm lateral to the midline and 2 cm medial to the ureters.[7] The parasympathetic nerves, or nervi erigenti, arise from the sacral splanchnic nerves (S2-S4) and travel anterolaterally along the pelvic wall. Together with the hypogastric nerves, they form the pelvic plexus. Neurovascular bundles from the pelvic plexus supply the distal rectum through the lateral stalks and supply the seminal vesicles, distal ureters, vasa deferentia, bladder, prostate, and cavernous bodies. Damage to the hypogastric nerves near the sacral promontory can result in primarily sympathetic dysfunction, including retrograde ejaculation, increased urinary frequency, nocturia, and incontinence. Injury to the mixed autonomic pelvic plexus can result in impotence and an atonic bladder.

BACKGROUND: ONCOLOGICAL PRINCIPLES
History of TME

Although TME was not popularized until the 1980s, its oncological significance was suspected as early as 1908 by Sir Ernest Miles. At a time when rectal resections were predominately performed via a perineal approach, Sir Miles noted that recurrences generally occurred in the proximal pelvic mesorectum and attributed this phenomenon to the upward spread of disease.[8] He consequently advocated for combined abdominoperineal resection (APR), whereby the upstream lymphatic drainage of the rectum would be removed *en bloc*.

In the 1940s, Claude Dixon called into question the significance of downward tumor spread, challenging the accepted standard of APRs for all rectal cancers. He proposed that a 4-5 cm distal margin with the restoration of intestinal continuity would be sufficient for local control. Dixon validated his hypothesis in a series of 426 restorative proctectomies, showing comparable oncological outcomes to APRs.[9] Shortly after, Goligher, Dukes, and Bussey demonstrated that only 2% of proctectomy specimens harbored microscopic tumor cells greater than 2 cm distal to the primary tumor, further validating the safety of a 5 cm distal resection margin.[10] By the mid-1950s, the concept of restorative proctectomy for mid to upper rectal cancers had become widely popularized.

The 1980s ushered in a new era in rectal cancer treatment, with TME emerging as the new gold standard for surgical management. At the time, R.J. Heald hypothesized that residual perirectal lymphovascular tissue harbored microscopic disease, and as such, complete mesorectal excision could reduce local recurrence rates. Heald advocated for sharp dissection in the potential space between the mesorectal fascia and the presacral fascia, the "holy plane," allowing for complete excision of the mesorectum (TME), while preserving the presacral plexus and hypogastric nerves (**Fig. 3**).[11] As such Heald described restorative proctectomy with TME as: (1) mobilization of the left colon from its retroperitoneal attachments; (2) *sharp dissection* along the relatively bloodless "holy plane" down to the levator muscle, separating the mesorectal fascia from the parietal endopelvic fascia; (3) sharp dissection anterior to Denonvilliers fascia; (4) ligation of IMA 1 cm from the aorta and ligation of the IMV 1 cm from the splenic vein; and (5) transection at the anorectum with the restoration of intestinal continuity.[12,13] Heald initially published a series of 50 patients who had undergone TME with curative intent, citing no evidence of locoregional recurrence at 2 years.[13] Over the next decade, TME alone would significantly outperform combined conventional surgery and chemoradiotherapy with respect to locoregional recurrence,[12] thereby emphasizing surgical technique as the cornerstone of rectal cancer management. The foundational work of Heald and colleagues marked a boom in the surgical literature, paving the way for present-day oncological principles and controversies with respect to proximal, distal, and circumferential resection margins.

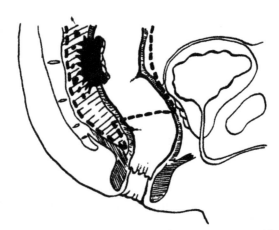

Fig. 3. The holy plane of total mesorectal excision. (*Permission granted from:* Heald RJ, Husband EM, Ryall RD. The mesorectum in rectal cancer surgery–the clue to pelvic recurrence? Br J Surg. 1982;69(10):613-616)

Principle 1: Proximal Ligation of the IMA

There remains ongoing debate as to whether ligation of the IMA at its root from the aorta (*high tie*) confers any oncological benefit, or if transection just distal to the take-off of the left colic artery (*low tie*) is sufficient.[14] Proponents of the former suggest that metastases to the para-aortic IMA nodes provide important prognostic value.[15] In addition, a high tie may increase mobility of the proximal colonic mesentery, facilitating a tension-free anastomosis.[16] However, there are theoretic concerns that a high tie may compromise proximal colonic blood flow,[17] and that dissection at this level may jeopardize the para-aortic autonomic nerve plexus. High ligation has been associated with an increased risk of genitourinary dysfunction in a recent randomized controlled trial (RCT).[18] To date, there remains no convincing evidence to suggest that a high tie confers any survival benefit,[18,19] and as such, in the absence of clinical concern for para-aortic nodal involvement, a low tie just distal to the take-off of the left colic artery remains acceptable practice.[14] However, even if a low tie is performed, it is paramount that the entire colon and rectal mesentery be removed en bloc with the bowel.

Principle 2: Distal Resection Margins

Before the adoption of TME, a 5 cm distal resection margin was deemed necessary to prevent local recurrence.[10] However, studies have shown that only 10% of rectal tumors exhibit distal intramural spread, and as few as 2% to 3% of stage I-III cancers extend beyond 1 cm from the primary tumor.[20] In fact, distal intramural spread is often associated with unfavorable tumor histology (such as poor differentiation), and its independent impact on local recurrence and overall survival are questionable.[20,21] Rather, it appears that spread into the mesorectum is significantly more important and can extend up to 3-4 cm from the primary tumor, forming the basis for TME.[12] In distal rectal cancers, when a TME is performed, a distal margin of 2 cm is considered ideal. However, in the absence of poor prognostic tumor characteristics, closer negative margins are acceptable, especially if there is a strong motivation for sphincter preservation.[14,22] In tumors of the mid and upper rectum, a partial mesorectal excision with 5 cm distal margins is deemed oncologically safe.[10,21]

Principle 3: Circumferential Resection Margins

In the 1980s, when surgical management of rectal cancer was garnering increased attention, Philip Quirke defined the importance of circumferential resection margins (CRMs). Upon careful reassessment of 52 proctectomy specimens, he found that 27% had microscopic lateral involvement, and among those, 85% developed local recurrence.[23] Since then, the importance of CRM involvement as a predictor of local recurrence and poor disease-free survival became well established.[24,25] At the same time, Heald's principles of TME of achieving an appropriate plane of dissection with an intact mesorectal fascia led to decreased CRM positivity and was shown to be an independent predictor of local recurrence.[25]

There has been some variability as to the definition of a clear CRM. In a series of 1,530 patients, Nagtegaal and colleagues showed that local recurrence rates were significantly lower when a 2 mm CRM was obtained compared with 1 mm (16% vs 10%), and thus advocated for more aggressive resection.[26] However, local recurrence rates have since decreased significantly worldwide. More recent landmark trials have considered 1 mm as an acceptable CRM, including the MERCURY and OCUM trials. Oncological data from the former showed a crude 5-year local recurrence rate of 7% when at least 1 mm pathologic CRM was achieved[27]; the latter showed a crude 3-year recurrence rate of 2.7%.[28] In addition, a recent Swedish population-based study of

8,392 patients found no difference in local recurrence when comparing 1 mm with 2 mm CRM.[24]

The MERCURY trial established preoperative MRI as an accurate and reproducible modality for predicting CRM involvement, with a specificity of 91% and a negative predictive value of 94%.[27] Moreover, mesorectal fascial involvement on MRI became a significant preoperative staging parameter in predicting overall survival, disease-free survival, and local recurrence.[27] Nonetheless, tumors extending into and beyond the mesorectal fascia may still be amenable to surgical resection. These locally advanced tumors often require multimodal therapy, and multivisceral resection to achieve negative margins.[29]

Current Controversy: Lateral Pelvic Node Dissection

The management of lateral pelvic lymph nodes, which include the internal iliac, external iliac, obturator, and common iliac nodes, is an area of active investigation. In Japan, all are considered regional and therefore reasonable targets for extended upfront resection. In North America, their involvement is considered metastatic and thus an indication for upfront systemic therapy.[30] Lateral node dissections have been associated with urinary and sexual dysfunction,[30] and, to date, have not been convincingly associated with any oncologic benefit.[31] The recent American Society of Colon and Rectal Surgeons (ASCRS) guidelines published in 2020 do not recommend routine lateral pelvic node dissection in the absence of clinically positive nodes.[14] Selective dissection in patients with clinically suspicious nodes or definitive involvement for local control may still be beneficial, and as such these guidelines recommend ipsilateral lateral pelvic node for clinically positive nodes.

OPERATIVE MANAGEMENT OF RECTAL CANCER

Regardless of the operative approach, oncological principles of rectal cancer surgery remain the same and largely reflect the early teachings of Professor Heald. Appropriate resection requires respect for embryologic planes with careful dissection of the mesorectum out of the pelvis, recognition of the anatomic principles which define the lymphatic drainage of the rectum, and preservation of the neurovascular supply to the closely associated urogenital structures.

Operative Approach

Open, laparoscopic, and robotic approaches can all be done safely in experienced hands, although true equivalence is still debated in the published literature. Although laparoscopic colon cancer surgery has been widely accepted as oncologically equivalent to open resection, with the added benefit of improved length of stay and reduced post-operative pain,[32,33] there have been conflicting findings on whether laparoscopic surgery obtains equivalent CRM results and rates of local recurrence as open surgery for rectal cancer (**Table 1**).[34–39] Despite these early concerns, recent meta-analyses suggest that a laparoscopic approach is noninferior with regard to oncologic outcomes.[40,41] The challenge of dissecting the distal rectum safely and efficiently continues to drive surgical innovation including the adoption of robotic and transanal approaches which are discussed in other sections.

The Procedure

Colonic mobilization
There are 2 main approaches to mobilizing the descending colon and sigmoid mesentery:

Table 1
Major trials comparing open to laparoscopic surgery for rectal cancer

Trials	Location	Year of Recruitment	Trial Design	Primary Outcome	Completed TME Rate	Locoregional Recurrence	CRM Positive	Conclusion
ACOSCOG Z6051[34]	US & Canada	2008–2013	Noninferiority	Successful resection	65% Lap vs 73.9% Open	Not reported	12.1% Lap vs 7.7% Open, P = .11	Failed to meet noninferiority target
COLOR II[37,38]	NA, Europe, Asia	2004–2010	Noninferiority	Local regional recurrence	88% Lap vs 95% open, P = .250	5% (CI −2.6 to 2.6) at 3 y	10% Lap vs 10% open, P = .85	Met noninferiority target
MRC CLASICC[33,35]	UK	1996–2002	Equivalence	OS, DFS, LR	NR	8.7% open vs 10.8% Lap at 5 y, (CI −7.3 to 2.3, P = .594)	7% Lap vs 5% open, P = .45	Met noninferiority targets
AlaCaRT[36]	Australia & New Zealand	2010–2014	Noninferiority	Adequate surgical resection*	87% Lap vs 92% Open, P = .06	Not reported	7% Lap vs 3% open	Failed to meet noninferiority target
COREAN[39]	South Korea	2006–2009	Noninferiority	DFS at 3 y	92% lap vs 88% open, P = .55	4.9% open vs 2.6% lap (CI −1.8 to 6.4)	3% lap vs 4% open, P = .77	Met noninferiority target

*Definitions of successful resection and adequate surgical resection were both composite endpoints.
Abbreviations: CRM, circumference resection margin; DFS, disease-free survival; LR, local recurrence; OS, overall survival; TME, total mesorectal excision.

1. Medial-to-lateral: the SRA is retracted superiorly, and the underlying peritoneum is incised in a transverse fashion entering the avascular plane between the mesentery and retroperitoneum. As the dissection proceeds laterally and superiorly, the left ureter is identified in the retroperitoneum. The pedicle can be traced backward to the IMA for a high ligation or the SRA is divided as the surgeon deems appropriate. During a high ligation, care must be taken to avoid damage to the sympathetic fibers of the superior hypogastric nerve plexus near the root of the IMA. The lateral attachments of the colon are then incised along the white line of Toldt, joining the medial dissection plane.
2. The lateral-to-medial approach starts with division of the white line of Toldt on the lateral sidewall, and dissection proceeds medially toward the vascular pedicle.

Once the descending colon and sigmoid colon mesenteries are mobilized off the retroperitoneum, the splenic flexure can be mobilized if deemed necessary for a tension-free anastomosis. Likewise, division of the IMV can be performed just distal to the inferior pancreatic border for maximal length or at the level of the mesenteric division if not needed for the conduit length.

Pelvic dissection
Pelvic dissection begins with partial circumferential division of the peritoneal reflection laterally and entry into the "holy plane." This is a precise millimetric plane. Exiting this plane posteriorly will result in diffuse and difficult to control bleeding from the sacral venous plexus, in addition to damage to the hypogastric nerve fibers. Similarly, exiting this plane anteriorly will result in an incomplete specimen and compromised oncologic outcomes.

The posterior aspect of the rectum lacks a peritoneal covering and is the easiest point of entry into the correct TME dissection plane. With the SRA pedicle retracted upward, sharp dissection allows for mobilization of the posterior TME plane. The dissection extends laterally toward the lateral stalks of the rectum. The middle rectal arteries, when present, may be encountered at this stage. Entry into the lateral sidewall is easy at this level and should be meticulously avoided, as the nervi erigenti running parallel in the lateral sidewall can be damaged. Anterior dissection is often approached last. The peritoneal reflection, between the rectum and bladder in men and between the rectum and vagina in women, is first divided, followed by careful dissection in the plane posterior to Denonvilliers fascia. Preserving this fascia, outside of selective anterior tumors with threatened margin at this level, significantly improves sexual and urinary function postoperatively, without increasing rates of local recurrence.[42] The parasympathetic nerves at the base of the prostate are easily damaged during this dissection. The prostatic urethra is also vulnerable to damage in the deep dissection in the pelvis, but this complication is primarily seen with the perineal approach where it is easier to enter the incorrect plane and dissect above the prostate. Deliberate effort must be made to avoid "coning" in early during dissection of the mesorectum. If the tumor is located in the upper rectum and a complete mesorectal excision is not planned, then the mesorectum must be divided perpendicular to the bowel wall at the level of the distal transection margin. For a complete mesorectal excision, dissection should be taken to the pelvic floor circumferentially. Completing this dissection circumferentially is often essential to achieve the mobility to place a stapler for distal transection.

Distal extent of resection
With limited distal intramural spread of rectal cancers and increasing evidence that 1 cm or even close shave margins are oncologically acceptable, there has been

increasing interest in sphincter-preserving surgery.[20–22] Rullier classification attempted to standardize patients being evaluated for sphincter preservation, dividing them into 4 groups based on distance from, and involvement of the sphincter complex (**Table 2**).[43] Although ultralow resections with coloanal anastomoses are possible, consideration must be given to the expected postoperative function (particularly in parous women).

An APR is performed when sphincter preservation is not possible for oncologic or functional reasons and involves resection of the entire rectum and anus. A standard APR is indicated for external sphincter involvement and involves excising a wide ellipse of perineal skin as well as the entire sphincter complex. An extralevator APR, with en bloc resection of the levator ani muscles, sphincter complex, anal canal, and mesorectum can be done for locally advanced tumors. This approach may result in reduced CRM positivity, local recurrence, and mortality at 3 years compared with the standard approach.[44] However, the data are limited with only one RCT that did not control for tumor characteristics, and thus further data are still required to identify the patients who will benefit most from this technique. The drawback of an extralevator APR is a large perineal defect often necessitating flap reconstruction, and potentially more extensive pelvic nerve damage.

Proximal extent of resections

The proximal resection margins for both restorative proctectomy and APR are identical from an oncological perspective and are generally determined by the vascular supply. If a high ligation is performed, some surgeons routinely resect the entire sigmoid, whereas if a low ligation of the IMA is performed, the proximal margin is often in the sigmoid colon at least 5 cm proximal from the tumor. Indocyanine green fluoroscopy (ICG) has been used to assess the blood supply to the colonic conduit after vascular ligation and before creation of the anastomosis to prevent relative ischemia. Insufficient perfusion was seen in 5% of cases but to date, the use of ICG has not been shown to reduce the rate of anastomotic leak.[45]

Colorectal anastomosis during rectal cancer surgery

Rectal surgery was transformed with the introduction of circular staplers in the 1980s and they have since become the mainstay of colorectal anastomoses. Although there is no conclusive evidence of the superiority of the stapled anastomosis, they are used almost exclusively due to technical ease in the pelvis, with one notable exception.[46] For ultra-LAR, there is often not sufficient distal rectum for a circular stapler firing, necessitating handsewn coloanal anastomoses. The handsewn coloanal anastomosis following ultralow restorative proctectomy is performed in a manner very similar to that initially described by Parks, with the rectum transected just above the anorectal ring and the proximal colon drawn down and sutured with interrupted stitches circumferentially at the level of the dentate line.[47]

Table 2
Rullier classification for low rectal cancer[42]

Classification	Distal of Tumor from Anal Ring	Distal Resection Margin	Anastomosis
Type 1—Supra-anal	>1 cm	Anal ring	Coloanal
Type 2—Juxta-anal	<1 cm	Partial intersphincteric	Coloanal
Type 3—Intra-anal	Invasion of internal sphincter	Total intersphincteric	Coloanal
Type 4—Transanal	Invasion of external sphincter	Complete resection	APR

The first described circular stapled technique for colorectal anastomosis involved a straight end-to-end anastomosis with purse string sutures holding the anvil in place proximally and surrounding the spike distally. The distal purse string was then replaced by a linear staple line forming a double stapled end-to-end anastomosis. Various techniques have since been trialed to reduce anastomotic leak and improve postoperative function.[48] The colonic J-pouch was used to recreate a colic reservoir in lieu of the lost rectum. There does not appear to be a benefit in terms of early post-operative complications, but the early functional outcomes for at least the first 18 months may be improved.[49,50] Coloplasty, a technique similar to strictureplasty, was introduced for use in the narrow pelvis which cannot accommodate the J-pouch. Despite early optimism surrounding this technique, it does not appear to confer any significant advantage over an end-to-end anastomosis, and thus it has largely been abandoned.[51] The side-to-end anastomosis was then introduced and seems to mimic many of the postoperative functional benefits of the colonic J-pouch without the additional time, colon length, and pelvic space required to create the pouch itself.[52]

Once the anastomosis is completed, it is assessed in the operating room with direct visualization using a flexible sigmoidoscope and an air leak test. If an air leak is detected, evidence suggests proximal diversion or revision of the anastomosis should be attempted rather than direct suture repair alone.[53]

Considerations for Anastomotic Leaks and Proximal Diversion

Proximal diversion is widely practiced to mitigate the clinical consequences of anastomotic leak,[54] but stoma creation has its own significant impact on quality of life, financial burden, and complications. Routine diversion for all patients following restorative

Table 3
Factors affecting the rate of anastomotic leak in colorectal anastomosis[54,55]

	Local Factors	Operative Factors	Patient Factors
Increase risk	Preoperative radiation Location (<6 cm) anastomosis from the anal verge Tension on anastomosis Local tissue ischemia Tumor >3 cm Advanced tumor stage	Intraoperative hypotension Blood loss, especially requiring transfusion Operative time >4 h Emergency vs elective surgery	Preoperative anemia Male ASA >11 Diabetes, pulmonary, renal, vascular disease Smoking Obesity Malnutrition Alcohol consumption Use of immunosuppressant agents, particularly steroids Crohn disease Bevacizumab
Inconclusive	Microbiome: presence of bacterial producing MMPs eg, *Enterococcus*, *pseudomonas*, *Serratia* species	Mechanical bowel preparation with oral antibiotics	Tacrolimus, everolimus
No impact on risk		Handsewn vs stapled anastomosis Placement of pelvic drains	

proctectomy had been widely debated and now generally abandoned.[54] Diversion may potentially be avoided in low-risk, proximal rectal resections in the absence of radiation, but is generally indicated for high-risk anastomoses. Risk factors can be divided into patient, disease, and operative factors (**Table 3**).[55,56] Patient factors include overall health, physiologic reserve in the face of a complication, and medications or diseases known to inhibit healing. For disease factors, a radiated field is considered a sufficient indication. In addition, a low pelvic anastomosis (<7 cm from the anal verge), a technically challenging anastomosis, or a positive air leak test are indications for diversion. Despite much literature on the topic, the need for proximal diversion is often subjective.

The ostomy can be safely reversed either after a 3 to 6 months period of healing, once all adjuvant treatments have been completed, or even in the early postoperative setting for well-selected patients.[57] Before reversal, the integrity of the anastomosis is tested with rectal contrast imaging and flexible sigmoidoscopy.[58]

SUMMARY

The management of rectal cancer continues to evolve, with ongoing improvements in multidisciplinary and multimodality treatment. Nonetheless, surgery remains the mainstay of treatment. Understanding anatomic and oncological principles of rectal cancer surgery remains essential to both current practice and future innovation.

CLINICS CARE POINTS

- Oncologically sound rectal cancer surgery requires respect for the embryonic planes surrounding the rectum and complete mesorectal excision.
- In the absence of high-risk features, distal intramural spread of rectal cancer appears to be minimal, thus expanding indications for sphincter-preserving surgery.
- High ligation of the IMA has not been proven to confer oncologic benefit but is often required to create a tension-free anastomosis in restorative proctectomy.
- Minimally invasive and open approaches are likely equivalent in experienced hands.

DISCLOSURE

The authors have nothing to disclose.

REFERENCES

1. Heald RJ, Moran BJ. Embryology and anatomy of the rectum. Semin Surg Oncol 1998;15(2):66–71.
2. Najarian MM, Belzer GE, Cogbill TH, et al. Determination of the peritoneal reflection using intraoperative proctoscopy. Dis Colon Rectum 2004;47(12):2080–5.
3. Gollub MJ, Maas M, Weiser M, et al. Recognition of the anterior peritoneal reflection at rectal MRI. AJR Am J Roentgenol 2013;200(1):97–101.
4. Sato K, Sato T. The vascular and neuronal composition of the lateral ligament of the rectum and the rectosacral fascia. Surg Radiol Anat 1991;13(1):17–22.
5. DiDio L, Diaz-Franco C, Schemainda R, et al. Morphology of the middle rectal arteries. Surg Radiol Anat 1986;8(4):229–36.
6. Bilhim T, Pereira JA, Tinto HR, et al. Middle rectal artery: myth or reality? Retrospective study with CT angiography and digital subtraction angiography. Surg Radiol Anat 2013;35(6):517–22.

7. Havenga K, DeRuiter MC, Enker WE, et al. Anatomical basis of autonomic nerve-preserving total mesorectal excision for rectal cancer. Br J Surg 1996;83(3):384-8.

8. Ernest Miles W. A method of performing abdomino-perineal excision for carcinoma of the rectum and of the terminal portion of the pelvic colon. Lancet 1908;172(4451):1812-3.

9. Dixon CF. Anterior resection for malignant lesions of the upper part of the rectum and lower part of the sigmoid. Ann Surg 1948;128(3):425-42.

10. Goligher JC, Dukes CE, Bussey HJ. Local recurrences after sphincter saving excisions for carcinoma of the rectum and rectosigmoid. Br J Surg 1951;39(155):199-211.

11. Heald RJ. The 'Holy Plane' of rectal surgery. J R Soc Med 1988;81(9):503-8.

12. MacFarlane JK, Ryall RD, Heald RJ. Mesorectal excision for rectal cancer. Lancet (London, England) 1993;341(8843):457-60.

13. Heald RJ, Husband EM, Ryall RD. The mesorectum in rectal cancer surgery-the clue to pelvic recurrence? Br J Surg 1982;69(10):613-6.

14. You YN, Hardiman KM, Bafford A, et al. The American Society of colon and rectal surgeons clinical practice guidelines for the management of rectal cancer. Dis Colon Rectum 2020;63(9):1191-222.

15. Kang J, Hur H, Min BS, et al. Prognostic impact of inferior mesenteric artery lymph node metastasis in colorectal cancer. Ann Surg Oncol 2011;18(3):704-10.

16. Bonnet S, Berger A, Hentati N, et al. High tie versus low tie vascular ligation of the inferior mesenteric artery in colorectal cancer surgery: impact on the gain in colon length and implications on the feasibility of anastomoses. Dis Colon Rectum 2012;55(5):515-21.

17. Komen N, Slieker J, De Kort P, et al. High tie versus low tie in rectal surgery: comparison of anastomotic perfusion. Int J Colorectal Dis 2011;26(8):1075-8.

18. Mari GM, Crippa J, Cocozza E, et al. Low ligation of inferior mesenteric artery in laparoscopic anterior resection for rectal cancer reduces genitourinary dysfunction: results from a randomized controlled trial (HIGHLOW Trial). Ann Surg 2019;269(6):1018-24.

19. Fujii S, Ishibe A, Ota M, et al. Short-term and long-term results of a randomized study comparing high tie and low tie inferior mesenteric artery ligation in laparoscopic rectal anterior resection: subanalysis of the HTLT (High tie vs. low tie) study. Surg Endosc 2019;33(4):1100-10.

20. Ueno H, Mochizuki H, Hashiguchi Y, et al. Preoperative parameters expanding the indication of sphincter preserving surgery in patients with advanced low rectal cancer. Ann Surg 2004;239(1):34-42.

21. Andreola S, Leo E, Belli F, et al. Distal intramural spread in adenocarcinoma of the lower third of the rectum treated with total rectal resection and coloanal anastomosis. Dis Colon Rectum 1997;40(1):25-9.

22. Bujko K, Rutkowski A, Chang GJ, et al. Is the 1-cm rule of distal bowel resection margin in rectal cancer based on clinical evidence? A systematic review. Ann Surg Oncol 2012;19(3):801-8.

23. Quirke P, Dixon MF, Durdey P, et al. Local recurrence of rectal adenocarcinoma due to inadequate surgical resection. Lancet 1986;328(8514):996-9.

24. Agger EA, Jorgren FH, Lydrup MA, et al. Risk of local recurrence of rectal cancer and circumferential resection margin: population-based cohort study. Br J Surg 2020;107(5):580-5.

25. Quirke P, Steele R, Monson J, et al. Effect of the plane of surgery achieved on local recurrence in patients with operable rectal cancer: a prospective study using data from the MRC CR07 and NCIC-CTG CO16 randomised clinical trial. Lancet 2009;373(9666):821–8.
26. Nagtegaal ID, Marijnen CA, Kranenbarg EK, et al. Circumferential margin involvement is still an important predictor of local recurrence in rectal carcinoma: not one millimeter but two millimeters is the limit. Am J Surg Pathol 2002;26(3):350–7.
27. Taylor FG, Quirke P, Heald RJ, et al. Preoperative magnetic resonance imaging assessment of circumferential resection margin predicts disease-free survival and local recurrence: 5-year follow-up results of the MERCURY study. J Clin Oncol 2014;32(1):34–43.
28. Ruppert R, Junginger T, Ptok H, et al. Oncological outcome after MRI-based selection for neoadjuvant chemoradiotherapy in the OCUM rectal cancer trial. Br J Surg 2018;105(11):1519–29.
29. Beyond TMEC. Consensus statement on the multidisciplinary management of patients with recurrent and primary rectal cancer beyond total mesorectal excision planes. Br J Surg 2013;100(8):1009–14.
30. Christou N, Meyer J, Toso C, et al. Lateral lymph node dissection for low rectal cancer: Is it necessary? World J Gastroenterol 2019;25(31):4294–9.
31. Kondo H, Yamaguchi S, Hirano Y, et al. Is prophylactic lateral lymph node dissection needed for lower rectal cancer? A single-center retrospective study. BMC Surg 2021;21(1):261.
32. Clinical Outcomes of Surgical Therapy Study G, Nelson H, Sargent DJ, Wieand HS, et al. A comparison of laparoscopically assisted and open colectomy for colon cancer. N Engl J Med 2004;350(20):2050–9.
33. Guillou PJ, Quirke P, Thorpe H, et al. Short-term endpoints of conventional versus laparoscopic-assisted surgery in patients with colorectal cancer (MRC CLASICC trial): multicentre, randomised controlled trial. Lancet (London, England) 2005;365(9472):1718–26.
34. Fleshman J, Branda M, Sargent DJ, et al. Effect of laparoscopic-assisted resection vs open resection of stage ii or iii rectal cancer on pathologic outcomes: the ACOSOG Z6051 randomized clinical trial. JAMA 2015;314(13):1346–55.
35. Jayne DG, Guillou PJ, Thorpe H, et al. Randomized trial of laparoscopic-assisted resection of colorectal carcinoma: 3-year results of the UK MRC CLASICC Trial Group. J Clin Oncol 2007;25(21):3061–8.
36. Stevenson AR, Solomon MJ, Lumley JW, et al. Effect of laparoscopic-assisted resection vs open resection on pathological outcomes in rectal cancer: the ALaCaRT randomized clinical trial. JAMA 2015;314(13):1356–63.
37. van der Pas MH, Haglind E, Cuesta MA, et al. Laparoscopic versus open surgery for rectal cancer (COLOR II): short-term outcomes of a randomised, phase 3 trial. Lancet Oncol 2013;14(3):210–8.
38. Bonjer HJ, Deijen CL, Abis GA, et al. A randomized trial of laparoscopic versus open surgery for rectal cancer. N Engl J Med 2015;372(14):1324–32.
39. Jeong SY, Park JW, Nam BH, et al. Open versus laparoscopic surgery for mid-rectal or low-rectal cancer after neoadjuvant chemoradiotherapy (COREAN trial): survival outcomes of an open-label, non-inferiority, randomised controlled trial. Lancet Oncol 2014;15(7):767–74.
40. Acuna SA, Chesney TR, Ramjist JK, et al. Laparoscopic versus open resection for rectal cancer: a noninferiority meta-analysis of quality of surgical resection outcomes. Ann Surg 2019;269(5):849–55.

41. Pędziwiatr M, Małczak P, Mizera M, et al. There is no difference in outcome between laparoscopic and open surgery for rectal cancer: a systematic review and meta-analysis on short- and long-term oncologic outcomes. Tech Coloproctol 2017;21(8):595–604.

42. Wei B, Zheng Z, Fang J, et al. Effect of denonvilliers' fascia preservation versus resection during laparoscopic total mesorectal excision on postoperative urogenital function of male rectal cancer patients: initial results of Chinese PUF-01 randomized clinical trial. Ann Surg 2021;274(6):e473–80.

43. Rullier E, Denost Q, Vendrely V, et al. Low rectal cancer: classification and standardization of surgery. Dis Colon Rectum 2013;56(5):560–7.

44. Tao Y, Han JG, Wang ZJ. Extralevator abdominoperineal excision for advanced low rectal cancer: where to go. World J Gastroenterol 2020;26(22):3012–23.

45. Jafari MD, Pigazzi A, McLemore EC, et al. Perfusion assessment in left-sided/low anterior resection (PILLAR III): a randomized, controlled, parallel, multicenter study assessing perfusion outcomes with PINPOINT near-infrared fluorescence imaging in low anterior resection. Dis Colon Rectum 2021;64(8):995–1002.

46. Neutzling CB, Lustosa SA, Proenca IM, et al. Stapled versus handsewn methods for colorectal anastomosis surgery. Cochrane Database Syst Rev 2012;(2):Cd003144.

47. Parks AG. Transanal technique in low rectal anastomosis. Proc R Soc Med 1972; 65(11):975–6.

48. Gordon PH. Chapter 23: Malignant neoplasms of the rectum. In: Gordon PH, Nivatvongs S, editors. Principles and Practice of Surgery for the Colon, Rectum, and Anus. 3rd. Boca Raton: CRC Press; 2007. p. 489–643.

49. Brown CJ, Fenech DS, McLeod RS. Reconstructive techniques after rectal resection for rectal cancer. Cochrane Database Syst Rev 2008;(2):Cd006040.

50. Heriot AG, Tekkis PP, Constantinides V, et al. Meta-analysis of colonic reservoirs versus straight coloanal anastomosis after anterior resection. Br J Surg 2006; 93(1):19–32.

51. Ho YH, Brown S, Heah SM, et al. Comparison of J-pouch and coloplasty pouch for low rectal cancers: a randomized, controlled trial investigating functional results and comparative anastomotic leak rates. Ann Surg 2002; 236(1):49–55.

52. Hou S, Wang Q, Zhao S, et al. Safety and efficacy of side-to-end anastomosis versus colonic J-pouch anastomosis in sphincter-preserving resections: an updated meta-analysis of randomized controlled trials. World J Surg Oncol 2021; 19(1):130.

53. Ricciardi R, Roberts PL, Marcello PW, et al. Anastomotic leak testing after colorectal resection: what are the data? Arch Surg 2009;144(5):407–11 [discussion 402–11].

54. Ahmad NZ, Abbas MH, Khan SU, et al. A meta-analysis of the role of diverting ileostomy after rectal cancer surgery. Int J Colorectal Dis 2021;36(3):445–55.

55. McDermott FD, Heeney A, Kelly ME, et al. Systematic review of preoperative, intraoperative and postoperative risk factors for colorectal anastomotic leaks. Br J Surg 2015;102(5):462–79.

56. Ambe PC, Zarras K, Stodolski M, et al. Routine preoperative mechanical bowel preparation with additive oral antibiotics is associated with a reduced risk of anastomotic leakage in patients undergoing elective oncologic resection for colorectal cancer. World J Surg Oncol 2019;17(1):20.

57. Menahem B, Lubrano J, Vallois A, et al. Early Closure of defunctioning loop ileostomy: is it beneficial for the patient? A meta-analysis. World J Surg 2018;42(10): 3171–8.

58. Habib K, Gupta A, White D, et al. Utility of contrast enema to assess anastomotic integrity and the natural history of radiological leaks after low rectal surgery: systematic review and meta-analysis. Int J Colorectal Dis 2015;30(8): 1007–14.

Targeted Therapy for Colorectal Cancer

Shinichiro Sakata, MBBS, PhD, FRACS, David W. Larson, MD, MBA*

KEYWORDS

- Metastatic colorectal cancer • Targeted therapy • Bevacizumab • EGFR

KEY POINTS

- Genomic profiling is used to detect specific genetic mutations that may offer selected patients a modest survival benefit with targeted therapy.
- Patients with mCRC with KRAS/NRAS/BRAF wild-type left-sided tumors may benefit from EGFR inhibition with either cetuximab or panitumumab in conjunction with chemotherapy.
- The VEGF inhibitor bevacizumab can be considered an alternative to EGFR inhibitors in right-sided tumors or second-line therapy.
- Many patients will have RAS mutations, and targeted therapies will not provide any benefit.
- Immunotherapy is recommended as first-line treatment of patients with MSI high and MMR deficient tumors, either due to Lynch syndrome or sporadic mutations.

INTRODUCTION

Over the last decade, there have been improvements in colorectal cancer (CRC) incidence and survival.[1-5] These outcomes are attributed to multidisciplinary advances, including the widespread adoption of colonoscopy in nationwide screening and surveillance programs,[6-10] accurate preoperative imaging and staging,[11-13] neoadjuvant chemoradiotherapy[14-16] and the adoption of total mesorectal excision (TME) as the standard of care for rectal cancer surgery.[17,18] Thus, in this current era of advanced cancer care, survival after early CRC is typically expected.

On the other hand, the projected 5-year survival rate for patients with metastatic colorectal cancer (mCRC) is only 14%.[5] In 2020, CRC was responsible for 930,000 deaths worldwide, making it the second leading cause of cancer-related death.[1-4] Metastatic disease is the overwhelming contributor to the death rate from CRC. More than 20% of patients with CRC in the United States will have metastatic disease

All authors provided intellectual contribution and have adhered to ICMJE guidelines on authorship.
Department of Surgery, Division of Colon and Rectal Surgery, Mayo Clinic, 200 first st sw, Rochester, MN 55905, USA
* Corresponding author.
E-mail address: larson.david2@mayo.edu

surgonc.theclinics.com

at the time of the first diagnosis, with a disproportionately high incidence of adults younger than 50 years.[19,20] Although complete surgical resection of the primary tumor and all sites of metastasis is the cornerstone for prolonged survival,[21–24] 80% of patients with mCRC will have unresectable disease.[25,26]

Palliative cytotoxic chemotherapy has been the mainstay for the treatment of mCRC. However, even the most effective regimens typically offer patients an overall survival of 12 to 24 months.[27–29] Significant investment into the understanding of CRC biology has paved the way to a modern era of targeted therapy, providing patients with a range of therapeutic antibodies that offer an improved overall survival compared with cytotoxic chemotherapy alone. Targeted therapy refers to small molecules, such as monoclonal antibodies, that can augment molecular pathways critical to cancer-specific growth and maintenance. Common examples of targeted therapy include antibodies against VEGF, the EGFR, B-type RAF (BRAF) V600E, and the human EGFR 2 (HER2). Targeted therapy is now almost exclusively used in patients with metastatic disease.

This review aims to provide colorectal surgeons' practical information on targeted therapies that are used for mCRC. In addition, this review discusses the indications and benefits of targeted therapy and provides an overview of critical molecular pathways.

BIOMARKERS FOR TARGETED THERAPY

Metastatic CRC is a heterogeneous disease with subtypes characterized by genetic mutations. Targeted therapies are not appropriate for all patients with mCRC, and their benefit relies on a proper pairing of medications with specific genetic mutations. Biomarkers are critical for tailoring individualized treatment by illuminating the mutations within individual tumors involved in oncogenesis.

The main molecular subtypes of mCRC are

1. KRAS/NRAS and BRAF wild type (wild type means that the tumor does not have a specific mutation)
2. KRAS/NRAS mutated
3. BRAF mutated
4. HER2 mutated
5. MSI high and MMR deficient

Based on the targeted therapies currently approved and available, the National Comprehensive Cancer Network (NCCN) recommends that all patients with mCRC have tumor tissue genotyped for rat sarcoma (RAS; specifically KRAS and NRAS) and BRAF mutations.[30] In addition, tumors should also be tested for HER2 amplification and MSI high/MMR deficient status.[30] Testing may be performed for individual genes or as part of a next-generation sequencing panel and no specific methodology is currently recommended.[30] In practice, if the tumor is already known to have either a KRAS/NRAS or BRAF mutation, HER2 testing is unnecessary.

PATHWAYS FOR COLORECTAL CANCER

CRC evolves from 3 main pathways: (1) chromosomal instability (CIN); (2) MSI; and (3) epigenetic instability via hypermethylation of the CPG island mutator phenotype (CIMP) promotor.[31,32] Aberrations within these molecular pathways are not mutually exclusive and occur in both sporadic and inherited CRCs. For example, CIN is present in 85%, CIMP in 20%, and MSI in 15% of tumors.[31,32]

Associated with CIN, the epidermal growth factor family is composed of 4 related receptors of tyrosine kinase within the cell membrane: the EGFR (EGFR; HER1),

HER2 (ErbB2), HER3 (ErbB3), and HER4 (ErbB4).[33,34] EGFR is a glycoprotein receptor that remains in a state of inhibition and regulates proliferation via signal transduction to the nucleus.[33,34] The pathway most connected with the pathogenesis, progression, and oncogenic behavior of CRC is the mitogen-activated protein kinase (MAPK) pathway activated by EGFR. The MAPK pathway is also known as the MAPK/extracellular signal-regulated kinase (ERK) pathway, as well as the rat sarcoma (RAS)- rapidly accelerated fibrosarcoma proto-oncogene serine/threonine-protein kinase (RAF)-MEK- ERK pathway. BRAF mutations are B-type RAF (BRAF) mutations and are considered part of the MAPK pathway.

The MAPK pathway involves the steps RAS-RAF-MEK-ERK, which are all downstream from the EGFR. The RAS-encoded proteins are a family of GTPase-related proteins involved in cell signal transduction. RAS mutations (including KRAS and NRAS mutations) result in abnormally high activity through MAPK pathways, and signal transduction is no longer reliant on receptor stimulation. Therefore, targeted therapy with EGFR receptor blockers does not benefit patients with RAS mutations.

Unlike breast and gastric cancer rates, HER2 mutations in CRC are relatively rare (4%–5%).[35,36] Contrary to other receptors in the epidermal growth factor family, HER2 does not directly bind to any known ligands to initiate signal transduction. Instead, heterodimerization activation of the HER2-mediated MAPK pathway occurs with ligand-activated EGFR (HER1) or Erb3 (HER3). HER2 mutations are receptor mutations and are upstream to RAS. Therefore, if a tumor is already known to have a RAS mutation, HER2 testing is generally not performed.

BRAF mutations activate BRAF kinase resulting in sustained signaling in the MAPK pathway. This mutation, in turn, leads to uncontrolled cell proliferation, migration, angiogenesis, escape from apoptosis and angiogenesis. Thus, the BRAF V600E gene mutation is an important biomarker in mCRC. BRAF V600E mutations are classically missense mutations occurring in codon 600, leading to an aminoacidic substitution of a valine for glutamic acid. They are more common in women, older patients, those with right-side, poorly differentiated tumors, and sessile serrated polyps. Biologically, these cancers are characterized by hypermethylation and a CIMP, and about 50% are MSI high.[37]

All mCRC should be screened for Lynch syndrome or sporadic mutations (MSI high and MMR deficient). MSI high mCRCs with BRAF V600E mutations are always sporadic, which rules out Lynch Syndrome. MSI occurs when tumors accumulate insertions or deletions at sites of repetitive DNA units called microsatellites. Typically, errors in base-pair matching during DNA replication are corrected, but a deficiency in MMR results in an accumulation of insertions or deletions that may result in malignancy. The MSI high and MMR deficient subtype of mCRC is essential to identify because tumors are susceptible to immune checkpoint inhibitor immunotherapy (discussed in more detail later in discussion).

TARGETED THERAPY FOR METASTATIC COLORECTAL CANCER: KEY CONCEPTS

Systemic chemotherapy is the principle treatment of metastatic CRC.[38] However, chemotherapy agents are cytotoxic to all rapidly dividing cells and do not distinguish between normal and malignant cells. These agents are further limited by unpredictable resistance and a narrow therapeutic index. Systemic toxicity is a common adverse effect of chemotherapy and includes peripheral neuropathy, myelosuppression, diarrhea, and mucosal inflammation. Established chemotherapy treatments for mCRC include the fluoropyrimidine 5-fluorouracil (5-FU) as a single agent and multichemotherapy regimens such as FOLFOX (leucovorin, 5-FU, and oxaliplatin), FOLFIRI (leucovorin, 5-FU, and irinotecan), and CAPOX/XELOX (capecitabine and oxaliplatin).

There is no cure for mCRC with unresectable disease. As discussed previously, there is strong evidence that complementing chemotherapy with systemic targeted therapy may help some patients survive longer, but targeted therapies will give no added benefit to others.

Based on the results of specific biomarkers, the principle treatment strategies for the 4 distinct molecular subtypes of mCRC are:

1. KRAS/NRAS and BRAF wild type (ie, nonmutant KRAS/NRAS/BRAF)

   Incidence: Between 30% and 50% of patients.

   Key concepts: In combination with chemotherapy, EGFR inhibitors, such as cetuximab and panitumumab, have been shown to extend median survival compared with chemotherapy alone. Furthermore, 2 meta-analyses have demonstrated that left-sided colon and rectal cancers are strongly associated with response to EGFR inhibition.[39,40] Therefore, current NCCN practice guidelines recommend that EGFR inhibitors be paired with chemotherapy as first-line treatment in KRAS/NRAS/BRAF wild-type tumors (ie, no mutations affecting KRAS/NRAS/BRAF), particularly in left-sided mCRC.[30] As an alternative to EGFR inhibitors, the VEGF inhibitor bevacizumab may be administered alongside systemic chemotherapy as a first-line treatment of mCRC. However, a recent meta-analysis has demonstrated that VEGF inhibitors may be inferior to EGFR inhibitors.[41] Therefore, bevacizumab may also be offered as a second-line treatment in cases that progress despite EGFR inhibition.

   Seminal trials:

   a. CRYSTAL trial[42]: This phase III trial randomized patients to either FOLFIRI plus cetuximab or FOLFIRI as first-line therapy. In patients without RAS (including KRAS), the addition of cetuximab improved median overall survival by 8 months ($P<.001$).

   b. PRIME trial[43]: This phase III trial randomized patients to either FOLFOX plus panitumumab or FOLFOX as first-line therapy. In patients without RAS (including KRAS), the addition of panitumumab improved median overall survival by 5.8 months ($P = .009$).

   c. FIRE-3 trial[44]: This phase III trial was the first head-to-head comparison of EGFR against VEGF inhibition, and randomized patients to either bevacizumab or cetuximab, in combined regimens with FOLFIRI. The proportion of patients who achieved an objective response did not significantly differ between groups. However, the FOLFIRI plus cetuximab group had a longer overall survival (28.7 vs 25 months, $P = .017$), suggesting that EGFR inhibition should be the preferred first-line regimen.

2. KRAS/NRAS mutated

   Incidence: Between 35% and 40% of patients.

   Key concepts: Targeted therapies are mainly ineffective and should not be offered to this group of patients, either alone or with other anticancer agents.[30]

   Seminal trials:

   a. CRYSTAL trial[42]: This phase III trial randomized patients to either FOLFIRI plus cetuximab or FOLFIRI as first-line therapy. In patients with RAS mutations, the addition of cetuximab provided no significant benefit.

   b. PRIME trial[43]: This phase III trial randomized patients to either FOLFOX plus panitumumab or FOLFOX as first-line therapy. In patients with RAS (including KRAS), the addition of panitumumab was associated with a *reduced* median overall survival by 3.2 months ($P = .04$).

3. BRAF mutated and RAS wild type

Incidence: Between 5% and 15% of patients. Approximately 90% of patients have a V600E mutation.

Key concepts: First-line therapy usually consists of either oxaliplatin-based chemotherapy (FOLFOX or CAPOX) or irinotecan-based chemotherapy (FOLFIRI or CAPIRI). As discussed previously, BRAF (B-type RAF) occurs downstream of RAS in the MAPK pathway involving the EGFR. In BRAF mutations, the mutated BRAF protein product is believed to be constitutively active and independent of EGFR inhibition by cetuximab or panitumumab. BRAF V600E mutations are, therefore, associated with inadequate response to the EGFR inhibitors cetuximab and panitumumab *unless* paired with a BRAF inhibitor. The combination of an EGFR inhibitor with a BRAF inhibitor (encorafenib) has been shown to extend overall survival.[45,46]

Seminal trial:

a. BEACON trial[47]: This phase III trial randomized patients with BRAF V600E mutations to either cetuximab plus encorafenib plus binimetinib or cetuximab plus encorafenib or cetuximab plus FOLFIRI/irinotecan in patients with disease progression on 1 or 2 prior regimens. Binimetinib inhibits the enzyme MEK kinase within tumor cells. The median overall survival was 9.0 months in the triplet-therapy group and 5.4 months in the control group (*P*<.001).

4. HER2 mutated and RAS/BRAF wildtype

Incidence: Between 3% and 4% of patients.

Key concept: First-line therapy consists of either an oxaliplatin-based regimen (FOLFOX or CAPOX) or irinotecan-based regimens (FOLFIRI or CAPIRI). NCCN recommends 3 different regimens as second-line options: trastuzumab monotherapy or trastuzumab combined with either pertuzumab or lapatinib.

Seminal trails:

a. MyPathway trial[48]: This ongoing phase II trial evaluates the activity of dual anti-HER2 agent therapy pertuzumab and trastuzumab in patients with HER2-amplified mCRC. At the interim analysis, among 57 evaluable patients, one patient had a complete response, and 17 (30%) had partial responses. The estimated progression-free survival was 2.9 months, and the estimated overall survival was 11.5 months.

b. HERACLES trial[49]: This phase II trial evaluated the activity of dual anti-HER2 agent therapy trastuzumab and lapatinib (a tyrosine kinase inhibitor that targets both EGFR and HER2) in patients with HER2-amplified mCRC. Among 27 evaluable patients, one patient had a complete response, and 7 (26%) had partial responses. The progression-free survival was 5.3 months and the overall survival was 11.5 months.

5. MSI high and MMR deficient

Incidence: 5% of patients have MSI and MMR deficiency due to Lynch syndrome or sporadic mutations.

K concept: Immunotherapy is the principle treatment. Chemotherapy and targeted therapies may have synergistic effects, and combination therapy has an extended median overall. On the other hand, CRC that is *not* MSI high and MMR deficient will *not* respond to immune checkpoint inhibitor immunotherapy.

Seminal trials:

a. KEYNOTE-177 trial.[50] This phase III trial randomized patients with untreated MSI-H/MMR-D metastatic CRC to the immune checkpoint inhibitor pembrolizumab or investigators' choice of FOLFOX or FOLFIRI with or without bevacizumab or cetuximab. The median progression-free survival was 16.5 months with pembrolizumab and 8.2 months without (P = .002). However, overall survival was challenging to interpret because patients who progressed in the chemotherapy group crossed over to the pembrolizumab group.[50]

TARGETED THERAPY IN PATIENTS WITH RESECTABLE COLORECTAL CANCER

The NCCN recommends targeted therapy for patients with unresectable metastatic disease. However, beyond this indication, the use of targeted therapy is controversial.

Following the successes of bevacizumab when added to chemotherapy in the palliative setting, clinical trials were launched to investigate its use in other settings. The National Surgical Adjuvant Breast and Bowel Project C-08 phase III randomized controlled trial evaluated 2672 patients.[51] It showed that bevacizumab for 1 year with FOLFOX did not significantly prolong disease-free or overall survival in stage II and III colon cancer. Likewise, the AVANT phase III randomized controlled trial evaluated 3451 patients.[52] It showed no benefit of the addition of bevacizumab to FOLFOX adjuvant therapy in patients with stage III colon cancer in terms of disease-free survival.[52] Updated results of this study demonstrated a significant adverse effect in 10-year overall survival with the addition of bevacizumab.[53] As such, bevacizumab was not recommended in the adjuvant setting.

The HEPATICA trial was a phase III randomized controlled trial that attempted to examine the efficacy of adding bevacizumab to CAPOX in patients with resectable colorectal liver metastasis.[54] This study closed prematurely from poor accrual, and the effect of VEGF inhibition on disease-free survival could not be determined. The study did suggest that quality of life was higher in patients receiving CAPEOX plus bevacizumab than those receiving CAPEOX alone after the resection of liver metastases.[54] The lack of positive data regarding adjuvant bevacizumab in stage II and III colon cancer has prompted the NCCN to not recommend bevacizumab in stage IV resectable colorectal metastases.[30] The New EPOC phase III randomized controlled trial evaluated patients with KRAS wild-type resectable colorectal liver metastases. This study randomized patients to chemotherapy alone or chemotherapy with cetuximab and demonstrated that the addition of cetuximab was associated with a significantly *worse* overall survival (81 vs 55.4) in the latest update.[55] The use of cetuximab in the perioperative setting in patients with operable disease confers a significant disadvantage and should not be used in this setting.

SUMMARY

MCRC is incurable for patients with unresectable diseases. For most patients, the primary treatment is palliative systemic chemotherapy. Genomic profiling is used to detect specific genetic mutations that may offer selected patients a modest survival benefit with targeted therapy. Patients with mCRC with KRAS/NRAS/BRAF wild-type left-sided tumors may benefit from EGFR inhibition with either cetuximab or panitumumab in conjunction with chemotherapy. EGFR inhibitors can extend survival by 6 months compared with chemotherapy alone. The VEGF inhibitor bevacizumab can be considered an alternative to EGFR inhibitors in right-sided tumors or second-line therapy. Many patients will have RAS mutations, and targeted therapies will not provide any benefit. The PRIME trial demonstrated that the addition of panitumumab to FOLFOX was associated with reduced overall survival. Patients with BRAF mutations do not benefit from targeted therapy unless a BRAF inhibitor supplements treatment. Triple combination therapy with cetuximab, the BRAF inhibitor encorafenib, and the MEK kinase inhibitor binimetinib have been shown to extend overall survival by about 3 months compared with chemotherapy alone. Finally, immunotherapy is recommended as first-line treatment of patients with MSI high and MMR deficient tumors, either due to Lynch syndrome or sporadic mutations. The KEYNOTE-177 trial demonstrated that therapy with single-agent pembrolizumab improved progression-free survival by 8 months compared with FOLFOX or FOLFIRI and with or without EGFR inhibition. At this time, targeted therapy should only be used in patients with unresectable metastatic disease.

DISCLOSURE

The authors have nothing to disclose.

REFERENCES

1. Sung H, Ferlay J, Siegel RL, et al. Global cancer statistics 2020: GLOBOCAN estimates of incidence and mortality worldwide for 36 cancers in 185 countries. CA Cancer J Clin. 2021 May;71(3):209–49.

2. The global, regional, and national burden of colorectal cancer and its attributable risk factors in 195 countries and territories, 1990-2017: a systematic analysis for the Global Burden of Disease Study 2017. Lancet Gastroenterol Hepatol 2019; 4(12):913–33.

3. Bray F, Ferlay J, Soerjomataram I, et al. Global cancer statistics 2018: GLOBOCAN estimates of incidence and mortality worldwide for 36 cancers in 185 countries. CA Cancer J Clin 2018;68(6):394–424.

4. Dekker E, Tanis PJ, Vleugels JLA, et al. Colorectal cancer. Lancet 2019; 394(10207):1467–80.

5. Siegel RL, Miller KD, Jemal A. Cancer statistics, 2020. CA Cancer J Clin 2020; 70(1):7–30.

6. Hewett DG, Rex DK. The big picture: does colonoscopy work? Gastrointest Endosc Clin North Am 2015;25(2):403–13.

7. Gupta S, Lieberman D, Anderson JC, et al. Spotlight: US multi-society task force on colorectal cancer recommendations for follow-up after colonoscopy and polypectomy. Gastroenterology 2020;158(4):1154.

8. Rex DK, Boland CR, Dominitz JA, et al. Colorectal cancer screening: recommendations for physicians and patients from the U.S. multi-society task force on colorectal cancer. Gastroenterology 2017;153(1):307–23.

9. Kahi CJ, Boland CR, Dominitz JA, et al. Colonoscopy surveillance after colorectal cancer resection: recommendations of the US multi-society task force on colorectal cancer. Gastroenterology 2016;150(3):758–68.e11.

10. Kahi CJ. Reviewing the evidence that polypectomy prevents cancer. Gastrointest Endosc Clin N Am 2019;29(4):577–85.

11. Salerno G, Daniels I, Heald RJ, et al. Management and imaging of low rectal carcinoma. Surg Oncol 2004;13(2–3):55–61.

12. Bhoday J, Balyasnikova S, Wale A, et al. How should imaging direct/orient management of rectal cancer? Clin Colon Rectal Surg 2017;30(5):297–312.

13. Diagnostic accuracy of preoperative magnetic resonance imaging in predicting curative resection of rectal cancer: prospective observational study. BMJ 2006; 333(7572):779.

14. Sauer R, Becker H, Hohenberger W, et al. Preoperative versus postoperative chemoradiotherapy for rectal cancer. N Engl J Med 2004;351(17):1731–40.

15. Bosset JF, Collette L, Calais G, et al. Chemotherapy with preoperative radiotherapy in rectal cancer. N Engl J Med 2006;355(11):1114–23.

16. Kong JC, Soucisse M, Michael M, et al. Total neoadjuvant therapy in locally advanced rectal cancer: a systematic review and metaanalysis of oncological and operative outcomes. Ann Surg Oncol. 2021 Nov;28(12):7476–86.
17. de Lacy FB, Chadi SA, Berho M, et al. The future of rectal cancer surgery: a narrative review of an international symposium. Surg Innov 2018;25(5):525–35.
18. Heald RJ, Husband EM, Ryall RD. The mesorectum in rectal cancer surgery–the clue to pelvic recurrence? Br J Surg 1982;69(10):613–6.
19. Siegel RL, Miller KD, Fuchs HE, et al. Cancer statistics, 2021. CA Cancer J Clin 2021;71(1):7–33.
20. You YN, Dozois EJ, Boardman LA, et al. Young-onset rectal cancer: presentation, pattern of care and long-term oncologic outcomes compared to a matched older-onset cohort. Ann Surg Oncol 2011;18(9):2469–76.
21. Kopetz S, Chang GJ, Overman MJ, et al. Improved survival in metastatic colorectal cancer is associated with adoption of hepatic resection and improved chemotherapy. J Clin Oncol 2009;27(22):3677–83.
22. Johnson B, Jin Z, Haddock MG, et al. A curative-intent trimodality approach for isolated abdominal nodal metastases in metastatic colorectal cancer: update of a single-institutional experience. Oncologist 2018;23(6):679–85.
23. Ali SM, Pawlik TM, Rodriguez-Bigas MA, et al. Timing of surgical resection for curative colorectal cancer with liver metastasis. Ann Surg Oncol 2018;25(1):32–7.
24. Jin Z, Sanhueza CT, Johnson B, et al. Outcome of mismatch repair-deficient metastatic colorectal cancer: the mayo clinic experience. Oncologist 2018;23(9):1083–91.
25. Grothey A, Fakih M, Tabernero J. Management of BRAF-mutant metastatic colorectal cancer: a review of treatment options and evidence-based guidelines. Ann Oncol. 2021 Aug;32(8):959–67.
26. Muratore A, Zorzi D, Bouzari H, et al. Asymptomatic colorectal cancer with unresectable liver metastases: immediate colorectal resection or up-front systemic chemotherapy? Ann Surg Oncol 2007;14(2):766–70.
27. Efficacy of intravenous continuous infusion of fluorouracil compared with bolus administration in advanced colorectal cancer. meta-analysis group in cancer. J Clin Oncol 1998;16(1):301–8.
28. Colucci G, Gebbia V, Paoletti G, et al. Phase III randomized trial of FOLFIRI versus FOLFOX4 in the treatment of advanced colorectal cancer: a multicenter study of the Gruppo Oncologico Dell'Italia Meridionale. J Clin Oncol 2005;23(22):4866–75.
29. Cassidy J, Tabernero J, Twelves C, et al. XELOX (capecitabine plus oxaliplatin): active first-line therapy for patients with metastatic colorectal cancer. J Clin Oncol 2004;22(11):2084–91.
30. Benson AB, Venook AP, Al-Hawary MM, et al. Colon cancer, version 2.2021, NCCN clinical practice guidelines in oncology. J Natl Compr Canc Netw 2021;19(3):329–59.
31. Requena DO, Garcia-Buitrago M. Molecular insights into colorectal carcinoma. Arch Med Res 2020;51(8):839–44.
32. Wright M, Beaty JS, Ternent CA. Molecular markers for colorectal cancer. Surg Clin North Am 2017;97(3):683–701.
33. Lai E, Liscia N, Donisi C, et al. Molecular-biology-driven treatment for metastatic colorectal cancer. Cancers 2020;12(5):1214.
34. Scaltriti M, Baselga J. The epidermal growth factor receptor pathway: a model for targeted therapy. Clin Cancer Res 2006;12(18):5268–72.

35. Laurent-Puig P, Balogoun R, Cayre A, et al. 459O - ERBB2 alterations a new prognostic biomarker in stage III colon cancer from a FOLFOX based adjuvant trial (PETACC8). Ann Oncol 2016;27:vi151.
36. Kavuri SM, Jain N, Galimi F, et al. HER2 activating mutations are targets for colorectal cancer treatment. Cancer Discov 2015;5(8):832–41.
37. Saridaki Z, Papadatos-Pastos D, Tzardi M, et al. BRAF mutations, microsatellite instability status and cyclin D1 expression predict metastatic colorectal patients' outcome. Br J Cancer 2010;102(12):1762–8.
38. Biller LH, Schrag D. Diagnosis and treatment of metastatic colorectal cancer: a review. JAMA 2021;325(7):669–85.
39. Holch JW, Ricard I, Stintzing S, et al. The relevance of primary tumour location in patients with metastatic colorectal cancer: a meta-analysis of first-line clinical trials. Eur J Cancer 2017;70:87–98.
40. Wang ZX, Wu HX, He MM, et al. Chemotherapy with or without anti-EGFR agents in left- and right-sided metastatic colorectal cancer: an updated meta-analysis. J Natl Compr Canc Netw 2019;17(7):805–11.
41. Khattak MA, Martin H, Davidson A, et al. Role of first-line anti-epidermal growth factor receptor therapy compared with anti-vascular endothelial growth factor therapy in advanced colorectal cancer: a meta-analysis of randomized clinical trials. Clin Colorectal Cancer 2015;14(2):81–90.
42. Van Cutsem E, Lenz HJ, Köhne CH, et al. Fluorouracil, leucovorin, and irinotecan plus cetuximab treatment and RAS mutations in colorectal cancer. J Clin Oncol 2015;33(7):692–700.
43. Douillard JY, Siena S, Cassidy J, et al. Randomized, phase III trial of panitumumab with infusional fluorouracil, leucovorin, and oxaliplatin (FOLFOX4) versus FOLFOX4 alone as first-line treatment in patients with previously untreated metastatic colorectal cancer: the PRIME study. J Clin Oncol 2010;28(31):4697–705.
44. Heinemann V, von Weikersthal LF, Decker T, et al. FOLFIRI plus cetuximab versus FOLFIRI plus bevacizumab as first-line treatment for patients with metastatic colorectal cancer (FIRE-3): a randomised, open-label, phase 3 trial. Lancet Oncol 2014;15(10):1065–75.
45. Al-Salama ZT. Encorafenib: a review in metastatic colorectal cancer with a BRAF V600E mutation. Drugs 2021;81(7):849–56.
46. Mauri G, Bonazzina E, Amatu A, et al. The evolutionary landscape of treatment for BRAF(V600E) mutant metastatic colorectal cancer. Cancers 2021;13(1):137.
47. Kopetz S, Grothey A, Yaeger R, et al. Encorafenib, binimetinib, and cetuximab in BRAF V600E-mutated colorectal cancer. N Engl J Med 2019;381(17):1632–43.
48. Meric-Bernstam F, Hurwitz H, Raghav KPS, et al. Pertuzumab plus trastuzumab for HER2-amplified metastatic colorectal cancer (MyPathway): an updated report from a multicentre, open-label, phase 2a, multiple basket study. Lancet Oncol 2019;20(4):518–30.
49. Sartore-Bianchi A, Trusolino L, Martino C, et al. Dual-targeted therapy with trastuzumab and lapatinib in treatment-refractory, KRAS codon 12/13 wild-type, HER2-positive metastatic colorectal cancer (HERACLES): a proof-of-concept, multicentre, open-label, phase 2 trial. Lancet Oncol 2016;17(6):738–46.
50. André T, Shiu KK, Kim TW, et al. Pembrolizumab in microsatellite-instability-high advanced colorectal cancer. N Engl J Med 2020;383(23):2207–18.
51. Allegra CJ, Yothers G, O'Connell MJ, et al. Phase III trial assessing bevacizumab in stages II and III carcinoma of the colon: results of NSABP protocol C-08. J Clin Oncol 2011;29(1):11–6.

52. de Gramont A, Van Cutsem E, Schmoll HJ, et al. Bevacizumab plus oxaliplatin-based chemotherapy as adjuvant treatment for colon cancer (AVANT): a phase 3 randomised controlled trial. Lancet Oncol 2012;13(12):1225–33.

53. André T, Vernerey D, Im SA, et al. Bevacizumab as adjuvant treatment of colon cancer: updated results from the S-AVANT phase III study by the GERCOR group. Ann Oncol 2020;31(2):246–56.

54. Snoeren N, van Hillegersberg R, Schouten SB, et al. Randomized Phase III study to assess efficacy and safety of adjuvant CAPOX with or without bevacizumab in patients after resection of colorectal liver metastases: HEPATICA study. Neoplasia 2017;19(2):93–9.

55. Bridgewater JA, Pugh SA, Maishman T, et al. Systemic chemotherapy with or without cetuximab in patients with resectable colorectal liver metastasis (New EPOC): long-term results of a multicentre, randomised, controlled, phase 3 trial. Lancet Oncol 2020;21(3):398–411.

Management of Synchronous Colorectal Cancer Metastases

Traci L. Hedrick, MD, MSc, FACRS*, Victor M. Zaydfudim, MD, MPH

KEYWORDS

- Colon cancer • Rectal cancer • Colorectal cancer • Metastases • Synchronous

KEY POINTS

- Recognizing the potential for long-term survival, management of patients presenting with synchronous colorectal metastases has evolved significantly over time reflecting a shift toward more aggressive therapy.
- The liver is the most common site of metastatic disease, accounting for 75% of CRC metastases.
- The functional status and primary goals of the patient, site, and volume of metastatic disease, as well as the degree of symptoms from the primary tumor determine treatment options in patients with synchronous CRC metastases.
- The patient with synchronous metastatic CRC requires a comprehensive multidisciplinary approach to develop an individualized treatment scheme integrating quality of life and patient needs.

INTRODUCTION

Up to 22% of patients with colorectal cancer (CRC) have evidence of metastatic disease at initial presentation (**Box 1**).[1,2] Most of the CRC-related deaths are attributable to metastatic disease with overall 5-year survival rates between 10% and 14% for patients with Stage IV CRC.[2–5] However, 5-year survival ranges between 24% and 58% (averaging 40%) in patients with resectable hepatic metastases, or patients converted to resectable status with systemic therapy, depending on the site and extent of disease. The liver accounts for 75% of patients with CRC metastases, followed by the lung in 22% with brain, bone, ovary, peritoneum, and adrenals making up the remaining less common sites of metastatic disease.[5] Prognosis is dictated by tumor biology (as currently measured by mutational/genetic profile), tumor volume, and site of

Division of General Surgery, Department of Surgery, University of Virginia Health, PO Box 800709, Charlottesville, VA 22901, USA
* Corresponding author.
E-mail address: Th8q@virginia.edu

Surg Oncol Clin N Am 31 (2022) 265–278
https://doi.org/10.1016/j.soc.2021.11.007
1055-3207/22/© 2021 Elsevier Inc. All rights reserved.

surgonc.theclinics.com

Box 1
NCCN guidelines for resectable synchronous liver and/or lung metastases

NCCN Guidelines for resectable synchronous liver and/or lung metastases only:

- Synchronous or staged colectomy with resection of metastatic disease followed by 6 months adjuvant chemotherapy.
- Neoadjuvant chemotherapy [2–3 months] followed by synchronous or staged colectomy and resection of metastatic disease followed by remaining 3 to 4 months of adjuvant therapy.
- Colectomy followed by chemotherapy (2–3 months) and staged resection of metastatic disease followed by 3 to 4 months remaining adjuvant chemotherapy.

---

metastases with single organ and metachronous metastases portending a better prognosis. .

The management of metastatic CRC depends on multiple factors, necessitating an individualized approach that takes into account oncologic principles, patient needs, and quality of life. Various treatment strategies are endorsed by the National Comprehensive Cancer Network (NCCN), American Society of Colon and Rectal Surgeons (ASCRS), and hepatobiliary and surgical oncology (AHPBA/SSO/SSAT) consensus guidelines.[6–10] Treatment of the patient with metastatic CRC hinges on a comprehensive multidisciplinary team using shared-decision making strategies to contemplate the different options and align medical decisions with patient care preferences.[6,11–13]

The patient with synchronous metastatic CRC presents a unique set of challenges. Treatment modalities are influenced by the degree of symptoms from the primary tumor, site, and volume of metastatic disease, as well as the functional status and primary goals of the patient. The algorithm presented in **Fig. 1** offers a framework for clinical decision making.

MANAGEMENT OF PRIMARY TUMOR

The degree of primary tumor-related symptoms often dictates the initial steps in the clinical management of the patient with synchronous metastatic disease.

Obstruction

Up to 30% of patients with CRC exhibit some type of obstructive symptoms related to the primary.[14] The inability to pass the endoscope past the primary lesion is an obvious indicator of pending obstruction. However, some patients (particularly those with proximal tumors) remain asymptomatic in the setting of a near-complete obstruction and do not require immediate intervention. Alternatively, patients may exhibit signs of obstruction despite the passage of the colonoscope. It can be difficult to accurately predict those at risk for obstruction during chemotherapy. This requires close attention to the patient's complaints combined with an objective evaluation of the endoscopic and radiographic images. In general, a stool column proximal to the primary lesion on cross-sectional imaging may indicate impending obstruction, even in the absence of colonic dilation.

Intervention is dictated by the degree of obstruction, stability of the patient, as well as the size and location of the primary tumor. Options include endoscopic stenting, diversion, and/or resection. In the stable patient without signs/symptoms of proximal perforation, ASCRS guidelines prioritize endoscopic stenting over surgery in the setting of incurable metastatic disease. Compared with surgery, stenting is associated with reduced short-term morbidity and time to chemotherapy initiation.[6,15–18]

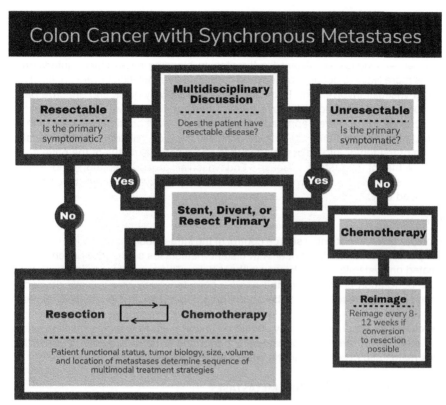

Fig. 1. Treatment algorithm to guide clinical decision making in patients with synchronous CRC metastases.

This depends on local capabilities and experience with colonic stenting, which anecdotally varies between institutions. The patient's overall life expectancy must also be considered given that the median duration of colonic stent patency is 106 (68–288) days.[19,20]

Resection may be appropriate for the easily resectable tumor in a patient with life expectancy greater than 6 months. In this setting, oncologic principles of resection should be applied when possible.[6] Diversion should be considered (either primary anastomosis with proximal diversion or Hartman) as the implications of an anastomotic leak are significant, particularly with regard to the initiation of chemotherapy.[6,21]

Proximal diversion is a viable option, specifically for locally invasive colonic or rectal cancers that are not easily amendable to resection. In patients with potentially resectable disease, one should consider the ultimate definitive resection so as not to sabotage future reconstructive options with a misplaced stoma. A distal transverse or mid/proximal descending loop colostomy in patients with rectal cancer may restrict future colonic mobility or damage the marginal artery, which could devascularize the distal colon following high ligation of the inferior mesenteric artery. As such, it is preferable to use the mid/distal sigmoid colon or the transverse colon proximal to the middle colic artery for the diversion of obstructing rectal tumors. Although the loop ileostomy has the least influence on the "next" operation, a loop ileostomy could potentially create a closed loop obstruction physiology within the colon in the setting of a competent ileocecal valve.

Bleeding

Ongoing blood loss from the primary tumor is typically low volume and managed non-operatively with iron replacement or blood transfusion. Occasionally, however, a patient can experience significant life-threatening bleeding necessitating intervention. This is more likely to occur in patients on chronic anticoagulation or rare cases of malignant vascular involvement. Radiation provides relatively quick and effective palliation for surface bleeding at the site of the tumor, particularly within the rectum.[22,23] Resection is the preferred approach, if possible, for more proximal cancers or in the setting of significant hemorrhage. However, this decision will depend on the local invasion of the tumor into adjacent structures, the functional status of the patient, and the volume of metastatic disease. Endovascular procedures (eg, embolization, covered stent placement) are also available in the palliative setting for bleeding from advanced CRC.[24,25]

Perforation

Priority is given to obtaining source control of the intra-abdominal infection in the case of a perforated colorectal cancer with distant metastases so that the patient may be initiated on systemic chemotherapy without delay. This may include simple diversion if the perforation is contained and can be percutaneously or surgically drained. In some situations, resection may be appropriate depending on the feasibility of resection according to the principles described above. When possible, a proper oncologic resection with lymphadenectomy should be undertaken. However, a multivisceral en bloc resection is rarely appropriate for a perforated tumor in the setting of synchronous metastatic disease given the overall poor prognosis.[26]

UNRESECTABLE SYNCHRONOUS METASTASES

In patients with Stage IV CRC, survival is closely linked to control of the distant disease. As such, initiation of systemic therapy for metastatic disease should be prioritized.[27] Early determination of curability is necessary to determine the appropriate treatment strategy (see **Fig. 1**).

All major guidelines recommend upfront systemic chemotherapy for patients with unresectable metastatic CRC and an asymptomatic primary tumor given that few patients (<20%) with metastatic CRC require the intervention of the primary during chemotherapy.[6,7,28] Systemic options include standard first and second line multimodality regimens (FOLFOX or FOLFIRI or CAPEOX or FOLFOXIRI; these can be administered ± bevacizumab).[7] Additionally, targeted epidermal growth factor receptor inhibitors (panitumumab, cetuximab) may be an option for patients with KRAS/NRAS/BRAF wild-type tumors. Patients with BRAF mutations have particularly poor prognoses and initiation of multi-agent targeted therapy should be considered early in the treatment course.[29] Re-evaluation with cross-sectional imaging to assess for conversion to resectable disease is recommended every 2 months if resectability is a possibility.[7] Conversion to resectability among patients with liver-only metastases treated with neaodjuvant systemic therapy occurs in up to 20% of patients depending on the initial definition of unresectability.[30] However, conversion to resection was reported in 48% of randomized patients with initially unresectable metastases in the latest CAIRO5 trial.[31] When surgery is indicated, it is typically delayed 4 weeks from the last dose of systemic therapy or 6 weeks from the last dose of bevacizumab with reinitiation of chemotherapy 6 to 8 weeks postoperatively.[7]

Upfront resection of an asymptomatic primary tumor in patients with synchronous metastases delays the initiation of systemic therapy without proven benefit to the patient. While historic retrospective data suggested greater survival among patients selected for the resection of primary tumor and systemic therapy as compared with systemic therapy alone in patients with unresectable synchronous CRC metastases, these studies are plagued by potential selection bias.[5,32,33] The recent JCOG 1007 randomized trial which enrolled patients with unresectable synchronous metastases from colon cancer demonstrated similar median OS (26 months) between patients enrolled in chemotherapy only versus patients assigned to the primary tumor resection followed by chemotherapy.[34] Several ongoing prospective clinical trials (CAIRO4 and GRECCAR 8) may further elucidate survival differences based on the resection of primary tumor in patients with unresectable metastases.[35–37] Current surgical management of the primary tumor should be individualized based on response to chemotherapy, estimated prognosis, and patient preference if presystemic diversion has been performed and resection would improve quality of life.

RESECTABLE SYNCHRONOUS METASTASES

Treatment with curative intent is possible in 20% to 25% of patients with CRC metastases through a number of different treatment sequences including chemotherapy and resection of the primary/metastatic disease.[38] There is no "one size fits all" approach for the sequencing of surgery and chemotherapy. The advantages and disadvantages of each approach must be carefully weighed by the multidisciplinary tumor board. Proponents of the resection first approach point to the theoretic elimination of metastatic cell tumor shedding from the primary tumor and avoidance for the need of emergent surgery during systemic treatment.[28] Additionally, oxaliplatin and irinotecan both can cause hepatotoxicity, particularly with long-term administration. There are numerous reports of liver toxicity (steatohepatitis, sinusoidal obstruction syndrome, noncirrhotic portal hypertension) that can predispose to increased operative risk following neoadjuvant therapy.[39–42] Alternatively, there are advantages of neoadjuvant chemotherapy including the elimination or detection of micrometastatic disease, cytoreduction facilitating an R0 resection or potentially converting a patient from unresectable to resectable disease. The avoidance of surgical complications from up-front surgery, which can significantly delay the initiation of chemotherapy, is another advantage to neoadjuvant chemotherapy.[21,43] Finally, initial treatment with chemotherapy may elucidate the phenotype of the patient's individual cancer with avoidance of futile surgery in patients with aggressive tumor biology who experience progression on therapy. Current NCCN guidelines recommend 2 to 3 months of neoadjuvant chemotherapy in the patient with resectable metastatic disease with the administration of the remaining 3 months of perioperative chemotherapy after surgery.[7]

SPECIAL CONSIDERATIONS IN RECTAL CANCER

The need for pelvic radiotherapy further complicates treatment considerations among patients with locally advanced rectal cancer and synchronous metastatic disease. Options include: up-front chemoradiation (short course or long course) followed by chemotherapy and then resection or up-front chemotherapy followed by short-course or long-course chemoradiation and then resection (synchronous or staged). With each of these approaches, there is some concern that delaying hepatic resection until the completion of systemic chemotherapy and long-course radiotherapy may worsen chemotherapy-induced liver injury leading to an increase in the risk of postoperative liver failure. In this setting, short-course radiotherapy followed by immediate surgery has emerged as the preferred option to shorten the time to resection.[7]

An additional option, in this case, is 2 to 3 months of neoadjuvant chemotherapy followed by liver resection, then 3 additional months of perioperative chemotherapy and chemoradiation before the resection of the rectal primary. This "liver first" approach allows for a full 12-week rest period following the completion of chemoradiotherapy, which may increase the odds of a complete clinical response of the primary tumor.[44] Certain patients with resectable metastases (particularly those facing an abdominoperineal resection with permanent colostomy) may elect to pursue a "wait and watch" approach in the event of a complete clinical response. However, one must recognize that each of the prior studies evaluating the "wait and watch" approach in rectal cancer excludes patients with Stage IV disease.[45–47] As such, the oncologic outcomes for a "wait and watch" approach in the setting of synchronous Stage IV disease are unknown, necessitating an in-depth discussion with the patient about their goals of treatment.[11–13]

LIVER METASTASES
Resection

Surgical resection in conjunction with perioperative systemic therapy is the recommended treatment of patients with potentially curable disease, and it is associated with the highest cure rates of the available treatment modalities. Five-year survival rates range between 24% and 58% (averaging 40%) with 30-day mortality rates less than 2% to 3%.[42] This is in comparison to 5-year survival rates of 5% to 10% for patients who received systemic chemotherapy alone. However, these data are obviously heavily influenced by selection bias.[48] Approximately 20% of patients are considered resectable at the time of initial presentation and another 20% to 48% may become resectable after induction chemotherapy.[30,31] The use of resection in patients with liver metastases has increased significantly in the past 3 decades,[49] though ongoing multi-disciplinary collaboration and surgical referrals to consider the resection of both primary tumor and liver metastases is required.

The definition of "resectable disease" has expanded significantly over time through the adoption of a more aggressive surgical approach in conjunction with advanced techniques that ensure both margin-negative resection and more precise assessment and optimization of the future liver remnant (FLR).[50,51] Aggressive resections can be pursued as long as vascular inflow and outflow, biliary outflow, and adequate FLR are assured. Some of these advanced technologies include three-dimensional (3-D) imaging, complex parenchymal and vascular sparing resections, preoperative portal vein embolization (PVE) to augment hypertrophy of contralateral liver and facilitate 1-stage hepatectomy or 2-stage hepatectomy, combined portal vein and ipsilateral hepatic vein embolization, and associating liver partition and portal vein ligation for staged hepatectomy (ALPPS).[51,52] Currently, patients meet the criteria for resection if they are fit, favorable disease biology can be assured, and an R0 resection can be achieved with the preservation of enough life-sustaining viable hepatic parenchyma.[50] While FLR ~ 25% can be considered in young and healthy patients without underlying liver disease who have not received preoperative systemic therapy, FLR greater than 30% of the total hepatic volume is generally regarded as the minimum liver remnant for patients who have received greater than 12 weeks of chemotherapy especially in growing proportion of U.S. population with underlying steatosis.[53]

The patient with extensive bilobar hepatic metastases presents the most significant challenge given the risks of inadequate resection, early recurrence, and postoperative liver failure. In the past, these patients were deemed unresectable. However, preoperative strategies to facilitate tumor downstaging and increase the safety of liver resection have evolved significantly in the past decade. PVE allows for hepatic hypertrophy of planned FLR, with at least 40% to 60% increase in the volume of planned remnant in most of the patients without underlying chronic liver disease, facilitating either 1-stage or 2-stage hepatectomy.[54] Recent expansion of embolization techniques to include both ipsilateral portal vein and hepatic vein embolization have facilitated planned FLR hypertrophy among selected patients.[55] Systemic therapy can be continued during the period of expected hepatic hypertrophy to reduce the risk of cancer progression. With a 2-stage approach, metastasectomy of the planned liver remnant is performed during the first stage to clear the FLR of metastases, and the portal vein to the contralateral liver is either ligated or embolized either during or after first stage operation. The primary tumor may be removed during this stage if appropriate based on the patient's individual risk profile. During the second stage, anatomic resection of the remaining diseased lobe is undertaken after adequate hypertrophy of the FLR has been achieved, assuming the metastatic disease has not progressed. Up to 38% of patients with initially unresectable bi-lobar hepatic metastases can progress during wait periods between different stages of liver-directed operative therapy and can fail to undergo curative-intent resection; however, in general, the chance of progression and failure to proceed with resection in the modern era of aggressive systemic therapy and aggressive operative approaches is lower.[54,56,57]

Initially developed to address potential challenges with PVE, the ALPPS approach combines in situ liver split and portal vein ligation with re-operation to complete resection, typically in a 5 to 14-day period.[58,59] While several variations have been developed, conceptually hepatic parenchyma is divided at the site of the planned transection margin and portal vein of the planned resection specimen is ligated at the time of index liver split. Theoretically, the combination of portal flow interruption and parenchymal transection results in more rapid hypertrophy of the planned liver remnant than portal vein occlusion alone, which may permit hypertrophy of the FLR in as little as 5 days. The patient undergoes repeat imaging and volumetric analysis with staged hepatectomy once adequate volume in the FLR is achieved.[58] Widespread adoption of the technique has been limited by increased rates of morbidity and mortality described initially compared with traditional complex hepatic resections. A recent multi-institutional trial of 510 patients from 22 ALPPS centers reported 4.9% 90-day mortality, 39 months median OS and 15 months median RFS.[60] The recently completed LIGRO randomized controlled trial demonstrated similar complication rates and resection rate (92% vs 80%, $P = .091$) and greater estimated median survival (46 months vs 26 months, $P = .028$) with ALPPS compared with 2-stage hepatectomy.[61] However, critics argue that 2-staged hepatectomy is not the standard of care for patients with bi-lobar metastases in whom 1-stage resection post-PVE can be performed, and are awaiting trial comparisons of ALPPS to PVE followed by 1-stage hepatectomy. Adoption of ALPPS seems to be more tempered in the United States than European centers, perhaps secondary to differences in practice patterns and utilization of venous embolization techniques. Transplant oncology has recently replaced ALPPS as the most controversial topic in liver surgery. Liver transplantation for extensive, unresectable, disseminated liver metastases is highly controversial and has been predominantly performed in highly selected patients in Europe. A few centers in the Americas have attempted this approach, few are considering developing protocols, and one center in Canada is currently prospectively enrolling patients.[51]

Predominantly, liver resections are performed via an open approach although minimally invasive approaches are being used increasingly. The OSLO-COMET trial demonstrated shorter hospital stays (2 days vs 4 days; $P<.001$), lower complication rates (19% vs 31%; $P = .021$), and better quality of life with the laparoscopic approach in patients with CRC metastases randomized to either laparoscopic or open liver resection with similar long-term oncologic outcomes [overall survival (OS) of 80 months (95% confidence interval (CI): 52–108) versus 81 months (95% CI: 42–120) ($P = .91$)]. When feasible, a minimally invasive approach should be considered. As liver recurrence after initial metastasectomy occurs in approximately 50% of patients, resection of recurrent metastases (including repeat sequential resection) can be pursued in selected patients with favorable disease biology.

Ablation and Locoregional Therapies

Resection is preferred over ablation and locoregional therapies in the management of hepatic CRC metastases given better DFS and OS.[62] However, patients who are not fit for surgery, patients with solitary small metastases which would require large anatomic resection, or patients with unresectable disease despite aggressive neoadjuvant therapy may benefit from alternative therapies including percutaneous ablative treatments (radiofrequency ablation, microwave ablation) or locoregional transcatheter intra-arterial therapies. Many of the image-guided ablative therapies can also be used in conjunction with resection in particular with parenchymal sparing approaches or during the management of metastases in planned FLR during 1-stage hepatectomy. **Box 2** provides an overview of the available ablative and locoregional treatment modalities in comparison with resection and systemic chemotherapy. Hepatic arterial infusion therapy has been advocated at select centers supported by retrospective institutional data[63]; however, prospective data are lacking and adoption of this method for drug delivery in general liver surgery practice has not been widely adopted.

LUNG METASTASES AND OTHER EXTRAHEPATIC DISEASE SITES

The lung is the second most common site of CRC metastatic disease, accounting for 22% of CRC metastases. Lung metastases are associated with a better prognosis than isolated liver metastases with 5-year OS up to 68%.[5,64] Surprisingly, despite the prevalence of surgical resection of pulmonary metastases, there has not been a single prospective trial to evaluate the effectiveness of pulmonary metastectomy (PM). Instead, practice patterns are based on retrospective series and several international registries, which are limited by variable follow-up length, selection bias, inconsistent systemic treatment, and a lack of comparative survival analyses.[65] The PulMiCC trial is an ongoing trial in patients with metastatic CRC, randomizing patients to resection or surveillance.[66] Until this and other prospective trials are available, management decisions will depend on expert consensus and retrospective series.[7,65]

The objective of PM for CRC is the complete resection of all viable tumors with the preservation of adequate functional lung. Most CRC metastases are amendable to metastastectomy as opposed to formal lobectomy, and pneumonectomy is generally discouraged. Ablative techniques and SBRT are options for patients with limited metastatic burden, particularly for high-risk patients or those who refuse resection.[7]

Resection of isolated peritoneal or ovarian metastases should be pursued if these are identified incidentally at the time of index resection or if favorable disease biology has been ascertained. Surgical management of extensive peritoneal disease remains controversial and is beyond the scope of the current article.

Box 2
Treatment options in patients with hepatic CRC metastases

Hepatic Resection

- Mechanism - Partial hepatectomy, lobectomy, portal vein occlusion, ALLPS
- Indication – If R0 resection can be achieved and patient medically fit for surgery
- Advantages/disadvantages - Only 20% of patients meet criteria for resection and are medically fit for surgery
- Overall survival - 5-year OS ranges from 24% to 58%
- Risks – 30-day morbidity less than 15%, 30-day mortality less than 3%

Radiofrequency ablation (RFA)

- Mechanism – Percutaneous procedure that induces thermal damage via high-frequency alternating current
- Indication - Unresectable, peripheral lesions <3 cm, patient not medically fit for surgery
- Advantages/disadvantages - Not effective near vascular structure or lesions >3 cm
- Overall survival - OS 28 to 53 months, 5-year OS 43%
- Risks – 30-day morbidity less than 2%, 30-day mortality less than 1%, postablation syndrome

Microwave ablation (MWA)

- Mechanism – Percutaneous procedure that uses electromagnetic signal to generate heat via molecular friction
- Indication - Unresectable, patient not medically fit for surgery
- Advantages/disadvantages - Effective for larger and more central lesions than RFA
- Overall survival - 5-year OS 37%
- Risks – 30-day morbidity less than 2%, 30-day mortality less than 1%, postablation syndrome

Transarterial chemoembolization ± drug eluding beads (TACE)

- Mechanism – Transcatheter intra-arterial technique that delivers chemotherapy into hepatic arteries supplying tumor
- Indication - Unresectable, patient not medically fit for surgery, not a candidate for ablation, failed chemotherapy
- Advantages/disadvantages – Significant toxicity with limited efficacy
- Overall survival - OS 8 to 14 months, 5-year OS 6%
- Risks – Postembolization syndrome (fever, pain, nausea) in 60% to 80%

Transarterial radioembolization (TARE) or selective internal radiotherapy (SIRT)

- Mechanism – Transcatheter intra-arterial technique that uses microspheres loaded with radioisotope (^{90}Y) to deliver high-dose radiation to tumor
- Indication - Unresectable, patient not medically fit for surgery, not a candidate for ablation, failed chemotherapy
- Advantages/disadvantages - significant toxicity with limited efficacy
- Overall survival - OS 8 to 14 mo, 5-year OS 4% to 7%
- Risks – Better tolerated than TACE

Stereotactic body radiation therapy (SBRT)

- Mechanism – Delivery of precise external beam radiation using 4-D imaging
- Indication - Unresectable, patient not medically fit for surgery

- Advantages/disadvantages - Unclear advantage over ablation or chemotherapy
- Overall survival - OS 24 to 27 months
- Risks – 20% hepatic toxicity

Chemotherapy

- Mechanism – FOLFOX or FOLFIRI or CAPEOX or FOLFOXIRI ± bevacizumab
- Indication - Unresectable, patient not medically fit for surgery
- Advantages/disadvantages - Noninvasive
- Overall survival - 5-year OS 20%, OS 23 months
- Risks – Neutropenia, neuropathy; perforation and bleeding (bevacizumab)

Abbreviations: ALLPS, liver partition and portal venous ligation for staged hepatectomy; OS, overall survival; yr, year; mo, month.

SUMMARY

Multidisciplinary management of patients with colorectal cancer and synchronous metastases is paramount to optimize long-term patient survival. Systemic therapy, resection of primary tumor, and resection of metastases should be planned from the time of diagnosis. Additional treatment complexity, such as the influence of molecular tumor profile on treatment and prognosis, radiotherapy for patients with rectal cancer, or venous embolization for patients requiring the augmentation of FLR, can further increase the complexity of treatment decisions re-enforcing the importance of multidisciplinary management. As systemic therapy and understanding of molecular markers of tumor biology continue to improve, aggressive resection will help achieve long-term survival in appropriately selected patients.

DISCLOSURE

T.L. Hedrick – consultant with Johnson and Johnson, V.M. Zaydfudim – none.

REFERENCES

1. Hu CY, Bailey CE, You YN, et al. Time trend analysis of primary tumor resection for stage IV colorectal cancer: less surgery, improved survival. JAMA Surg 2015; 150(3):245–51.

2. Brouwer NPM, Bos A, Lemmens V, et al. An overview of 25 years of incidence, treatment and outcome of colorectal cancer patients. Int J Cancer 2018; 143(11):2758–66.

3. Siegel RL, Miller KD, Jemal A. Cancer statistics, 2019. CA Cancer J Clin 2019; 69(1):7–34.

4. Ansa BE, Coughlin SS, Alema-Mensah E, et al. Evaluation of colorectal cancer incidence trends in the United States (2000-2014). J Clin Med 2018;7(2):22.

5. Wang J, Li S, Liu Y, et al. Metastatic patterns and survival outcomes in patients with stage IV colon cancer: a population-based analysis. Cancer Med 2020; 9(1):361–73.

6. Vogel JD, Eskicioglu C, Weiser MR, et al. The American Society of Colon and rectal surgeons clinical practice guidelines for the treatment of colon cancer. Dis Colon Rectum 2017;60(10):999–1017.

7. Benson AB 3rd, Venook AP, Cederquist L, et al. Colon cancer, version 1.2017, NCCN clinical practice guidelines in oncology. J Natl Compr Canc Netw 2017; 15(3):370–98.

8. Adams RB, Aloia TA, Loyer E, et al. Selection for hepatic resection of colorectal liver metastases: expert consensus statement. HPB (Oxford) 2013;15(2):91–103.

9. Abdalla EK, Bauer TW, Chun YS, et al. Locoregional surgical and interventional therapies for advanced colorectal cancer liver metastases: expert consensus statements. HPB (Oxford) 2013;15(2):119–30.

10. Schwarz RE, Berlin JD, Lenz HJ, et al. Systemic cytotoxic and biological therapies of colorectal liver metastases: expert consensus statement. HPB (Oxford) 2013;15(2):106–15.

11. Morris AM. Shared decision making for rectal cancer care: a long way forward. Dis Colon Rectum 2016;59(10):905–6.

12. Hawley ST, Jagsi R. Shared decision making in cancer care: does one size fit all? JAMA Oncol 2015;1(1):58–9.

13. Ellis PG, O'Neil BH, Earle MF, et al. Clinical pathways: management of quality and cost in oncology networks in the metastatic colorectal cancer setting. J Oncol Pract 2017;13(5):e522–9.

14. Deans GT, Krukowski ZH, Irwin ST. Malignant obstruction of the left colon. Br J Surg 1994;81(9):1270–6.

15. van Hooft JE, van Halsema EE, Vanbiervliet G, et al. Self-expandable metal stents for obstructing colonic and extracolonic cancer: European Society of Gastrointestinal Endoscopy (ESGE) clinical guideline. Endoscopy 2014;46(11):990–1053.

16. Fiori E, Lamazza A, Schillaci A, et al. Palliative management for patients with subacute obstruction and stage IV unresectable rectosigmoid cancer: colostomy versus endoscopic stenting: final results of a prospective randomized trial. Am J Surg 2012;204(3):321–6.

17. Gianotti L, Tamini N, Nespoli L, et al. A prospective evaluation of short-term and long-term results from colonic stenting for palliation or as a bridge to elective operation versus immediate surgery for large-bowel obstruction. Surg Endosc 2013;27(3):832–42.

18. Young CJ, De-Loyde KJ, Young JM, et al. Improving quality of life for people with incurable large-bowel obstruction: randomized control trial of colonic stent insertion. Dis Colon Rectum 2015;58(9):838–49.

19. van den Berg MW, Ledeboer M, Dijkgraaf MG, et al. Long-term results of palliative stent placement for acute malignant colonic obstruction. Surg Endosc 2015; 29(6):1580–5.

20. Watt AM, Faragher IG, Griffin TT, et al. Self-expanding metallic stents for relieving malignant colorectal obstruction: a systematic review. Ann Surg 2007;246(1): 24–30.

21. Gao P, Huang XZ, Song YX, et al. Impact of timing of adjuvant chemotherapy on survival in stage III colon cancer: a population-based study. BMC Cancer 2018; 18(1):234.

22. Cameron MG, Kersten C, Vistad I, et al. Palliative pelvic radiotherapy of symptomatic incurable rectal cancer - a systematic review. Acta Oncol 2014;53(2): 164–73.

23. Cameron MG, Kersten C, Vistad I, et al. Palliative pelvic radiotherapy for symptomatic rectal cancer - a prospective multicenter study. Acta Oncol 2016; 55(12):1400–7.

24. Corvino F, Giurazza F, Cangiano G, et al. Endovascular treatment of peripheral vascular blowout syndrome in end-stage malignancies. Ann Vasc Surg 2019; 58:382.e1–5.
25. Tan KK, Strong DH, Shore T, et al. The safety and efficacy of mesenteric embolization in the management of acute lower gastrointestinal hemorrhage. Ann Coloproctol 2013;29(5):205–8.
26. Daniels M, Merkel S, Agaimy A, et al. Treatment of perforated colon carcinomas-outcomes of radical surgery. Int J Colorectal Dis 2015;30(11):1505–13.
27. Lam VW, Laurence JM, Pang T, et al. A systematic review of a liver-first approach in patients with colorectal cancer and synchronous colorectal liver metastases. HPB (Oxford) 2014;16(2):101–8.
28. Poultsides GA, Servais EL, Saltz LB, et al. Outcome of primary tumor in patients with synchronous stage IV colorectal cancer receiving combination chemotherapy without surgery as initial treatment. J Clin Oncol 2009;27(20):3379–84.
29. Kopetz S, Grothey A, Yaeger R, et al. Encorafenib, binimetinib, and cetuximab in BRAF V600E-mutated colorectal cancer. N Engl J Med 2019;381(17):1632–43.
30. Adam R, De Gramont A, Figueras J, et al. The oncosurgery approach to managing liver metastases from colorectal cancer: a multidisciplinary international consensus. Oncologist 2012;17(10):1225–39.
31. Bolhuis K, Grosheide L, Wesdorp NJ, et al, for the Dutch Colorectal Cancer Group Liver Expert Panel. Short-term outcomes of secondary liver surgery for initially unresectable colorectal liver metastases following modern induction systemic therapy in the dutch CAIRO5 trial. Ann Surg Open 2021;2(3):e081.
32. Faron M, Pignon JP, Malka D, et al. Is primary tumour resection associated with survival improvement in patients with colorectal cancer and unresectable synchronous metastases? A pooled analysis of individual data from four randomised trials. Eur J Cancer 2015;51(2):166–76.
33. Shida D, Boku N, Tanabe T, et al. Primary tumor resection for stage IV colorectal cancer in the era of targeted chemotherapy. J Gastrointest Surg 2019;23(11): 2144–50.
34. Kanemitsu Y, Shitara K, Mizusawa J, et al. Primary tumor resection plus chemotherapy versus chemotherapy alone for colorectal cancer patients with asymptomatic, synchronous unresectable metastases (JCOG1007; iPACS): a randomized clinical trial. J Clin Oncol 2021;39(10):1098–107.
35. Moritani K, Kanemitsu Y, Shida D, et al. A randomized controlled trial comparing primary tumour resection plus chemotherapy with chemotherapy alone in incurable stage IV colorectal cancer: JCOG1007 (iPACS study). Jpn J Clin Oncol 2020;50(1):89–93.
36. Cotte E, Villeneuve L, Passot G, et al. GRECCAR 8: impact on survival of the primary tumor resection in rectal cancer with unresectable synchronous metastasis: a randomized multicentre study. BMC Cancer 2015;15:47.
37. Lam-Boer J, Mol L, Verhoef C, et al. The CAIRO4 study: the role of surgery of the primary tumour with few or absent symptoms in patients with synchronous unresectable metastases of colorectal cancer-a randomized phase III study of the Dutch Colorectal Cancer Group (DCCG). BMC Cancer 2014;14:741.
38. Creasy JM, Sadot E, Koerkamp BG, et al. Actual 10-year survival after hepatic resection of colorectal liver metastases: what factors preclude cure? Surgery 2018;163(6):1238–44.
39. Fernandez FG, Ritter J, Goodwin JW, et al. Effect of steatohepatitis associated with irinotecan or oxaliplatin pretreatment on resectability of hepatic colorectal metastases. J Am Coll Surg 2005;200(6):845–53.

40. Simpson AL, Leal JN, Pugalenthi A, et al. Chemotherapy-induced splenic volume increase is independently associated with major complications after hepatic resection for metastatic colorectal cancer. J Am Coll Surg 2015;220(3):271–80.

41. Khan AZ, Morris-Stiff G, Makuuchi M. Patterns of chemotherapy-induced hepatic injury and their implications for patients undergoing liver resection for colorectal liver metastases. J Hepatobiliary Pancreat Surg 2009;16(2):137–44.

42. Duwe G, Knitter S, Pesthy S, et al. Hepatotoxicity following systemic therapy for colorectal liver metastases and the impact of chemotherapy-associated liver injury on outcomes after curative liver resection. Eur J Surg Oncol 2017;43(9): 1668–81.

43. Jamnagerwalla M, Tay R, Steel M, et al. Impact of surgical complications following resection of locally advanced rectal adenocarcinoma on adjuvant chemotherapy delivery and survival outcomes. Dis Colon Rectum 2016;59(10): 916–24.

44. Habr-Gama A, Sao Juliao GP, Fernandez LM, et al. Achieving a complete clinical response after neoadjuvant chemoradiation that does not require surgical resection: it may take longer than you think! Dis Colon Rectum 2019;62(7):802–8.

45. Dattani M, Heald RJ, Goussous G, et al. Oncological and survival outcomes in watch and wait patients with a clinical complete response after neoadjuvant chemoradiotherapy for rectal cancer: a systematic review and pooled analysis. Ann Surg 2018;268(6):955–67.

46. Renehan AG, Malcomson L, Emsley R, et al. Watch-and-wait approach versus surgical resection after chemoradiotherapy for patients with rectal cancer (the OnCoRe project): a propensity-score matched cohort analysis. Lancet Oncol 2016;17(2):174–83.

47. Smith JJ, Strombom P, Chow OS, et al. Assessment of a watch-and-wait strategy for rectal cancer in patients with a complete response after neoadjuvant therapy. JAMA Oncol 2019;5(4):e185896.

48. Ferrarotto R, Pathak P, Maru D, et al. Durable complete responses in metastatic colorectal cancer treated with chemotherapy alone. Clin Colorectal Cancer 2011; 10(3):178–82.

49. Zaydfudim VM, McMurry TL, Harrigan AM, et al. Improving treatment and survival: a population-based study of current outcomes after a hepatic resection in patients with metastatic colorectal cancer. HPB (Oxford) 2015;17(11):1019–24.

50. Venook AC. Management of potentially resectable colorectal liver metastases. UpToDate; 2020. Available at: https://www-uptodate-com/management-of-potentially-resectable-colorectal-cancer-liver-metastases?search=colorectal%20metastases&source=search_result&selectedTitle=1~150&usage_type=default&display_rank=1. [Accessed 14 August 2021], Accessed 2020.

51. Kambakamba P, Hoti E, Cremen S, et al. The evolution of surgery for colorectal liver metastases: a persistent challenge to improve survival. Surgery 2021 Dec; 170(6):1732–40.

52. Takamoto T, Sano K, Hashimoto T, et al. Practical contribution of virtual hepatectomy for colorectal liver metastases: a propensity-matched analysis of clinical outcome. J Gastrointest Surg 2018;22(12):2037–44.

53. Ethun CG, Maithel SK. Determination of resectability. Surg Clin North Am 2016; 96(2):163–81.

54. Shindoh J, Truty MJ, Aloia TA, et al. Kinetic growth rate after portal vein embolization predicts posthepatectomy outcomes: toward zero liver-related mortality in patients with colorectal liver metastases and small future liver remnant. J Am Coll Surg 2013;216(2):201–9.

55. Laurent C, Fernandez B, Marichez A, et al. Radiological simultaneous portohepatic vein embolization (RASPE) before major hepatectomy: a better way to optimize liver hypertrophy compared to portal vein embolization. Ann Surg 2020; 272(2):199–205.

56. Shindoh J, Vauthey JN, Zimmitti G, et al. Analysis of the efficacy of portal vein embolization for patients with extensive liver malignancy and very low future liver remnant volume, including a comparison with the associating liver partition with portal vein ligation for staged hepatectomy approach. J Am Coll Surg 2013; 217(1):126–33 [discussion 124–33].

57. Capussotti L, Muratore A, Baracchi F, et al. Portal vein ligation as an efficient method of increasing the future liver remnant volume in the surgical treatment of colorectal metastases. Arch Surg 2008;143(10):978–82 [discussion 982].

58. Schnitzbauer AA, Lang SA, Goessmann H, et al. Right portal vein ligation combined with in situ splitting induces rapid left lateral liver lobe hypertrophy enabling 2-staged extended right hepatic resection in small-for-size settings. Ann Surg 2012;255(3):405–14.

59. Olthof PB, Schnitzbauer AA, Schadde E. The HPB controversy of the decade: 2007-2017 - Ten years of ALPPS. Eur J Surg Oncol 2018;44(10):1624–7.

60. Petrowsky H, Linecker M, Raptis DA, et al. First long-term oncologic results of the ALPPS procedure in a large cohort of patients with colorectal liver metastases. Ann Surg 2020;272(5):793–800.

61. Hasselgren K, Rosok BI, Larsen PN, et al. ALPPS improves survival compared with TSH in patients affected of CRLM: survival analysis from the randomized controlled trial LIGRO. Ann Surg. 2021 Mar 1;273(3):442–8.

62. Di Martino M, Rompianesi G, Mora-Guzman I, et al. Systematic review and meta-analysis of local ablative therapies for resectable colorectal liver metastases. Eur J Surg Oncol. 2020 May;46(5):772–81.

63. Gholami S, Kemeny NE, Boucher TM, et al. Adjuvant hepatic artery infusion chemotherapy is associated with improved survival regardless of KRAS mutation status in patients with resected colorectal liver metastases: a retrospective analysis of 674 patients. Ann Surg 2020;272(2):352–6.

64. Okumura T, Boku N, Hishida T, et al. Surgical outcome and prognostic stratification for pulmonary metastasis from colorectal cancer. Ann Thorac Surg 2017; 104(3):979–87.

65. Handy JR, Bremner RM, Crocenzi TS, et al. Expert consensus document on pulmonary metastasectomy. Ann Thorac Surg 2019;107(2):631–49.

66. Treasure T, Fallowfield L, Lees B. Pulmonary metastasectomy in colorectal cancer: the PulMiCC trial. J Thorac Oncol 2010;5(6 Suppl 2):S203–6.

Neoadjuvant Therapy for Rectal Cancer

Felipe F. Quezada-Diaz, MD[a], J. Joshua Smith, MD, PhD[b],*

KEYWORDS

- Neoadjuvant therapy • Rectal cancer • Total neoadjuvant therapy • Chemoradiation
- Short-course radiotherapy

KEY POINTS

- Locally advanced rectal cancer treatment requires a multidisciplinary approach
- Neoadjuvant treatment of rectal cancer has improved local control and enhanced sphincter preservation but has not improved overall survival.
- Short-course radiotherapy and long-course chemoradiation have shown similar oncological results in terms of overall survival, local recurrence, and surgical complications
- The addition of neoadjuvant chemotherapy may prevent distant failure and benefit overall survival
- Total neoadjuvant therapy may be associated with reduction in the risk of systemic recurrence while enhancing the rates of pathological and clinical response, providing a chance for organ preservation in selected patients.

INTRODUCTION

Colorectal cancer is the third most frequent cancer diagnosed worldwide and it is the fourth cause of cancer-related deaths in the world.[1] It is estimated globally that 1.6 million patients with colorectal cancer are diagnosed per year[2] with patients with rectal cancer corresponding to 28% of all cases in the United States[3] and 35% in Europe.[4]

The treatment of locally advanced rectal cancer (LARC, AJCC TNM cT3-4 with or without secondary lymph nodes) has historically been considered a challenge due to complex pelvic anatomy. Specific anatomic difficulties such as limited pelvic space, autonomic nerve involvement, and anal sphincter proximity, may elevate the risk of local recurrence[5] and/or late functional sequelae[6] after a proper oncological resection.

[a] Colorectal Unit, Department of Surgery, Complejo Asistencial Doctor Sótero del Río, Avenida Concha y Toro#3459, Santiago, Puente Alto, RM 8207257, Chile; [b] Colorectal Service, Department of Surgery, Memorial Sloan Kettering Cancer Center, 1275 York Avenue, SR-201, New York, NY 10065, USA
* Corresponding author.
E-mail address: smithj5@mskcc.org
Twitter: @ffquezad (F.F.Q.-D.); @JoshSmithMDPhD (J.J.S.)

Surg Oncol Clin N Am 31 (2022) 279–291
https://doi.org/10.1016/j.soc.2021.11.008

Table 1
Summary of important neoadjuvant treatment studies for locally advanced rectal cancer

	Study	n	Interventions	Local Recurrence	Overall Survival	Disease-Free Survival	pCR/cCR
SCRT	Swedish Rectal Cancer Trial,[13] 1997	1168	25 Gy × 5 d + following week surgery vs surgery alone	25% vs 11%	58% vs 48%	74% vs 65%	N/A
	Dutch Rectal Cancer Trial, 2001[14]	1861	25 Gy × 5 d + following week TME vs TME alone	2.4% vs 8.2%	82% vs 81.8%	N/A	ypT0 1% vs 2%
	Stockholm III, 2017[29]	840	SCRT wo TME delay vs SCRT 4-8 wk TME delay vs LCRT	2.2% vs 2.8% vs 5.5%	73% vs 76% vs 78%	65% vs 64% vs 65%	pCR: 0.3% vs 10.4% vs 2.2%
LCRT	CAO/ARO-094, 2004[7]	850	Preoperative 50.4 Gy over 5 wk with 5-FU + TME surgery vs postoperative	6% vs 13% (40% grade 3-4 toxicity in postoperative CRT group)	76% vs 74%	68% vs 65%	pCR: 8% vs 0%
	FFCD9203, 2006[17]	733	Preoperative chemoradiation + TME vs RT alone	8.1% vs 16.5%	67.4% vs 66.9%	N/A	pCR: 11.4% vs 3.6%
	EORTC22921, 2006[18]	1011	Preoperative RT alone/CRT + TME vs preoperative RT alone/CRT + TME + adjuvant chemo	7.6% vs 17.1%	65.8% (preoperative CRT w/wo adjuvant chemo) vs 64.8% (preoperative radiotherapy w/wo adjuvant chemo)	58.2% (with adjuvant chemotherapy) vs 52.2% (no adjuvant chemotherapy)	pCR = 13.7% (RT alone/CRT + postoperative chemotherapy) vs 5.3% (RT alone/CRT)

	Trial	N	Treatment				Outcomes
TNT SCRT	Polish Colorectal Study Group, 2016[41]	515	SCRT + 3 cycles consolidation FOLFOX4 + TME vs LCRT + TME	22 vs 21% Distant failure (no resection + R2 resection + local recurrence)	73% vs 65%	53 vs 52%	pCR: 16% vs 12%
	RAPIDO Trial, 2021[52]	920	SCRT + 6 cycles CAPOX or 9 cycles FOLFOX4 vs LCRT	23.7% vs 30.4% Disease Treatment Failure at 3 y (local recurrence + distant metastasis + new primary CRC and/or treatment related death)			pCR:28% vs 14%
	STELLAR Trial, 2021[53]	591	SCRT + 4 cycles CAPOX vs LCRT	N/A	86.5% vs 75.1%	64.5% vs 62.3%	pCR: 16.6% vs 11.8% pCR + cCR: 22%, 5% vs 12.6%
TNT LCRT	GCR-3, 2015[48]	108	LCRT + TME + 4 cycles CAPOX vs 4 cycles CAPOX + LCRT + TME	2% vs 5%	78% vs 75%	64% vs 62%	pCR: 13% vs 14%
	CAO/ARO/AIO 12, 2019[49]	306	3 cycles of FOLFOX + LCRT + TME vs LCRT + 3 cycles FOLFOX + TME	N/A	N/A	N/A	pCR: 17% vs 25%
	OPRA Trial, 2020[50]	307	4m of FOLFOX + LCRT + TME vs LCRT + 4m FOLFOX + TME	N/A	N/A	78% vs 77%	Organ Preservation: 43% vs 58%
TNT + Immunotherapy	NRG-GI002, 2021[56]	137	4m FOLFOX + CRT + Pembrolizumab + TME vs 4m FOLFOX + LCRT + TME	N/A	N/A	N/A	pCR: 31.9% vs 29.4% cCR: 13.9% vs 13.6%

(continued on next page)

Table 1
(continued)

Study	n	Interventions	Local Recurrence	Overall Survival	Disease-Free Survival	pCR/cCR
Neoadjuvant Chemotherapy						
Schrag et al, 2014[43]	30	6 cycles FOLFOX/ Bevacizumab + TME	0%	N/A	84%	pCR: 25%
PROSPECT Trial, *ongoing*[44]	1194	6 cycles FOLFOX + selective surgery vs CRT according to MRI response	TBA	TBA	TBA	TBA

Abbreviations: 5-FU, 5-Fluorouracil; cCR, clinical complete response; CRT, chemoradiation; FOLFOX, folinic acid; Fluorouracil, Oxaliplatin; FU, fluorouracil; LCRT, long-course radiotherapy; N/A, Nonavailable; pCR, pathologic complete response; RT, radiotherapy; SCRT, short-course radiotherapy; TME, total mesorectal excision; TNT, total neoadjuvant therapy.

As its implementation, neoadjuvant treatment (NAT) for LARC has enhanced sphincter preservation and improved local control.[7,8] Current multimodal NAT treatment of LARC using radiotherapy (RT) with or without the association of systemic chemo-therapy is associated with local recurrences rates of 5% to 7% and overall survival of 65%.[9]

Currently, different types of NAT strategies have raised the question about which one is the optimal strategy for LARC treatment (**Table 1**). In this article, we explore the different NAT regimens currently available, along with associated benefits and tox-icities and novel approaches in this area.

STANDARD NEOADJUVANT TREATMENT FOR LOCALLY ADVANCED RECTAL CANCER

Classically, the standard surgical approach for LARC has been total mesorectal exci-sion (TME). First described by Heald and colleagues,[5] it corresponds to a en-bloc resection of the rectum with the surrounding lymphovascular fatty tissue.

As TME has been adopted, rates of local recurrence in LARC have steadily declined.[10,11] To further enhance the rates of locoregional control, patients with LARC have been classically treated with 2 NAT modalities.

SHORT-COURSE RADIOTHERAPY

Short-course RT (SCRT) consists of 25 Gy in 5 doses (5 × 5 Gy) in addition to TME in the following 7 days or can be delayed similar to what is conducted with standard long-course RT.[12] This approach has shown a significant reduction in local recurrence in at least 3 Phase III Trials.[13–15] The first evidence came from the Swedish Trial,[13] which found an absolute reduction of 14% in favor of the SCRT and surgery arm (9% vs 23%). However, it should be noted that this trial was developed before TME principles were widespread in the surgical community, which explains the higher rate of local recurrence in the surgery alone group.

Most of the evidence supporting the use of SCRT came from the Dutch Colorectal Cancer Group Trial.[14] This trial showed that adding neoadjuvant SCRT to TME was associated with a reduction in local recurrence rates from 8.2% to 2.4% when compared with the TME group alone, without adding major morbidity. Also, sub-group analysis suggests that the major benefit was for tumors located in the low-middle rectum. These findings were sustained over time, with a 6-year local recurrence rate of 5.6% in the SCRT plus TME group versus 10.9% in the TME alone group[16]

LONG-COURSE CHEMORADIATION

After the findings of the Dutch Trial, several trials evaluated different types of RT reg-imens with or without concomitant sensitizing chemotherapeutics.[7,8,17,18]

Currently, standard long-course chemo-RT (LCRT) frequently consists of 5040 cGy in 28 fractions over a 5- to 6-weeks period and sensitizing fluorouracil or capecitabine for the duration of the RT. After this NAT is complete, surgery is performed between 8 and 12 weeks.

This approach was adopted after the results of the German Rectal Cancer Group Study[7] that demonstrated the superiority of neoadjuvant LCRT versus adjuvant LCRT with better local control and a higher rate of sphincter preservation. Multiple studies support the use of neoadjuvant LCRT based on a reduction in the local recur-rence rate[19,20] and the possibility to identify good responders[18] who have a better course of disease.[21–23]

SHORT-COURSE RADIOTHERAPY VERSUS LONG-COURSE CHEMO-RADIOTHERAPY

When compared with each other, both strategies have shown similar oncological results in terms of overall survival, local recurrence, and surgical complications.[24] In an attempt to search for the best NAT strategy for LARC, the EORTC 22921 trial[25] assigned patients with clinical stage T3 or T4 rectal cancer to receive preoperative RT with or without concomitant chemotherapy before surgery followed by either adjuvant chemotherapy or surveillance. Local recurrence rates were lower in the preoperative LCRT and postoperative chemotherapy group (7.6%) and highest in the preoperative RT group only (22.4%), suggesting that fluorouracil-based chemotherapy helped reduce local recurrence rates.

It has been suggested that tumor regression rates are lower in the SCRT strategy when compared with LCRT.[26,27] This may be due to the recommendation of immediate surgery after the completion of treatment and lack of waiting for a response in the early trials. Bujko and colleagues[28] conducted a trial comparing SCRT and immediate surgery versus LCRT followed by surgery between 4 and 6 weeks. The oncologic outcomes (overall survival, disease-free survival, and local recurrence) at 4 years were similar between the 2 groups, but patients with LCRT had higher rates of pathologic complete response and lower rates of positive circumferential margins.

This raises the question as to the best timing to perform surgery after SCRT. Surprisingly, the results of the Stockholm III trial[29] showed that waiting 4 to 8 weeks after SCRT had higher rates of pathologic complete response rates compared with LCRT (10.4% vs 2.2%, respectively),[30] without adding more surgical morbidity.

Despite all the favorable results of NAT for locoregional control, none of these strategies have demonstrated any association with improved overall survival rates.[31] Systemic recurrence remains the main problem in patients with LARC and 25% of the patients with LARC develop distant metastasis during follow-up.[32–34]

In the light of these findings, it has been proposed to add systemic chemotherapy as a part of the NAT regimen to diminish the risk of distant failure and address potential micrometastases.

NEOADJUVANT SYSTEMIC CHEMOTHERAPY

The addition of chemotherapy as part of NAT has the potential advantages of treating systemic disease upfront and improving treatment compliance.

Several phase III studies such as PETACC6, NSABP R-04, STAR 01, and ACCORD 12 explored the benefit of adding oxaliplatin to LCRT as a way to optimize NAT treatment with no benefits in terms of pathologic complete response, disease-free and overall survival. [32,35–37] However, the German Study CAO/ARO/AIO-04 showed an increase in the pathologic complete response rate in patients that received neoadjuvant LCRT with additional oxaliplatin (17 vs 13%).[38] This effect was also associated with better 3-year disease-free survival (75.9 vs 71.2%).[39]

In this context, the tendency has been to adopt the use of LCRT with additional oxaliplatin as the standard of care in patients with LARC.

Notably, there is evidence supporting the use of neoadjuvant chemotherapy in addition to SCRT, with favorable initial overall survival results. The phase II study COPERNICUS reported 73% tumor regression using 4 cycles of chemotherapy based on 5-fluorouracil and Oxaliplatin (FOLFOX) followed by SCRT.[40] The phase III Polish Trial II has demonstrated that the combination of SCRT and FOLFOX versus LCRT was associated with a better 3-year overall survival, without differences in the rate of pathologic complete.[41] However, this difference was not maintained at the 8-year follow-up report.[42]

As a way to avoid potential RT toxicities, prevent distant failure and benefit overall survival, the use of neoadjuvant chemotherapy alone has been proposed. A single-institution phase II trial[43] with 32 patients demonstrated that the selective elimination of preoperative RT might be feasible in patients with LARC using 6 cycles of FOLFOX plus bevacizumab. All patients with neoadjuvant chemotherapy had an adequate clinical response allowing TME without adding RT. The authors reported a 25% of pathologic complete response. Disease-free survival at 4 years was 84%. Recently, the multicenter phase II/III trial PROSPECT Trial investigated the selective use of RT in patients with intermediate-risk LARC (T1/2N1, T3N0, or T3N1) with a negative preoperative circumferential margin and who are eligible for sphincter-preserving surgery.[44] The trial completed accrual in late 2019 and results will be available as soon as the prespecified endpoints are met as measured by the Alliance for Clinical Trials study team (Dr Schrag, Dr Shi, and colleagues). Overall, these data have led to the consideration of transferring the use of adjuvant systemic chemotherapy to the NAT setting to improve survival and to actively search for optimal ways in which to improve both pathologic and clinical complete response (cCR) rates in patients with LARC.

TOTAL NEOADJUVANT THERAPY

The concept of total neoadjuvant therapy (TNT) implies the use of SCRT or LCRT and the full adjuvant dose of chemotherapy as part of NAT. It has been proposed that TNT may have the potential ability to reduce the risk of systemic recurrence and to enhance the rate of pathologic and clinical response,[45] in addition to giving the chance for organ preservation in selected patients.

One of the largest series published about the adoption of TNT came from the Memorial Sloan Kettering group.[45] This retrospective cohort of 608 patients of which half received TNT, reported a 35,7% complete response rate (pathological complete response/sustained clinical complete response) without differences in overall survival or distant metastasis, better adherence to systemic therapy and early loop ileostomy closure. Using a consolidation TNT approach (LCRT followed by consolidation chemotherapy), Garcia-Aguilar and colleagues published the phase II TIMING trial using LCRT followed by 2,4 and 6 cycles of FOLFOX, reporting a 38% pathologic complete response rate in the last group[46] and a better 5-year disease-free survival.[47] Another Spanish phase II trial (GCR-3) compared the use of standard of care (LCRT + surgery + adjuvant chemotherapy) versus 4 cycles of neoadjuvant CAPOX followed by LCRT and surgery. The authors did not report differences in overall and disease-free survival, but noted a higher compliance to neoadjuvant chemotherapy (94% vs 57%).[48]

Currently, there is no consensus as to the best TNT strategy. The phase II German trial CAO/ARO/AIO-12 compared 4 cycles of FOLFOX before (induction) or after (consolidation) LCRT. They reported 17% (induction) and 25% (consolidation) pathologic complete response rates, respectively.[49] The OPRA trial compared the use of induction versus consolidation chemotherapy in addition to LCRT.[50] This trial is the first to address the effect of the sequence of NAT in the context of modern TNT approaches, while incorporating a watch-and-wait (WW) option for patients who achieved a cCR to TNT. Preliminary results showed similar rates of disease-free survival and distant metastasis for both arms, but with a higher rate of organ preservation for those managed by a WW strategy at 3 years in the consolidation chemotherapy group (58% vs 43%).

The PRODIGE 23 trial[51] randomized patients with LARC to either 6 cycles of neoadjuvant mFOLFIRINOX followed by LCRT and surgery and 3 months of adjuvant chemotherapy or standard of care (LCRT + surgery + adjuvant chemotherapy).

Patients in the mFOLFIRINOX arm had a higher rate of pathologic complete response (27.5% vs 11.7%, P-value<.001) and better 3-year rates of disease-free survival (75.7% vs 68.5%, P-value = .034).

Of note, 2-phase III studies using SCRT and consolidation chemotherapy have shown higher rates of pathologic complete response and potential benefits in overall survival. The RAPIDO Trial evaluated 920 patients with high-risk LARC (cT4c, cN2, compromised radial margin and/or enlarged lateral pelvic lymph nodes), who were randomized to either SCRT followed by consolidation systemic chemotherapy (6 cycles of CAPOX or 9 cycles of FOLFOX) and TME surgery or standard of care (LCRT, TME then adjuvant chemotherapy).[52] Patients in the experimental arm had higher rate of pathologic complete response (27.7% vs 13.8%, P-value<.01) and a lower 3-year rate of disease-related treatment failure (23.7% vs 30.4%, P-value = .02).

Recently, the STELLAR trial showed results comparing SCRT plus 4 cycles of CAPOX versus standard LCRT followed by surgery. Both groups received adjuvant CAPOX as well. The SCRT group had higher rates of pathologic complete response rates plus cCR (22.5% vs 12.6% in the control group) and higher rates of 3-year overall survival (86.5% vs 75.1%).[53]

Novel agents such as PD-L1 blockers have gained interest in the treatment of CRC.[54,55] The recent NRG-GI002 study[56] evaluated the addition of neoadjuvant and adjuvant pembrolizumab in the context of TNT (4 months of induction FOLFOX followed by LCRT) for distal, bulky, and high risk of metastasis LARC. There were no differences in rates of pathologic complete response (31.9 vs 29.4%, P = .75) and cCR (13.9 vs 13.6%, P = .95) between the TNT plus pembrolizumab versus TNT alone group. Even in the absence of long-term results of phase III trials comparing TNT versus standard of care, NCCN guidelines now recommend FOLFOX or CAPOX followed by LCRT as an alternative treatment of patients with stage III rectal cancer.[9]

TOXICITY AND FUNCTIONAL OUTCOMES OF NEOADJUVANT TREATMENT

Although NAT and surgery are part of the standard of care in patients with LARC, the combination of both of them is associated with significant morbidity (as high as 30%).[57] This includes, among others, postoperative complications such as anastomotic leaks, pelvic sepsis, and the need of a temporary/definitive stoma. In addition, oncological rectal resections are frequently associated with late sequelae such as bowel, sexual and urinary dysfunction, all of which significantly affect the quality of life of patients with LARC.[6]

LCRT has been associated as one of the major risk factors in developing low anterior resection syndrome (LARS).[58] In the Memorial Sloan Kettering published experience, the addition of neoadjuvant chemotherapy alone or in association with LCRT was not associated with a negative impact on bowel function.[59] TNT may be associated with better bowel function, especially if a nonoperative management is achieved. Patients under a WW protocol have better bowel function when compared with those who underwent sphincter-preserving TME.[60,61] Nonetheless, neoadjuvant RT seems to exert a detrimental effect on bowel function in patients who undergo rectal preservation.[62]

SUMMARY

The treatment of LARC is challenging and requires a multidisciplinary approach. NAT has improved local control by appropriate use of neoadjuvant RT, meticulous surgical technique, and chemotherapy. However, NAT using LCRT or SCRT prior TME has not yet improved overall survival and it is associated with toxicities and late sequelae that may impair the quality of life of patients with LARC.

TNT may reduce the likelihood of distant metastasis by introducing systemic chemotherapy early in the course of treatment, while enhancing the rates of complete response. Use of the optimal TNT regimen may give patients with LARC a chance for organ preservation in the case of a cCR which may also reduce treatment morbidity without compromising oncologic outcomes in selected patients.

The upcoming results of ongoing trials (eg, OPRA, PROSPECT) will hopefully lead to a more personalized treatment of rectal cancer, based on tumor characteristics and patient preferences.

CLINICS CARE POINTS

- Local recurrence rates have been markedly reduced with the use of preoperative neoadjuvant therapy in patients with locally advanced rectal cancer.
- Despite the current trend to add systemic chemotherapy as part of the neoadjuvant treatment regimen, no clear benefit has been observed in long-term overall survival data (5-year endpoints) in patients with locally advanced rectal cancer.
- Use of mFOLFIRINOX in the recent PRODIGE23 study seems promising relative to 3-year DFS outcomes, but longer term follow-up is required.
- Total Neoadjuvant Therapy using consolidation chemotherapy may be the strategy of choice if higher rates of rectal preservation are desired, but long-term outcomes relative to survival are to be determined with this approach.

DISCLOSURE

The authors have nothing to disclose.

REFERENCES

1. Arnold M, Sierra MS, Laversanne M, et al. Global patterns and trends in colorectal cancer incidence and mortality. Gut 2017;66(4):683–91.
2. Salem ME, Hartley M, Unger K, et al. Neoadjuvant combined-modality therapy for locally advanced rectal cancer and its future direction. Oncology (Williston Park) 2016;30(6):546–62.
3. Monson JRT, Weiser MR, Buie WD, et al. Practice parameters for the management of rectal cancer (revised). Dis Colon Rectum 2013;56(5):535–50.
4. Glynne-Jones R, Wyrwicz L, Tiret E, et al. Rectal cancer: ESMO clinical practice guidelines for diagnosis, treatment and follow-up. Ann Oncol 2017;28(suppl_4): iv22–40.
5. Heald RJ, Husband EM, Ryall RD. The mesorectum in rectal cancer surgery–the clue to pelvic recurrence? Br J Surg 1982;69(10):613–6.
6. Chen TY-T, Wiltink LM, Nout RA, et al. Bowel function 14 years after preoperative short-course radiotherapy and total mesorectal excision for rectal cancer: report of a multicenter randomized trial. Clin Colorectal Cancer 2015;14(2):106–14.
7. Sauer R, Becker H, Hohenberger W, et al. Preoperative versus postoperative chemoradiotherapy for rectal cancer. N Engl J Med 2004;351(17):1731–40.
8. Sauer R, Liersch T, Merkel S, et al. Preoperative versus postoperative chemoradiotherapy for locally advanced rectal cancer: results of the German CAO/ARO/AIO-94 randomized phase III trial after a median follow-up of 11 years. J Clin Oncol 2012;30(16):1926–33.

9. National Comprehensive Cancer Network. NCCN guidelines: rectal cancer. Available at: https://www.nccn.org/professionals/physician_gls/pdf/rectal.pdf. Accessed December 30, 2021.

10. Heald RJ, Ryall RD. Recurrence and survival after total mesorectal excision for rectal cancer. Lancet 1986;1(8496):1479–82.

11. MacFarlane JK, Ryall RD, Heald RJ. Mesorectal excision for rectal cancer. Lancet 1993;341(8843):457–60.

12. Pettersson D, Lörinc E, Holm T, et al. Tumour regression in the randomized Stockholm III Trial of radiotherapy regimens for rectal cancer. Br J Surg 2015;102(8):972–8 [discussion 978].

13. Swedish Rectal Cancer Trial, Cedermark B, Dahlberg M, et al. Improved survival with preoperative radiotherapy in resectable rectal cancer. N Engl J Med 1997;336(14):980–7.

14. Kapiteijn E, Marijnen CA, Nagtegaal ID, et al. Preoperative radiotherapy combined with total mesorectal excision for resectable rectal cancer. N Engl J Med 2001;345(9):638–46.

15. Sebag-Montefiore D, Stephens RJ, Steele R, et al. Preoperative radiotherapy versus selective postoperative chemoradiotherapy in patients with rectal cancer (MRC CR07 and NCIC-CTG C016): a multicentre, randomised trial. Lancet 2009;373(9666):811–20.

16. Peeters KCMJ, Marijnen CAM, Nagtegaal ID, et al. The TME trial after a median follow-up of 6 years: increased local control but no survival benefit in irradiated patients with resectable rectal carcinoma. Ann Surg 2007;246(5):693–701.

17. Gérard J-P, Conroy T, Bonnetain F, et al. Preoperative radiotherapy with or without concurrent fluorouracil and leucovorin in T3-4 rectal cancers: results of FFCD 9203. J Clin Oncol 2006;24(28):4620–5.

18. Bosset J-F, Collette L, Calais G, et al. Chemotherapy with preoperative radiotherapy in rectal cancer. N Engl J Med 2006;355(11):1114–23.

19. Roh MS, Colangelo LH, O'Connell MJ, et al. Preoperative multimodality therapy improves disease-free survival in patients with carcinoma of the rectum: NSABP R-03. J Clin Oncol 2009;27(31):5124–30.

20. Park J, Yoon SM, Yu CS, et al. Randomized phase 3 trial comparing preoperative and postoperative chemoradiotherapy with capecitabine for locally advanced rectal cancer. Cancer 2011;117(16):3703–12.

21. Rödel C, Martus P, Papadoupolos T, et al. Prognostic significance of tumor regression after preoperative chemoradiotherapy for rectal cancer. J Clin Oncol 2005;23(34):8688–96.

22. Park IJ, You YN, Agarwal A, et al. Neoadjuvant treatment response as an early response indicator for patients with rectal cancer. J Clin Oncol 2012;30(15):1770–6.

23. Fokas E, Liersch T, Fietkau R, et al. Tumor regression grading after preoperative chemoradiotherapy for locally advanced rectal carcinoma revisited: updated results of the CAO/ARO/AIO-94 trial. J Clin Oncol 2014;32(15):1554–62.

24. Ngan SY, Burmeister B, Fisher RJ, et al. Randomized trial of short-course radiotherapy versus long-course chemoradiation comparing rates of local recurrence in patients with T3 rectal cancer: Trans-Tasman Radiation Oncology Group trial 01.04. J Clin Oncol 2012;30(31):3827–33.

25. Bosset J-F, Calais G, Mineur L, et al. Fluorouracil-based adjuvant chemotherapy after preoperative chemoradiotherapy in rectal cancer: long-term results of the EORTC 22921 randomised study. Lancet Oncol 2014;15(2):184–90.

26. Maas M, Nelemans PJ, Valentini V, et al. Long-term outcome in patients with a pathological complete response after chemoradiation for rectal cancer: a pooled analysis of individual patient data. Lancet Oncol 2010;11(9):835–44.

27. Martin ST, Heneghan HM, Winter DC. Systematic review and meta-analysis of outcomes following pathological complete response to neoadjuvant chemoradiotherapy for rectal cancer. Br J Surg 2012;99(7):918–28.

28. Bujko K, Nowacki MP, Nasierowska-Guttmejer A, et al. Long-term results of a randomized trial comparing preoperative short-course radiotherapy with preoperative conventionally fractionated chemoradiation for rectal cancer. Br J Surg 2006;93(10):1215–23.

29. Erlandsson J, Holm T, Pettersson D, et al. Optimal fractionation of preoperative radiotherapy and timing to surgery for rectal cancer (Stockholm III): a multicentre, randomised, non-blinded, phase 3, non-inferiority trial. Lancet Oncol 2017;18(3):336–46.

30. Erlandsson J, Lörinc E, Ahlberg M, et al. Tumour regression after radiotherapy for rectal cancer - Results from the randomised Stockholm III trial,. Radiother Oncol, 135, 2019;178–86.

31. De Caluwé L, Van Nieuwenhove Y, Ceelen WP. Preoperative chemoradiation versus radiation alone for stage II and III resectable rectal cancer. Cochrane Database Syst Rev 2013;(2):CD006041.

32. Schmoll H-J, Haustermans K, Price TJ, et al. Preoperative chemoradiotherapy and postoperative chemotherapy with capecitabine +/- oxaliplatin in locally advanced rectal cancer: final results of PETACC-6. J Clin Orthod 2018;36(15_suppl):3500.

33. Banwell VC, Phillips HA, Duff MJ, et al. Five-year oncological outcomes after selective neoadjuvant radiotherapy for resectable rectal cancer. Acta Oncol 2019;58(9):1267–72.

34. Rahbari NN, Elbers H, Askoxylakis V, et al. Neoadjuvant radiotherapy for rectal cancer: meta-analysis of randomized controlled trials. Ann Surg Oncol 2013;20(13):4169–82.

35. Gérard J-P, Azria D, Gourgou-Bourgade S, et al. Comparison of two neoadjuvant chemoradiotherapy regimens for locally advanced rectal cancer: results of the phase III trial ACCORD 12/0405-Prodige 2. J Clin Oncol 2010;28(10):1638–44.

36. O'Connell MJ, Colangelo LH, Beart RW, et al. Capecitabine and oxaliplatin in the preoperative multimodality treatment of rectal cancer: surgical end points from National Surgical Adjuvant Breast and Bowel Project trial R-04. J Clin Oncol 2014;32(18):1927–34.

37. Aschele C, Lonardi S, Cionini L, et al. Final results of STAR-01: a randomized phase III trial comparing preoperative chemoradiation with or without oxaliplatin in locally advanced rectal cancer. J Clin Orthod 2016;34(15_suppl):3521.

38. Rödel C, Liersch T, Becker H, et al. Preoperative chemoradiotherapy and postoperative chemotherapy with fluorouracil and oxaliplatin versus fluorouracil alone in locally advanced rectal cancer: initial results of the German CAO/ARO/AIO-04 randomised phase 3 trial. Lancet Oncol 2012;13(7):679–87.

39. Rödel C, Graeven U, Fietkau R, et al. Oxaliplatin added to fluorouracil-based preoperative chemoradiotherapy and postoperative chemotherapy of locally advanced rectal cancer (the German CAO/ARO/AIO-04 study): final results of the multicentre, open-label, randomised, phase 3 trial. Lancet Oncol 2015;16(8):979–89.

40. Gollins S, West N, Sebag-Montefiore D, et al. A prospective phase II study of pre-operative chemotherapy then short-course radiotherapy for high risk rectal cancer: COPERNICUS. Br J Cancer 2018;119(6):697–706.
41. Bujko K, Wyrwicz L, Rutkowski A, et al. Long-course oxaliplatin-based preoperative chemoradiation versus 5 × 5 Gy and consolidation chemotherapy for cT4 or fixed cT3 rectal cancer: results of a randomized phase III study. Ann Oncol 2016; 27(5):834–42.
42. Cisel B, Pietrzak L, Michalski W, et al. Long-course preoperative chemoradiation versus 5 × 5 Gy and consolidation chemotherapy for clinical T4 and fixed clinical T3 rectal cancer: long-term results of the randomized Polish II study. Ann Oncol 2019;30(8):1298–303.
43. Schrag D, Weiser MR, Goodman KA, et al. Neoadjuvant chemotherapy without routine use of radiation therapy for patients with locally advanced rectal cancer: a pilot trial. J Clin Oncol 2014;32(6):513–8.
44. Schrag D, Weiser M, Saltz L, et al. Challenges and solutions in the design and execution of the PROSPECT Phase II/III neoadjuvant rectal cancer trial (NCCTG N1048/Alliance). Clin Trials 2019;16(2):165–75.
45. Cercek A, Roxburgh CSD, Strombom P, et al. Adoption of total neoadjuvant therapy for locally advanced rectal cancer. JAMA Oncol 2018;4(6):e180071.
46. Garcia-Aguilar J, Chow OS, Smith DD, et al. Effect of adding mFOLFOX6 after neoadjuvant chemoradiation in locally advanced rectal cancer: a multicentre, phase 2 trial. Lancet Oncol 2015;16(8):957–66.
47. Marco MR, Zhou L, Patil S, et al. Consolidation mFOLFOX6 chemotherapy after chemoradiotherapy improves survival in patients with locally advanced rectal cancer: final results of a multicenter phase II trial. Dis Colon Rectum 2018; 61(10):1146–55.
48. Fernandez-Martos C, Garcia-Albeniz X, Pericay C, et al. Chemoradiation, surgery and adjuvant chemotherapy versus induction chemotherapy followed by chemoradiation and surgery: long-term results of the Spanish GCR-3 phase II randomized trial. Ann Oncol 2015;26(8):1722–8.
49. Fokas E, Allgäuer M, Polat B, et al. Randomized phase II trial of chemoradiotherapy plus induction or consolidation chemotherapy as total neoadjuvant therapy for locally advanced rectal cancer: CAO/ARO/AIO-12. J Clin Oncol 2019; 37(34):3212–22.
50. Garcia-Aguilar J, Patil S, Jin Kim, et al. Preliminary results of the organ preservation of rectal adenocarcinoma (OPRA) trial. Journal of Clinical Oncology 2020 38:15_suppl, 4008-4008.
51. Conroy T, Bosset J-F, Etienne P-L, et al. Neoadjuvant chemotherapy with FOLFIRINOX and preoperative chemoradiotherapy for patients with locally advanced rectal cancer (UNICANCER-PRODIGE 23): a multicentre, randomised, open-label, phase 3 trial. Lancet Oncol 2021;22(5):702–15.
52. Bahadoer RR, Dijkstra EA, van Etten B, et al. Short-course radiotherapy followed by chemotherapy before total mesorectal excision (TME) versus preoperative chemoradiotherapy, TME, and optional adjuvant chemotherapy in locally advanced rectal cancer (RAPIDO): a randomised, open-label, phase 3 trial. Lancet Oncol 2021;22(1):29–42.
53. A multicenter, randomized, phase III trial of short-term radiotherapy plus chemotherapy versus long-term chemoradiotherapy in locally advanced rectal cancer (STELLAR): The final reports. J Clin Oncol.
54. Le DT, Uram JN, Wang H, et al. PD-1 blockade in tumors with mismatch-repair deficiency. N Engl J Med 2015;372(26):2509–20.

55. André T, Shiu K-K, Kim TW, et al. Pembrolizumab in microsatellite-instability-high advanced colorectal cancer. N Engl J Med 2020;383(23):2207–18.
56. Rahma OE, Yothers G, Hong TS, et al. Use of total neoadjuvant therapy for locally advanced rectal cancer: initial results from the pembrolizumab arm of a phase 2 randomized clinical trial. JAMA Oncol 2021;7(8):1225–30.
57. Longo WE, Virgo KS, Johnson FE, et al. Risk factors for morbidity and mortality after colectomy for colon cancer. Dis Colon Rectum 2000;43(1):83–91.
58. Bregendahl S, Emmertsen KJ, Lous J, et al. Bowel dysfunction after low anterior resection with and without neoadjuvant therapy for rectal cancer: a population-based cross-sectional study. Colorectal Dis 2013;15(9):1130–9.
59. Quezada-Diaz F, Jimenez-Rodriguez RM, Pappou EP, et al. Effect of neoadjuvant systemic chemotherapy with or without chemoradiation on bowel function in rectal cancer patients treated with total mesorectal excision. J Gastrointest Surg 2019;23(4):800–7.
60. Hupkens BJP, Martens MH, Stoot JH, et al. Quality of life in rectal cancer patients after chemoradiation: watch-and-wait policy versus standard resection - a matched-controlled study. Dis Colon Rectum 2017;60(10):1032–40.
61. Quezada-Diaz FF, Smith JJ, Jimenez-Rodriguez RM, et al. Patient-reported bowel function in patients with rectal cancer managed by a watch-and-wait strategy after neoadjuvant therapy: a case-control study. Dis Colon Rectum 2020;63(7): 897–902.
62. Wang K, Tepper JE. Radiation therapy-associated toxicity: etiology, management, and prevention. CA Cancer J Clin 2021;71(5):437–54.

Complete Mesocolic Excision and Extent of Lymphadenectomy for the Treatment of Colon Cancer

Tsuyoshi Konishi, MD, PhD*, Y. Nancy You, MD, MHSc

KEYWORDS

- Colon cancer • Complete mesocolic excision • Central vascular ligation
- D3 dissection

KEY POINTS

- CME with CVL emphasizes an anatomy-based approach to the resection of tumor and regional lymph nodes that does not breach the embryonic visceral fascia and ensures complete lymph node dissection up to the mesenteric root.
- Adoption of CME with CVL has been associated with improved oncologic outcomes for stage II–III colon cancer in multiple retrospective observational studies. Oncologic outcome data from prospective trials are currently lacking.
- Completeness of mesocolic plane dissection, lymph nodes harvested, and circumferential resection margin in the surgical specimen impact oncologic outcomes.
- D3 dissection is an overlapping concept to CME with CVL that involves the same surgical technical principles but can be associated with shorter length of bowel resection.
- There is limited evidence to support an absolute superiority of a particular approach for CME among the open, laparoscopic or robotic approaches, and the approach must be determined by surgeon's technical experiences.

INTRODUCTION

The primary curative-intent treatment of patients diagnosed with nonmetastatic colon cancer is colectomy ensuring R0 tumor resection with en-bloc removal of the regional lymph nodes.[1,2] Optimal oncologic principles of colectomy for colon cancer include embryonic plane-based anatomic dissection, en-bloc specimen in a visceral package

Department of Colon and Rectal Surgery, Division of Surgery, The University of Texas MD Anderson Cancer Center, 1400 Pressler Street, Unit 1484, PO Box 301402, Houston, TX 77230, USA
* Corresponding author. Department of Colon and Rectal Surgery, Division of Surgery, The University of Texas MD Anderson Cancer Center, 1400 Pressler Street, Unit 1484, PO Box 301402, Houston, TX 77230.
E-mail address: tkonishi@mdanderson.org

Surg Oncol Clin N Am 31 (2022) 293–306
https://doi.org/10.1016/j.soc.2021.11.009
1055-3207/22/© 2021 Elsevier Inc. All rights reserved.
surgonc.theclinics.com

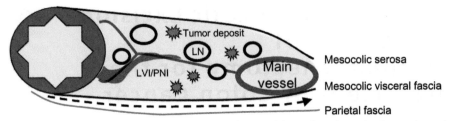

Fig. 1. Concept of CME with CVL. The concept of CME with CVL is embryonic plane-oriented dissection that achieves the resection of primary tumor and regional mesocolic spread within an en-bloc visceral package of the mesocolon. Dissection follows the plane between the mesocolic visceral fascia and parietal fascia (*arrow*). LN, lymph node; LVI, lymphovascular invasion; PNI, perineural invasion

with appropriate circumferential tumor-free margin and vascular-oriented lymph node dissection.

The extent of colectomy is defined by the tumor location and feeding/draining vessels that contain regional lymph nodes within the mesentery. Over the past decades, adoption of a standardized, anatomically based surgical technique called complete mesocolic excision (CME) with central vascular ligation (CVL) has been described as a technique to increase the thoroughness of tumor resection and lymph node dissection, theoretically leading to more accurate staging and improved survival outcomes.[3–7] In the East, radical and meticulous regional lymph node dissection (ie, D3 dissection) has been standardized and performed under established guidelines for decades.[8] Greater than 90% overall survival for stage II–III colon cancers has been reported with the D3 dissection.[9] In recent years, adoption of minimally invasive approaches within an enhanced recovery program further improved short term outcomes including length of hospital stay and postoperative complication rates.[10–12] These surgical techniques have yet to be universally adopted in oncology care guidelines.[13,14] However, surgeons have recently focused more attention to and have shown wider uptake of these technical advances in the United States[15,16] This article aims to review the modern surgical oncologic principles for nonmetastatic locoregional colon cancer, particularly focusing on the West and East approaches.

MODERN ONCOLOGIC PRINCIPLES OF SURGERY FOR COLON CANCER IN THE WEST: COMPLETE MESOCOLIC EXCISION WITH CENTRAL VASCULAR LIGATION

As first reported by Hohenberger and colleagues,[5] CME with CVL is the sharp dissection of the visceral mesocolic fascia from the parietal retroperitoneal fascia that achieves the complete mobilization of the entire mesocolon. The key concept of CME is that the embryonic visceral fascia is not breached during sharp dissection. Thus, this technique provides anatomy-based resection of tumor and regional lymph nodes, and avoids tumor spillage and spread within the peritoneal cavity (**Fig. 1**). The concept is quite similar to that of total mesorectal excision (TME) which is an established surgical principle in rectal cancer that ensures the resection of the tumor and regional lymph nodes within the visceral package of the mesorectum.[17]

Whereas CME represents mesocolic plane-based sharp dissection, CVL emphasizes adequate proximal lymph node dissection to the root of the mesocolon and ensures complete lymph node dissection up to the central nodes. In general, lymphatic spread of colon cancer first arrives in the pericolic lymph nodes, typically within 8 cm from the primary tumor, then toward the lymph nodes following along the feeding

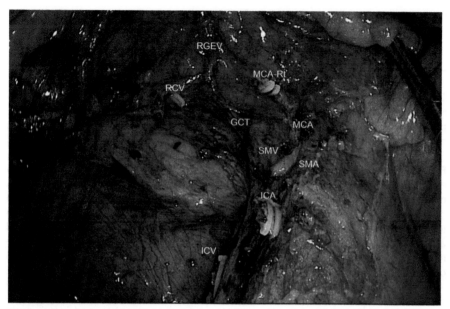

Fig. 2. Surgical view after CME with CVL or D3 dissection for right colon cancer Regional feeding arteries and drainage veins are divided at the root from the superior mesenteric artery/vein. *Abbreviations:* GCT, gastrocolic trunk (Henle's trunk); ICA, ileocolic artery; ICV, ileocolic vein; MCA, middle colic artery; MCA-Rt, right branch of the middle colic artery; RCV, right colic vein; RGEV, right gastroepiploic vein; SMA, superior mesenteric artery; SMV, superior mesenteric vein.

arteries centripedally.[18,19] In CME with CVL, supplying vessels are divided at their origin to ensure proximal lymph node dissection.

For right colon cancer, the original procedure by Hohenberger describes division of the feeding vessels at their origin from the superior mesenteric artery (SMA) and vein (SMV) with exposure of these superior mesenteric vessels to ensure central lymph node dissection (**Fig. 2**). For left colon cancer, the inferior mesenteric artery (IMA) is divided at the root.

ONCOLOGIC IMPACT OF COMPLETE MESOCOLIC EXCISION WITH CENTRAL VASCULAR LIGATION

A retrospective observational cohort study by the Hohenberger's group reported a significant improvement of oncologic outcomes in stage III colon cancer after the implementation of CME with CVL.[20] Although the oncologic improvements in this study likely reflect advancements along the spectrum of care including surgery, staging and adjuvant chemotherapy, the study reported improvement in 5-year cancer-specific survival from 62% to 81% and 5-year local recurrence rate from 15% to 4.1%. The population-based observational cohort study by the Danish Colorectal Cancer Group[21] suggested a 10% improvement in 4-year disease-free survival after the adoption of CME than conventional colectomy for stage I–III colon cancers (86% after CME vs 76% after non-CME), and CME was independently associated with improved outcomes irrespective of the stage. Similar findings of improved survival and reduction of local recurrence without major increase in morbidity and mortality were reported in observational studies from China and Sweden,[22,23] and have been demonstrated in several meta-analyses and systematic reviews.[24–26] Although the current data are all retrospective and are yet to be validated through prospective randomization, improved outcomes through the adoption of this surgical technique deserves attention.[14]

PATHOLOGY GRADING OF SURGICAL SPECIMEN

The mesocolon has recently gained attention for its oncologic importance beyond lymph node metastasis to include pathologic evidence of venous invasion, tumor deposits and perineural invasion. The most fundamental concept in the CME with CVL is embryonic plane-oriented dissection that achieves the resection of primary tumor and regional mesocolic spread within an en-bloc visceral package of the mesocolon (see **Fig. 1**). In keeping with this principle, the quality of the mesocolic plane dissection as measured by the degree of breaching of the visceral fascia may be a key determinant of outcomes in colon cancer similar to the TME concept in rectal cancer. West and colleagues[27] proposed the pathology grading of the colon cancer specimen according to the plane of mesocolic dissection. This study found a 15% 5-year overall survival advantage with surgical resection carried out along the mesocolic plane versus the muscularis propria plane. Another study that compared surgical specimens from colectomy with CME with CVL versus conventional approach revealed that CME with CVL removed more tissue compared with conventional colectomy, including 4 cm wider span distance from the tumor to the high vascular tie, greater than 10 cm longer length of resected bowel and more than 1.5 times larger area of mesentery, resulting in a greater lymph node yield (30 vs 18) with a higher proportion of nonbreached mesocolic plane resections (92% vs 40%).[2]

D3 DISSECTION: CONCEPT FROM THE EAST

D3 dissection is a radical regional lymph node dissection that has been routinely conducted as standard of care in Japan for decades.[8] Technically, D3 dissection is an overlapping concept with CME with CVL and also emphasizes the principle of resecting the entire mesocolon within embryonic fascia up to the root of feeding vessels. In the Japanese classification, anatomic location of each harvested lymph node in the surgical specimen is mapped and coded per the predefined location number (**Fig. 3**).[28] With such meticulous vascular-oriented anatomic mapping, the regional lymph nodes are classified into pericolic (along the marginal artery), intermediate (along the feeding artery) and central (along the surface of the SMV/SMA in the right colon cancer and at the root of IMA in the left colon cancer).

The Japanese Classification defines the extent of lymph node dissection from D0 to D3 as follows.

D0: incomplete dissection of pericolic lymph nodes D1: complete dissection of pericolic lymph nodes.

D2: complete dissection of pericolic and intermediate lymph nodes up to the root of feeding arteries that runs into the bowel within 10 cm from the tumor.

D3: complete dissection of regional lymph nodes including pericolic, intermediate and central lymph nodes.

Besides proximal extent of the lymphatic spread, the Japanese classification defines horizontal lymphatic spread within 10 cm from the tumors as regional. This is based on the Japanese studies showing that longitudinal spread greater than 10 cm beyond the tumor is extremely rare, occurring in 1% to 4% for right-sided tumors and 0% for left-sided tumors.[18,19] All the feeding vessels within 10 cm from the tumors are regarded as regional and are to be resected to achieve complete regional lymph node dissection (**Fig. 4**).

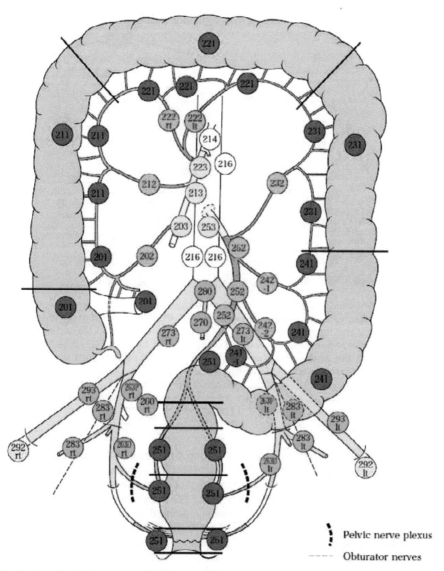

Fig. 3. Lymph node groups and station numbers in the Japanese Classification of Colorectal, Appendiceal, and Anal Carcinoma: the 3d English Edition. Red: Pericolic/perirectal lymph nodes; Blue: Intermediate lymph nodes; Yellow: Main lymph nodes; Green: Lateral lymph nodes (for rectum); White: Lymph nodes proximal to the main lymph nodes. (*Reprinted with permission from* the Japanese Society for Cancer of the Colon and Rectum and Kanehara & Co., Ltd.: Japanese Classification of Colorectal, Appendiceal, and Anal Carcinoma-the 3rd English edition, 2019.)

D3 DISSECTION VERSUS COMPLETE MESOCOLIC EXCISION WITH CENTRAL VASCULAR LIGATION

In principle, D3 dissection and CME with CVL are overlapping technical concepts that both emphasize the need to resect the entire mesocolon in a visceral package with

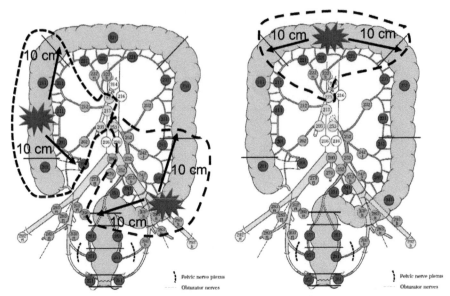

Fig. 4. Extent of lymph node dissection in D3 dissection. Central extent of the lymph node dissection is similar, whereas horizontal extent (length of bowel resection) is shorter in D3 dissection, taking the feeding arteries within 10 cm proximal distal to the tumor. For the right colon cancer and left colon cancer, feeding arteries taken by D3 dissection is the same as CME with CVL as the vessels are within 10 cm from the tumor (*left*). For transverse colon cancer, D3 dissection is defined as transverse colectomy as ileocolic artery is beyond 10 cm from the tumor (*right*). (*Reprinted with permission from* the Japanese Society for Cancer of the Colon and Rectum and Kanehara & Co., Ltd.: Japanese Classification of Colorectal, Appendiceal, and Anal Carcinoma-the 3rd English edition, 2019.)

proximal lymph node dissection along the feeding arteries up to the root of the mesenteric artery. Despite such similarity, there are a few differences worth highlighting between the 2 procedures (**Table 1**). An international collaborative group from Europe and Japan compared the surgical specimen of D3 dissection and CME with CVL.[7] Both techniques showed high rates of resection along the mesocolic plane resection rates and similarly high rates of specimens showing long distances between the bowel wall to the high vascular tie. However, Japanese D3 specimens were significantly shorter in bowel length (162 versus 324 mm, $P<.001$), resulting in a smaller amount of resected mesentery (8309 vs 17,957 mm^2). Lymph node yield was higher in the CME with CVL (median, 18 vs 32), but the number of metastatic nodes was equivalent between the 2 techniques. As shown in the Japanese studies,[18,19] significant longitudinal lymphatic spread is rare in colon cancer, and therefore, it is not surprising that the CME with CVL did not have an increased number of positive nodes compared with D3 dissection. Importantly, the distance between the high vascular tie and the closest bowel wall was equivalent in the 2 techniques, suggesting a similar degree of central radicality of resection. This translated to oncologically superior pathologic outcomes associated with both techniques as compared with those previously reported from other countries. Another study that focused on stage III disease confirmed similar trends.[29] In summary, D3 dissection is identical to CME with CVL in the principles of mesocolic plane-oriented dissection and central lymph node dissection, but differs in resulting a specimen of shorter length of resected bowel.

Table 1
Comparison of CME with CVL versus D3 dissection

	Tumor Location	CME with CVL	D3
Dissection plane		Mesocolic	Mesocolic
Proximal extent of LN dissection	Right-Transverse colon	SMV/SMA	SMV/SMA
	Left colon	IMA root	IMA root
Horizontal extent of bowel resection		Longer	10 cm each from the tumor
Resected arteries	Right colon	ICA, RCA, MCA-Rt	ICA, RCA, (MCA-Rt if within 10 cm)
	Transverse	ICA, RCA, MCA, (RGEA)	MCA
	Left colon	IMA	IMA

Abbreviations: ICA, ileocolic artery; IMA, inferior mesenteric artery; MCA, middle colic artery; RCA, right colic artery (if present); RGEA, right gastroepiploic artery; SMV/SMA, superior mesenteric vein/artery.

ONCOLOGIC OUTCOMES OF D3 DISSECTION

Along with meticulous anatomic mapping of regional lymph nodes, data from Japanese D3 dissection showed several important findings. First, central location of positive lymph nodes is independently prognostic in addition to the number of positive lymph nodes in stage III disease.[30,31] Central lymph node metastasis has been shown to correlate with poorer outcomes: after D3 right hemicolectomy, the 5-year overall survival rates with and without central nodal metastasis were 85% and 60% in stage IIIB disease.[30] Second, the incidence of central lymph node metastasis (D3 area) is 3% (overall; 5% in T4 tumors),[8,30,32] whereas the incidence of the intermediate lymph node metastasis (D2 area along the feeding arteries) exceeds 10%. Thus, ensuring adequate D2 dissection and extending to include D3 dissection is critically important for the resection of stage II–III disease. Finally, D3 dissection has been associated with over 50% survival in patients with positive central nodes, suggesting a potential oncological benefit from D3 dissection.[31] A propensity score-matched study from a Japanese multicenter prospective registry revealed that for pathologic T3-4 colon cancer, D3 dissection offered overall survival advantage when compared with D2 dissection (hazard ratio 0.827, 95% confidence interval 0.76–0.90).[33] Excellent oncological outcomes and safety of D3 dissection have also been reported in a multicenter prospective study regardless of laparoscopic or open approaches.[9] Based on these data, the Japanese treatment guidelines recommend D3 dissection for T3-4 colon cancers. Many Japanese surgeons postulate that the benefit of D3 dissection exists in ensuring central radicality with complete D2 dissection up to the root of the mesentery by exposing SMV/SMA or the root of IMA.

Prospective Studies

While retrospective studies have consistently suggested oncologic advantage and surgical safety of CME with CVL and of D3 dissection, there has been no oncologic outcome data from prospective randomized controlled trial that have compared these techniques against "conventional" colectomy. Currently, the Chinese RELARC trial and the Russian COLD trial have reported short term outcomes only.[34,35] The final oncologic results are still awaited.

The RELARC trial is a multicenter phase III randomized superiority trial that assesses the safety and oncologic impact of CME with CVL versus D2 dissection without central node dissection (ClinicalTrials.gov, NCT02619942). The primary endpoint is 3-year disease-free survival. A total of 995 patients were included in the modified intention-to-treat analyses of short-term outcomes (495 in the CME group, 500 in D2 dissection group). The overall postoperative surgical complications were similar (20% in CME, 22% in D2), but Clavien-Dindo grade III–IV complications were less frequent in the CME group than in the D2 group (1% vs 3%, $P = .022$), and there was no mortality in either group. Among intraoperative complications, vascular injury was more frequently observed in the CME group (3% vs 1%, $P = .045$). Metastases in the central lymph nodes were detected in 3.3% in the CME group. Pathologic examination of the specimen revealed larger area of removed mesocolon (115 vs 108 cm^2) with larger number of lymph node yield (26 vs 23) in the CME group.

The COLD trial is a multicenter phase III superiority randomized controlled trial that assesses oncologic advantage and safety of D3 dissection versus D2 dissection (ClinicalTrials.gov, NCT03009227). The primary endpoint is 5-year overall survival. Nine-two among the first 100 randomized patients were included in the per-protocol analyses of short-term outcomes (53 in the D3 group, 39 in the D2 group). The overall 30-day postoperative surgical complications were similar (47% in D2, 48% in D3) with similar Clavien-Dindo grade III–IV complications (12% in D2, 7% in D3) including 2 cases (5%) of anastomotic leaks in the D2 group. Postoperative recovery and read-mission rates did not differ. The mean lymph node yield was also similar (27 in D2, 28 in D3). Interestingly, good quality of CME was more frequently observed in the D3 group (76% in D2, 92% in D3, $P = .048$). Central nodal metastasis was observed in 5% of the D3 group, while overall nodal positivity was more frequently observed in the D3 group (46% vs 26%, $P = .044$). These results highlight the safety and feasibility of CME with CVL or D3 dissection by experienced surgeons, and suggest potential improvements in surgical pathology outcomes.

The T-REX study is a currently ongoing prospective international multicenter observational study (ClinicalTrials.gov, NCT02938481) designed to define the optimal length of bowel resection and extent of lymph node dissection.[36] This study aims to include a total of 4000 patients with stage I–III colon cancer from 35 specialized centers in 6 Asian and European countries. The anatomic distribution of lymph node metastasis and its relation to the feeding arteries are precisely marked intraoperatively and investigated in surgical specimens, and all patients are followed for long-term oncologic outcomes. The findings of this study are expected to provide fundamental evidence for the international standardization of colon cancer resection through in-depth lymph node mapping.

MINIMALLY INVASIVE APPROACH IN THE ERA OF COMPLETE MESOCOLIC EXCISION WITH CENTRAL VASCULAR LIGATION AND D3 DISSECTION

In the United States, laparoscopic surgery is currently accepted as a standard treatment approach for colon cancer. Laparoscopic colon cancer surgery has been shown to have comparable long-term oncologic outcomes as open surgery in multiple randomized controlled trials and meta-analyses, while also offering more favorable short term outcomes including reduced postoperative pain, reduced ileus, reduced wound infection, faster recovery, and shorter hospital stay.[37–42] The Enroll trial (ISRCTN48516968) is a randomized controlled trial that compared the outcomes of laparoscopic versus open surgery within an enhanced recovery program.[10] The study showed shorter hospital stay in the laparoscopic arm (5 vs 7 days), but other outcomes were similar including complications, physical function such as fatigue, and other patient reported outcomes. However, these trials were conducted before the era of CME with CV and/or did not specify the plane of dissection or extent of vascular tie in the protocol.

The JCOG 0404 trial (UMIN-CTR number C000000105) is the only randomized trial that has specifically mandated D3 dissection per protocol.[9,43] Given the technical similarity and overlap between D3 dissection and CME with CVL as discussed above, the results of this trial are also relevant and valuable for the Western countries. The trial randomized a total of 1057 patients with clinical stage II–III colon cancer to laparoscopic versus open D3 dissection arms. The study ensured quality control through intraoperative photo documentation, which confirmed greater than 98% technical compliance to the D3 dissection in both arms.[44] Conversion to open surgery was observed in 5.4%. The laparoscopic surgery arm had more favorable short-term outcomes including less blood loss, earlier bowel recovery, reduced postoperative pain and a shorter hospital stay, despite longer operative time. The overall perioperative adverse event rate was lower in the laparoscopic arm (14% vs 22%; $P<.001$). The 5-year overall survival was similarly high in the 2 arms (90·4%, 95% CI: 87·5–92·6 for open vs, 91·8%, 95% CI: 89·1–93·8% for laparoscopic). Although the study failed to show noninferiority of the laparoscopic D3 dissection in terms of OS, the more favorable short-term outcomes and the excellent overall survival for stage II–III disease make it a reasonable treatment option.

Robotic assistance is another minimally invasive option for colectomy.[16] Retrospective observational studies suggested less blood loss, earlier bowel recovery, shorter hospital stay and lower postoperative complication rates when compared with laparoscopic colectomy despite longer operative time and higher cost.[45–47] More comparative data regarding long-term outcomes are awaited.

While minimally invasive techniques are generally accepted for curative-intent resection of colon cancer, there is limited evidence to support a superiority of a particular approach for CME/CVL, among open, laparoscopic or robotic options.[48] Thus, CME is feasible by all 3 approaches, and the optimal approach should be determined by the individual surgeon's preference and technical experiences.[14]

CIRCUMFERENTIAL RESECTION MARGIN

Circumferential resection margin (CRM) is defined as the radial margin created during the dissection of colon cancer from the retroperitoneum whereby the adventitial soft tissue is closest to the furthest penetrant edge of the tumor.[14] It is relevant for the aspect of the colon cancer that is secondarily re-retroperitonealized during embryologic development and is determined during surgical pathology assessment. A positive CRM has generally been defined as the presence of malignant tumor within 1 mm of the edge of the resected tumor. While the status of the CRM has been shown to be the most important determinant of outcomes for patients with rectal cancer, its oncologic importance in colon cancer has only recently been gaining attention. In a retrospective series of 148 patients,[49] those with positive CRM (13%) after colectomy experienced significantly lower disease-free and overall survival. Indeed, in a recent audit of the data from the U.S. National Cancer Database, the overall rate of positive CRM after colon cancer resection (2010–2015) was 11.6%, with the highest rates observed for pT4 tumors (25.8%), versus pT1(4.5%), pT2(6.3%) and pT3 (10.9%, $P<.001$).[50] Similarly, another analysis of nearly 190,000 stage II and III colon cancers resected during 2004 to 2015 reported in the NCDB revealed that a positive CRM could be identified in 10.7% of the specimens, with 9% in stage II and 12% in stage III tumors, respectively.[51] Furthermore, after adjusting for available confounders, having a positive CRM was associated with a 1.1-fold risk of death. Importantly, both of these studies identified that positive CRM was independently associated with other high risk pathologic features such as inadequate nodal harvest (fewer than 12 nodes resected) and positive proximal or distal resection margin.

SUMMARY AND FUTURE DIRECTIONS

For curative intent resection of colon cancer, there has been emerging attention focused on complete (nonviolated) mesocolic excision, adequate nodal resection through CVL or D3 dissection and tumor resection with negative CRM. CME with CVL is a modern surgical technique for colon cancer that parallels the TME concept of dissection following the embryologic planes. The procedure appreciates mesocolic plane dissection (iI.e. CME) with lymph node dissection along the feeding artery up to the mesocolic root (ie, CVL). Japanese D3 dissection is an almost identical procedure to CME with CVL except the shorter length of bowel resection (10 cm proximal and distal to the tumor). Improved oncologic outcomes by the adoption of these techniques have been widely reported in large retrospective studies and meta-analyses from both the Western and Eastern countries. However, oncologic outcome data from prospective trials are currently lacking. Despite the lack of randomized trials, encouraging oncologic results have led to wider adoption of these techniques for colon cancer, similar to the case of TME for rectal cancer. Although prospective studies from Asia and Russia showed safety and feasibility of CME with CVL and D3 dissection,[9,34,35] some studies reported high morbidity with these procedures, suggesting potential technical difficulties during the adoption phase.[52-54] Proper surgical training programs and anatomic knowledge are required to establish these techniques as the standard of care for curative-intent treatment of colon cancer.

CLINICS CARE POINTS

- Improved oncologic outcomes by adoption of CME with CVL and D3 dissection have been widely reported in large retrospective studies and meta-analyses from both the Western and Eastern countries, despite prospective trials are currently lacking.
- Although prospective studies showed safety and feasibility of CME with CVL and D3 dissection, some studies reported high morbidity with these procedures suggesting potential technical difficulties during the adoption phase.
- Completeness of the mesocolic plane, number of harvested nodes, and circumferential resection margin in the surgical specimen are pathologic parameters that impact oncologic outcome.
- There is limited evidence to support an absolute superiority of a particular approach for CME among the open, laparoscopic or robotic approaches, and the approach must be determined by surgeon's technical experiences.

DISCLOSURE

The authors have nothing to disclose.

REFERENCES

1. Bass EM, Del Pino A, Tan A, et al. Does preoperative stoma marking and education by the enterostomal therapist affect outcome? Dis Colon Rectum 1997;40(4): 440–2.

2. West NP, Hohenberger W, Weber K, et al. Complete mesocolic excision with central vascular ligation produces an oncologically superior specimen compared with standard surgery for carcinoma of the colon. J Clin Oncol 2010;28(2):272–8.
3. Bertelsen CA, Neuenschwander AU, Jansen JE, et al. Disease-free survival after complete mesocolic excision compared with conventional colon cancer surgery: a retrospective, population-based study. Lancet Oncol 2015;16(2):161–8.
4. Cho MS, Baek SJ, Hur H, et al. Modified complete mesocolic excision with central vascular ligation for the treatment of right-sided colon cancer: long-term outcomes and prognostic factors. Ann Surg 2015;261(4):708–15.
5. Hohenberger W, Weber K, Matzel K, et al. Standardized surgery for colonic cancer: complete mesocolic excision and central ligation–technical notes and outcome. Colorectal Dis 2009;11(4):354–64 [discussion 355–64].
6. Konishi T, Shimada Y, Hsu M, et al. Contemporary validation of a nomogram predicting colon cancer recurrence, revealing all-stage improved outcomes. JNCI Cancer Spectr 2019;3(2):pkz015.
7. West NP, Kobayashi H, Takahashi K, et al. Understanding optimal colonic cancer surgery: comparison of Japanese D3 resection and European complete mesocolic excision with central vascular ligation. J Clin Oncol 2012;30(15):1763–9.
8. Hashiguchi Y, Muro K, Saito Y, et al. Japanese Society for Cancer of the Colon and Rectum (JSCCR) guidelines 2019 for the treatment of colorectal cancer. Int J Clin Oncol 2020;25(1):1–42.
9. Kitano S, Inomata M, Mizusawa J, et al. Survival outcomes following laparoscopic versus open D3 dissection for stage II or III colon cancer (JCOG0404): a phase 3, randomised controlled trial. Lancet Gastroenterol Hepatol 2017;2(4):261–8.
10. Kennedy RH, Francis EA, Wharton R, et al. Multicenter randomized controlled trial of conventional versus laparoscopic surgery for colorectal cancer within an enhanced recovery programme: EnROL. J Clin Oncol 2014;32(17):1804–11.
11. Nelson G, Kiyang LN, Crumley ET, et al. Implementation of enhanced recovery after surgery (ERAS) across a provincial healthcare system: the ERAS Alberta colorectal surgery experience. World J Surg 2016;40(5):1092–103.
12. Varadhan KK, Lobo DN, Ljungqvist O. Enhanced recovery after surgery: the future of improving surgical care. Crit Care Clin 2010;26(3):527–47, x.
13. Argiles G, Tabernero J, Labianca R, et al. Localised colon cancer: ESMO clinical practice guidelines for diagnosis, treatment and follow-up. Ann Oncol 2020;31(10):1291–305.
14. Benson AB, Venook AP, Al-Hawary MM, et al. Colon cancer, version 2.2021, NCCN clinical practice guidelines in oncology. J Natl Compr Canc Netw 2021;19(3):329–59.
15. Hameed I, Aggarwal P, Weiser MR. Robotic extended right hemicolectomy with complete mesocolic excision and D3 lymph node dissection. Ann Surg Oncol 2019;26(12):3990–1.
16. Yang Y, Peacock O, Malakorn S, et al. Superior mesenteric vein-first approach for robotic salvage surgery with indocyanine green fluorescence angiography. Ann Surg Oncol 2020;27(9):3500.
17. Heald RJ, Ryall RD. Recurrence and survival after total mesorectal excision for rectal cancer. Lancet 1986;1(8496):1479–82.
18. Morikawa E, Yasutomi M, Shindou K, et al. Distribution of metastatic lymph nodes in colorectal cancer by the modified clearing method. Dis Colon Rectum 1994;37(3):219–23.
19. Toyota S, Ohta H, Anazawa S. Rationale for extent of lymph node dissection for right colon cancer. Dis Colon Rectum 1995;38(7):705–11.

20. Merkel S, Weber K, Matzel KE, et al. Prognosis of patients with colonic carcinoma before, during and after implementation of complete mesocolic excision. Br J Surg Aug 2016;103(9):1220–9.
21. Bertelsen CA, Neuenschwander AU, Jansen JE, et al. 5-year outcome after complete mesocolic excision for right-sided colon cancer: a population-based cohort study. Lancet Oncol 2019;20(11):1556–65.
22. Bernhoff R, Martling A, Sjovall A, et al. Improved survival after an educational project on colon cancer management in the county of Stockholm–a population based cohort study. Eur J Surg Oncol 2015;41(11):1479–84.
23. Gao Z, Wang C, Cui Y, et al. Efficacy and safety of complete mesocolic excision in patients with colon cancer: three-year results from a prospective, nonrandomized, double-blind, controlled trial. Ann Surg 2020;271(3):519–26.
24. Crane J, Hamed M, Borucki JP, et al. Complete mesocolic excision versus conventional surgery for colon cancer: a systematic review and meta-analysis. Colorectal Dis 2021;23(7):1670–86.
25. Emmanuel A, Haji A. Complete mesocolic excision and extended (D3) lymphadenectomy for colonic cancer: is it worth that extra effort? A review of the literature. Int J Colorectal Dis 2016;31(4):797–804.
26. Mazzarella G, Muttillo EM, Picardi B, et al. Complete mesocolic excision and D3 lymphadenectomy with central vascular ligation in right-sided colon cancer: a systematic review of postoperative outcomes, tumor recurrence and overall survival. Surg Endosc 2021;35(9):4945–55.
27. West NP, Morris EJ, Rotimi O, et al. Pathology grading of colon cancer surgical resection and its association with survival: a retrospective observational study. Lancet Oncol 2008;9(9):857–65.
28. Japanese classification of colorectal, appendiceal, and anal carcinoma: the 3d english edition [Secondary Publication]. J Anus Rectum Colon 2019;3(4):175–95.
29. Kobayashi H, West NP, Takahashi K, et al. Quality of surgery for stage III colon cancer: comparison between England, Germany, and Japan. Ann Surg Oncol 2014;21(Suppl 3):S398–404.
30. Kanemitsu Y, Komori K, Kimura K, et al. D3 lymph node dissection in right hemicolectomy with a no-touch isolation technique in patients with colon cancer. Dis Colon Rectum 2013;56(7):815–24.
31. Nagasaki T, Akiyoshi T, Fujimoto Y, et al. Prognostic impact of distribution of lymph node metastases in stage III colon cancer. World J Surg 2015;39(12):3008–15.
32. Yamaoka Y, Kinugasa Y, Shiomi A, et al. The distribution of lymph node metastases and their size in colon cancer. Langenbecks Arch Surg 2017;402(8):1213–21.
33. Kotake K, Mizuguchi T, Moritani K, et al. Impact of D3 lymph node dissection on survival for patients with T3 and T4 colon cancer. Int J Colorectal Dis 2014;29(7):847–52.
34. Karachun A, Panaiotti L, Chernikovskiy I, et al. Short-term outcomes of a multicentre randomized clinical trial comparing D2 versus D3 lymph node dissection for colonic cancer (COLD trial). Br J Surg 2020;107(5):499–508.
35. Xu L, Su X, He Z, et al. Short-term outcomes of complete mesocolic excision versus D2 dissection in patients undergoing laparoscopic colectomy for right colon cancer (RELARC): a randomised, controlled, phase 3, superiority trial. Lancet Oncol 2021;22(3):391–401.
36. Shiozawa M, Ueno H, Shiomi A, et al. Study protocol for an international prospective observational cohort study for optimal bowel resection extent and central radicality for colon cancer (T-REX study). Jpn J Clin Oncol 2021;51(1):145–55.

37. Jayne DG, Thorpe HC, Copeland J, et al. Five-year follow-up of the Medical Research Council CLASICC trial of laparoscopically assisted versus open surgery for colorectal cancer. Br J Surg 2010;97(11):1638–45.

38. Buunen M, Veldkamp R, Hop WC, et al. Survival after laparoscopic surgery versus open surgery for colon cancer: long-term outcome of a randomised clinical trial. Lancet Oncol 2009;10(1):44–52.

39. Fleshman J, Sargent DJ, Green E, et al. Laparoscopic colectomy for cancer is not inferior to open surgery based on 5-year data from the COST Study Group trial. Ann Surg 2007;246(4):655–62 [discussion 654–62].

40. Lacy AM, Delgado S, Castells A, et al. The long-term results of a randomized clinical trial of laparoscopy-assisted versus open surgery for colon cancer. Ann Surg 2008;248(1):1–7.

41. Schiphorst AH, Verweij NM, Pronk A, et al. Non-surgical complications after laparoscopic and open surgery for colorectal cancer - A systematic review of randomised controlled trials. Eur J Surg Oncol 2015;41(9):1118–27.

42. Sammour T, Malakorn S, Thampy R, et al. Selective central vascular ligation (D3 lymphadenectomy) in patients undergoing minimally invasive complete mesocolic excision for colon cancer: optimizing the risk-benefit equation. Colorectal Dis 2020;22(1):53–61.

43. Yamamoto S, Inomata M, Katayama H, et al. Short-term surgical outcomes from a randomized controlled trial to evaluate laparoscopic and open D3 dissection for stage II/III colon cancer: Japan Clinical Oncology Group Study JCOG 0404. Ann Surg 2014;260(1):23–30.

44. Nakajima K, Inomata M, Akagi T, et al. Quality control by photo documentation for evaluation of laparoscopic and open colectomy with D3 resection for stage II/III colorectal cancer: Japan Clinical Oncology Group Study JCOG 0404. Jpn J Clin Oncol 2014;44(9):799–806.

45. Chang YS, Wang JX, Chang DW. A meta-analysis of robotic versus laparoscopic colectomy. J Surg Res 2015;195(2):465–74.

46. Lim S, Kim JH, Baek SJ, et al. Comparison of perioperative and short-term outcomes between robotic and conventional laparoscopic surgery for colonic cancer: a systematic review and meta-analysis. Ann Surg Treat Res 2016;90(6):328–39.

47. Zarak A, Castillo A, Kichler K, et al. Robotic versus laparoscopic surgery for colonic disease: a meta-analysis of postoperative variables. Surg Endosc 2015;29(6):1341–7.

48. Athanasiou CD, Markides GA, Kotb A, et al. Open compared with laparoscopic complete mesocolic excision with central lymphadenectomy for colon cancer: a systematic review and meta-analysis. Colorectal Dis 2016;18(7):O224–35.

49. Khan MA, Hakeem AR, Scott N, et al. Significance of R1 resection margin in colon cancer resections in the modern era. Colorectal Dis 2015;17(11):943–53.

50. Healy MA, Peacock O, Hu CY, et al. High rate of positive circumferential resection margin in colon cancer: a national appraisal and call for action. Ann Surg 2020;262(6):891–8.

51. Goffredo P, Zhou P, Ginader T, et al. Positive circumferential resection margins following locally advanced colon cancer surgery: risk factors and survival impact. J Surg Oncol 2020;121(3):538–46.

52. Prevost GA, Odermatt M, Furrer M, et al. Postoperative morbidity of complete mesocolic excision and central vascular ligation in right colectomy: a retrospective comparative cohort study. World J Surg Oncol 2018;16(1):214.

53. Bertelsen CA, Neuenschwander AU, Jansen JE, et al. Short-term outcomes after complete mesocolic excision compared with 'conventional' colonic cancer surgery. Br J Surg 2016;103(5):581–9.
54. Wang C, Gao Z, Shen K, et al. Safety, quality and effect of complete mesocolic excision vs non-complete mesocolic excision in patients with colon cancer: a systemic review and meta-analysis. Colorectal Dis 2017;19(11):962–72.

Management of Colorectal Cancer in Hereditary Syndromes

Lisa A. Cunningham, MD[a], Alessandra Gasior, DO[a,b],
Matthew F. Kalady, MD[a,c,*]

KEYWORDS

- Hereditary colon and rectal cancer • Lynch syndrome
- Hereditary nonpolyposis colorectal cancer • Familial adenomatous polyposis

KEY POINTS

- Approximately 5% of colorectal cancers arise within a known hereditary syndrome. Diagnosis and classification is essential to provide appropriate management and risk-reduction.
- Hereditary colorectal cancer syndromes can be broadly classified as polyposis or non-polyposis. The more common polyposis syndromes characterized by adenomas are familial adenomatous polyposis (FAP) and MYH-associated polyposis. Hamartomatous polyp syndromes include juvenile polyposis syndrome, Peutz-Jeghers syndrome, and PTEN-hamartoma tumor syndrome.
- The most common hereditary colorectal cancer syndrome is Lynch syndrome, which is a non-polyposis phenotype. Lynch syndrome is a genetic diagnosis and should be differentiated from Hereditary Non-polyposis Colorectal Cancer (HNPCC) which is defined by clinical criteria (Amsterdam criteria). Although there is overlap between the 2, there are differences in risk and thus management recommendations vary.
- The risk of developing colorectal cancer in FAP approaches 100% and patients ultimately will require surgery to remove their colon and possibly rectum.
- Colorectal cancer risk in Lynch syndrome varies by the pathogenic variant and patient gender. Management principles include minimizing colorectal cancer risk and death from cancer, while trying to preserve bowel function and quality of life.

INTRODUCTION

Colorectal cancers (CRCs) arise via a series of sequential genetic and molecular changes. Similar genetic alterations occur in both sporadic and inherited CRC, but

[a] Division of Colorectal Surgery, Department of Surgery, The Ohio State University Medical Center, N737B Doan Hall, 410 West 10th Avenue, Columbus, OH 43210, USA; [b] Pediatric and Adult Colorectal Surgery, The Ohio State University Medical Center, Nationwide Children's Hospital, N747 Doan Hall, 410 West 10th Avenue, Columbus, OH 43210, USA; [c] Clinical Cancer Genetics Program, The James Comprehensive Cancer Center, Columbus, OH 43201, USA
* Corresponding author.
E-mail address: matthew.kalady@osumc.edu

Surg Oncol Clin N Am 31 (2022) 307–319
https://doi.org/10.1016/j.soc.2021.11.010
1055-3207/22/© 2021 Elsevier Inc. All rights reserved.

patients born with an inherited pathogenic gene variant develop CRC and specific extracolonic cancers at a higher incidence and an accelerated rate. Approximately 15% of all CRCs are associated with a defined germline pathogenic variant, and about 5% arise within a known hereditary cancer syndrome.[1] Therefore, it is critical to have a high index of suspicion to identify those at risk and diagnose the syndrome. Patients and families with an inherited syndrome need to be educated and managed according to their risks to minimize the development of and death from cancer. This article will cover the general approach and classification of inherited CRC syndromes and focus on the clinical and surgical management of familial adenomatous polyposis (FAP) and Lynch syndrome (LS).

OVERVIEW OF HEREDITARY CRC SYNDROMES

Hereditary CRC syndromes can be broadly classified as polyposis or nonpolyposis. Within these broad classifications, the syndromes can be further delineated by the histology of the polyps, numbers of polyps, and ultimately the underlying genetic pathogenic variant. Polyposis syndromes are separated by the predominant polyp type: adenomas, hamartomas, or serrated polyps. Within adenomatous syndromes, FAP is the most common, followed by MYH-associated polyposis (MAP), and the extremely rare polymerase proofreading-associated polyposis. Juvenile polyposis syndrome, Peutz-Jeghers syndrome, and PTEN-hamartoma tumor syndrome are characterized by hamartomatous polyps. A predominance of serrated colorectal polyps might lead to a diagnosis of serrated polyposis syndrome (SPS). SPS is a clinical definition and although believed to be somewhat inherited, no known heritable pathogenic variant has yet to be identified. The 2 main nonpolyposis CRC syndromes are LS and hereditary colorectal cancer type X (HCC-X). These are defined by germline variants, molecular, and clinical criteria and discussed in more detail in the section on nonpolyposis syndromes. An overview of the hereditary CRC syndromes is outlined in **Table 1**.

POLYPOSIS SYNDROMES
Familial Adenomatous Polyposis

FAP is an autosomal dominant condition caused by a pathogenic variant of the *APC* gene.[2] The clinical phenotype varies, but the basis is diffuse colorectal adenomatous polyps, as well as extracolonic manifestations, including duodenal adenomas, desmoid disease, osteomas, thyroid cancer, and congenital hypertrophy of retinal pigment epithelium. Patients with a clinical phenotype consistent with FAP but without an identified pathogenic variant are still diagnosed and managed as FAP if the clinical picture and family history fit. Approximately 25% of proband cases arise without a known family history of FAP due to a founder germline mutation.[3] Without intervention, FAP patients have a lifetime CRC risk approaching 100% that increases with age, ranging from 7% by age 21 years to as high as 95% by age 50 years.[4] Therefore, early diagnosis and surveillance is critical.

CRC surveillance and timing of surgery

Patients with FAP are recommended to undergo colonoscopy starting at age 10 to 12 years.[5] Earlier screening may be considered based on family history. Colonoscopy with polypectomy serves to decrease CRC risk and should be repeated annually.[6] Absolute indications for surgery include the development of CRC or significant colorectal-related symptoms. Other factors that should push toward surgical intervention include increasing number or distribution of polyps, multiple polyps that are larger

Table 1
An overview of the hereditary CRC syndromes

Syndrome	Main Polyp Histology	Pathogenic Variant
Polyposis		
FAP	Adenoma	*APC*
MAP	Adenoma	*Mut-YH*
JPS	Hamartoma (juvenile polyps)	*SMAD4, BMPR1A*
PJS	Hamartoma (Peutz-Jeghers polyps)	*STK11*
PHTS	Hamartomas	*PTEN*
SPS	Serrated polyps	Unknown
Nonpolyposis		
Lynch syndrome	Adenoma	*MLH1, MSH2, MSH6, PMS2, EPCAM*
HNPCC	Adenoma	Unknown
Familial CRC Type X	Adenoma	Unknown

Abbreviation: JPS, Juvenile polyposis syndrome; PJS, Peutz-Jeghers syndrome.

than 10 mm in size, and polyps with high-grade dysplasia. Passage of blood with bowel motions is associated with the presence of high-grade dysplasia and cancer[7] and surgery should be recommended.

The decision of when to proceed with the surgery is complex and individualized based on patient and family experience, and management of risk. The risk for CRC before 18 years of age is rare and delaying until patients are physically and emotionally mature is reasonable, unless there is a clear indication for surgery as discussed above before that time. Patients will often choose to have prophylactic surgery during life transitions such as between high school and college, or between school and starting a job, or between jobs. One group recently published an online predictive model that incorporates factors such as genotype, age, gender, history of desmoids, number and size of polyps on initial colonoscopy, and the percent of polyps removed during colonoscopy. Based on these variables, the model predicts the need for surgery within 2 or 5 years with accuracy greater than 80%.[8] Female patients may wish to delay proctectomy until after family planning is completed because of the risk of decreased fecundity after pelvic surgery. Decreased ability to conceive was found in 50% of FAP patients who underwent ileal pouch-anal anastomosis (IPAA) compared with controls.[9] Obesity also may factor into the timing of surgery, particularly if the patient has a phenotype that would require a total proctocolectomy (TPC) and IPAA. Morbid obesity may technically preclude the creation of an IPAA and in these situations, surgery may be delayed until adequate weight loss is achieved. Attempts at weight loss may not be successful and indications for surgery may supersede weight loss. Another significant factor to consider in the timing of surgery is desmoid disease. As most desmoids form after surgery,[10] patients who are at an increased risk of desmoid disease (eg, those with a personal or family history)[11] should delay surgery as long as feasible. It is important to note that these are all relative considerations and the ultimate decision of when to undergo surgery is driven by the principle to decrease CRC risk. If a patient is to delay surgery for the aforementioned reasons, strict colorectal surveillance by colonoscopy is required at least annually.

Patients with attenuated FAP (aFAP) have a decreased polyp burden and often have a later onset of the development of colorectal adenomas and subsequently CRC.

aFAP may present with minimal to 100 adenomas and the lifetime risk of CRC is 70%, with an average age of around 30 years.[4,6] Because of this, the polyp burden is often easier to manage endoscopically and surgery often is not needed or performed until patients are in their 30s.

Surgical options and extent of resection

Determining the extent of surgical resection relies on a balance of managing CRC risk against bowel function and quality of life. Surgical options include TPC with end ileostomy or with restoration via an IPAA, or total abdominal colectomy (TAC) with an ileorectal anastomosis (IRA). As the goal of prophylactic surgery is minimizing or eliminating CRC risk, the first branch in decision-making is the presence of cancer and polyp burden, with particular attention to the rectum. One commonly used recommendation is to offer TPC if the polyp burden in the rectum is $\geq$20 adenomas.[12] When meeting this recommendation along with a modest colon polyp burden (<1000 polyps), the rate of subsequent proctectomy was zero at a median follow-up of 12 years in one study.[13] Again, surgical decision-making should be individualized and it may be reasonable to offer an IRA even when the rectal polyp burden is more than 20; such as patients with high risk for desmoids as discussed earlier. In either situation, if the rectum is preserved, annual surveillance and polypectomies are required to prevent rectal cancer development.

If a patient has rectal cancer, rectal polyps with high-grade dysplasia, uncontrollable rectal polyp burden, or diffuse colonic polyposis, TPC with end ileostomy or IPAA is recommended. This more extensive resection lowers future CRC risk compared with TAC/IRA, but is associated with increased surgical morbidity and increased number of bowel movements. TPC and IPAA are associated with an increased risk of urinary and sexual dysfunction including impotence in men and decreased fecundity in women as well as decreased quality of life scores compared with patients undergoing IRA.[9,14,15] The average number of bowel movements after an IPAA is approximately 6 compared to 4 after an IRA, and there is also an increase in nighttime leakage and need for antimotility agents. Patients with locally advanced rectal cancer who require neoadjuvant chemoradiation often have more challenges with bowel function due to the radiation effect on the small bowel that will become the pouch. This needs to be discussed with the patient in terms of expectations.

Another consideration in determining the extent of resection is the risk of desmoid disease. For patients who have a personal or family history of desmoids, it is prudent to try to minimize surgical stressors that could lead to desmoid development. There has been debate regarding the influence of extent of surgery and surgical approach (ie, laparoscopic vs laparotomy). Recent data show that TPC and IPAA are more desmoidogenic than a TAC/IRA and that an open approach is more desmoidogenic than laparoscopic.[16]

Double-stapled versus handsewn mucosectomy anastomosis in IPAA

The debate between patients with FAP undergoing an IPAA with a handsewn versus stapled anastomosis is ongoing. Proponents of the handsewn anastomosis support removal of all of the anorectal mucosa to the dentate line to remove all at-risk mucosa. This comes at the cost of decreased function such as anal seepage and incontinence.[17,18] Leaving a small anorectal cuff in the anal transition zone (ATZ) during a double-stapled anastomosis results in better function, but leaves mucosa at risk for future polyp and cancer development. For patients undergoing an IPAA, 34% of those who had a double-stapled technique developed ATZ adenomas, compared to 21% of patients in the mucosectomy group.[19] On longer follow-up, the rate of ATZ neoplasia is as high as 52% after a double-stapled IPAA.[20] It is also important to note that polyps and cancer can develop in the ileal pouch as well and lifelong annual surveillance is still required after either operation.[21]

MUTYH-Associated Polyposis

MAP is an adenomatous polyposis syndrome caused by a pathogenic variant in the *MUTYH* gene and is inherited in an autosomal recessive pattern. The clinical phenotype varies widely and can present with only the incident cancer, or with hundreds of adenomas. The lifetime risk of developing CRC is approximately 60%, with 19% by age 50 years and 43% by age 60 years.[22] The average age of CRC diagnosis is about 47 years.[23] Because of the common lack of polyposis, the diagnosis is often missed. Surgeons must have a high suspicion of inherited syndromes particularly in younger patients which warrants gene-panel testing, which would detect a biallelic *MYH* pathogenic variant. Like FAP, germline defects make every cell susceptible to developing neoplasia and consideration should be given to extended resection in patients who have CRC. Indications for surgery include CRC, uncontrolled polyp burden, uncontrolled symptoms, or the inability to adequately survey the colon. Surgical considerations for MAP patients are similar to FAP with total colectomy and IRA. If there is rectal cancer or if the rectum is significantly involved, TPC and end ileostomy or IPAA should be performed.

Hamartomatous Polyposis Syndromes

A detailed discussion of each of the hamartomatous syndromes is outside the scope of this article. An overview is provided in **Table 2**. Like other syndromes, management is founded in the prevention of cancer. Patients undergo annual colonoscopy with polypectomy to control symptoms and neoplasia risk. Surgery is indicated if CRC develops or if polyp-related symptoms or neoplasia risk cannot be controlled endoscopically. TAC/IRA is the recommended procedure or TPC/IPAA or end ileostomy if the rectum is involved. These are based on low-quality evidence but strongly recommended.[5] Patients with any colorectal mucosa remaining are at risk for future neoplasia and the rectum or pouch should be endoscopically surveyed annually.[27]

Serrated Polyposis Syndrome

There is no known pathogenic variant that is responsible for SPS and it is diagnosed by clinical criteria. Recently updated World Health Organization criteria[28] are given below and patients must meet one of the following criteria:

1. More than 5 serrated lesion/polyps proximal to the rectum, all being ≥5 mm in size, with at least 2 being ≥10 mm; or
2. More than 20 serrated lesions/polyps of any size distributed throughout the large bowel with at least 5 being proximal to the rectum.

As this is a clinical diagnosis, patients are identified at colonoscopy performed to evaluate symptoms or for routine screening. The lifetime risk of CRC remains debated and is difficult to characterize because of the lack of genetic underpinnings and changing clinical definitions. Approximately 30% of patients with SPS developed CRC at a median age of 61 years in a large European study.[29] Patients with SPS should undergo surveillance colonoscopy with polypectomy every 1 to 2 years depending on the findings. Indications for surgery include the development of CRC or a polyp burden that cannot adequately be controlled endoscopically. In cases where surgery is indicated, consideration should be given to TAC and IRA due to CRC risk throughout the colon, although this is not supported by level 1 evidence.[5,30]

Table 2
Hamartomatous polyposis syndromes

Syndrome	Polyp Type	Pathogenic Variant	Clinical Diagnosis	Inheritance Pattern	Typical Clinical Presentation	Other Systems	Estimated CRC Risk
JPS	Juvenile polyps	*SMAD4, BMPR1A*	5 ≥ juvenile polyps in colon and rectum Family history of juvenile polyposis Juvenile polyposis throughout GI system	Autosomal dominant	Infancy in severe form associated with macrocephaly and hypotonia Later in adolescence or adulthood	Confined to GI tract	40%[24]
PJS	Peutz-Jeghers polyps	*STK11*	2 ≥ histologic JPS polyp 1 ≥ polyp and family history of JPS 1 ≥ polyp with mucocutaneous pigmentation	Autosomal dominant	Multiple polyps in GI tract, mucocutaneous pigmentation	Biliary tract Bladder Lungs Genitourinary system	40%[25]
PHTS	Hamartomas	*PTEN*	3 ≥ major[a] criteria including macrocephaly, GI hamartomas, Lhermitte-Duclos disease or Two major and 3 minor[b] criteria	Autosomal dominant	Variable clinical presentation	Brain lesions Breast Thyroid Renal Skin	9%–16%[26]

Abbreviation: GI, gastrointestinal; JPS, Juvenile polyposis syndrome; PJS, Peutz-Jeghers syndrome.
[a] Major criteria: breast cancer, endometrial cancer, thyroid cancer, GI hamartomas, macrocephaly, macular pigmentation of glans penis, multiple mucocutaneous lesions, multiple trichilemmomas, acral keratoses, mucocutaneous neuromas, and oral papillomas.
[b] Minor criteria: autism, colon cancer, esophageal glycogenic acanthosis, lipomas, developmental delay, renal cell carcinoma, testicular lipomatosis, thyroid cancer, thyroid structural lesions, and vascular anomalies.

NONPOLYPOSIS COLORECTAL CANCER

The term hereditary nonpolyposis colorectal cancer (HNPCC) was first developed to describe an autosomal dominant inheritance pattern of colorectal and extracolonic cancers; mainly to distinguish it from the well-known and genetically characterized syndrome FAP. The specific diagnostic criteria for HNPCC were first outlined following a consensus meeting in Amsterdam in 1991, and thus bear the name Amsterdam criteria.[31] The Amsterdam criteria were broadened to include non-CRC cancers in 1999.[32] Definitions of Amsterdam criteria are given in **Box 1**. The main goal of developing such criteria was to identify and classify patients and families that were believed to have a similar underlying etiology for their syndrome, and thus be able to study these defined families. With the discovery of the DNA mismatch repair genes (*MSH1, MSH2, MSH6,* and *PMS2*) responsible for this hereditary predisposition, a more precise definition of this syndrome was borne. Now, patients with a pathogenic variant in one of the above genes are diagnosed with LS, named after the oncologist Henry Lynch who propelled the field by his study of these families. Only about half of the patients who have LS meet formal Amsterdam criteria, and only about half of the patients who meet Amsterdam criteria (HNPCC) will have LS. Patients who fulfill Amsterdam criteria but do not have microsatellite unstable tumors are classified as Familial CRC Type X (FCC X). Each diagnosis is associated with specific cancer risks and the management is different, as discussed below.

Lynch Syndrome

LS is an autosomal dominant hereditary predisposition to develop colorectal and certain extracolonic cancers due to a germline mutation in one of the DNA mismatch repair genes *MSH2, MLH1, MSH6, PMS2,* or the nonmismatch repair gene *EPCAM* that leads to epigenetic downstream silencing of the promoter region of *MSH2*.[33–37] Sporadic loss of the corresponding other allele results in loss of mismatch repair protein function, which leads to an accumulation of unrepaired DNA mismatches that occur during cell division and DNA replication. These areas of mismatch tend to occur in highly repetitive DNA sequences called microsatellites, leading to the term microsatellite instability. A high level of microsatellite instability means that DNA mismatch

---

Box 1
Amsterdam criteria for HNPCC

Amsterdam I[31]

- Three relatives with pathologically verified colorectal cancer
  - At least one should be a first degree relative to the other two

- FAP is excluded
  - At least 2 successive generations are affected
  - In one relative, colorectal cancer should be diagnosed before age 50 years
  - FAP is excluded

Amsterdam II[32]

- At least 3 relatives with HNPCC-associated cancer (CRC, endometrial cancer, small bowel cancer, renal pelvis, or ureteral cancer)
  - At least one should be a first degree relative to the other two

- FAP is excluded
  - At least 2 successive generations are affected
  - In on relative, colorectal cancer should be diagnosed before age 50 years

repair is deficient (dMMR). dMMR or microsatellite instability is the molecular hallmark of LS and is present in approximately 93% of Lynch tumors.

LS is the most common inherited form of CRC, accounting for nearly 3% of diagnosed cases.[1,38,39] The lifetime risk of CRC continues to evolve and be defined as more information is accumulated in large databases. The risk varies by the pathogenic variant and increases with age.[40] This is summarized in **Table 3**. LS is a multisystem disease. Other associated cancers include endometrial, gastric, and ovarian, each with a differing lifetime risk depending on the pathologic variant.[40,41] There is also an association with small intestine, biliary tract, brain, and cancer of the upper urogenital tract.[41] In a review of 1942 patients with known LS MMR mutations, Moller and colleagues found the highest rates of colon cancer and ovarian cancer associated with *MLH1* and *MSH 2* cancers, with *MSH2* and *MSH6* having a higher cumulative incidence for endometrial cancer due to differences in gene penetrance and expression.[42] In a later, large prospective database, Dominguez-Valentin and colleagues studied 6350 patients with LS and the highest cancer rates were again found associated with *MLH1* and *MSH2* carriers, with a lifetime risk of CRC approaching 50% regardless of attempts at prevention with colonoscopy and polypectomy.[40] Similar findings were also found for *MSH6* in this larger study, with decreased penetrance in men versus women and there being a high risk for gynecologic cancers with a modest increase in the risk of CRC on both sexes.[40] In this cohort, there were also no LS-associated cancers in patients with PMS2 before age 50 years, which is less than previously reported.[40]

Surveillance and intervention are critical to reducing mortality. Regular colonoscopy with polypectomy reduces the risk of developing CRC by 62% and reduces CRC-associated mortality by approximately 65%.[43] Colonoscopy is recommended every 1 to 2 years starting between ages 20 and 25 or 2 and 5 years before the youngest age of CRC diagnosis.[44] There is lower-quality evidence to support endometrial and ovarian cancer screening but current recommendations include pelvic examination with endometrial sampling and transvaginal ultrasound starting between ages 30 and 35 years.[44] As mentioned earlier, more data about risk stratification are being delineated based on the specific MMR gene variant, which may have implications in the future toward personalized surveillance recommendations.

Indications for surgical intervention are the same as for patients without LS: CRC or a high-risk lesion that cannot be removed endoscopically. Once it is determined to proceed with surgery, decision-making in LS should incorporate treatment of the incident tumor, extended prophylactic resection as risk reduction, and expected future bowel function and quality of life. Clinical Practice Guidelines set forth by the American

Table 3
Percentile risk of developing CRC in Lynch syndrome according to age, gender, and pathogenic variant

Age	MLH1		MSH2		MSH6		PMS2	
	Male	Female	Male	Female	Male	Female	Both	
30	4.5	0	2.6	1.9	0	0	0	0
50	33.6	20.8	18.1	16.9	6.3	4.4	0	0
75	57.1	48.3	51.4	46.6	18.2	20.3	10.4	10.4

Adapted from Dominguez-Valentin M, Sampson JR, Seppälä TT, et al. Cancer risks by gene, age, and gender in 6350 carriers of pathogenic mismatch repair variants: findings from the Prospective Lynch Syndrome Database [published correction appears in Genet Med. 2020 Sep;22(9):1569]. Genet Med. 2020;22(1):15-25. https://doi.org/10.1038/s41436-019-0596-9.

Society of Colon and Rectal Surgeons recommend a total colectomy for LS patients who develop colon cancer.[45] These recommendations are supported by retrospective studies reporting significantly increased risk of metachronous colorectal cancer following segmental versus extended resections. In a multicenter study of 382 LS patients with CRC, of those treated with segmental resection, 22% developed a metachronous CRC, whereas no patients developed a metachronous CRC if extended colectomy was performed.[46] As expected, the risk increases with time from surgery and the metachronous CRC rate was as high as 72% at 40 years.[46] Extended resection for risk reduction is associated with changes in bowel function and this needs to be discussed with the patient and taken into consideration. Patients undergoing a subtotal or total colectomy compared with segmental colectomy have more frequent bowel movements daily (about 4 compared with 2), have some perceived impact on social functions, but these findings did not translate into a worse quality of life.[47,48] Consideration should be given to segmental resection if patients prefer or if there are medical conditions that preclude a total colectomy. Patients and surgeons must be aware of the metachronous risk and annual colonoscopy needs to be performed.

Rectal cancer in LS presents a clinical challenge as extended resection would entail a TPC with or without restoration of the gastrointestinal tract with an IPAA. Rectal cancer must be treated with oncologic principles of appropriate staging, neoadjuvant therapy as indicated, and surgical mesorectal excision. Proctectomy alone has a significant metachronous colon cancer risk. One study reported 39.4% high-risk adenoma and 15.2% colon cancer development after proctectomy alone at a median follow-up of 8.5 years.[49] Another study projected increasing metachronous colon cancer risk over time: 19% at 10 years, 47% at 20 years, and 69% at 30 years.[50] In terms of function, patients after an IPAA can expect to have more frequent bowel movements and a higher incidence of incontinence and seepage compared with a coloanal anastomosis. IPAA is a technically challenging procedure and should only be performed by those with specialized surgical training and expertise. The effect of creating an IPAA after radiation also should be considered. Although there is no increased rate of postoperative complications after preoperative radiation,[51,52] there is a higher frequency of stools noted, along with urgency and the greater need for antidiarrheal medication.[51]

Familial Colorectal Cancer Type X

Familial Colorectal Cancer Type X (FCC X) describes cases of CRC that meet Amsterdam 1 criteria but whose tumors do not have the characteristic dMMR or germline mutations seen in LS, thus the tumors are MMR proficient.[31,53] These families have an approximately 2-fold increased risk of CRC compared with the general population, but less than what is seen in LS families. In addition, FCC X has a later onset of CRC than LS, is not associated with typical LS extracolonic malignancies, and tumors are more likely to be left-sided.[53,54] Multiple genes have been implicated, but none have been able to explain this syndrome consistently.[55] It is suspected that FCC X results from more than one genetic cause and may have many different clinical variants.[54,56]

Patients with FCC X should be managed with more frequent colonoscopic evaluations than the general public, but not as intensely as those with LS. Initial colonoscopy for asymptomatic individuals should begin at age 40 years, or 10 years younger than the youngest CRC in the family, whichever is earlier. Intervals between normal colonoscopy are 3 to 5 years.[57,58] No extracolonic screening is indicated. For patients who develop CRC, a segmental colectomy is recommended, given the lack of data on increased metachronous CRC risk and the desire to preserve bowel length and function.[59]

DISCLOSURE

The authors have nothing to disclose.

REFERENCES

1. Pearlman R, Frankel WL, Swanson BJ, et al. Prospective statewide study of universal screening for hereditary colorectal cancer: the Ohio Colorectal Cancer Prevention Initiative. JCO Precis Oncol 2021;5. https://doi.org/10.1200/PO.20.00525. PO.20.00525.
2. Kinzler KW, Nilbert MC, Su LK, et al. Identification of FAP locus genes from chromosome 5q21. Science 1991;253(5020):661–5. https://doi.org/10.1126/science. 1651562.
3. Bisgaard ML, Fenger K, Bülow S, et al. Familial adenomatous polyposis (FAP): frequency, penetrance, and mutation rate. Hum Mutat 1994;3(2):121–5. https:// doi.org/10.1002/humu.1380030206.
4. Kanth P, Grimmett J, Champine M, et al. Hereditary colorectal polyposis and cancer syndromes: a primer on diagnosis and management. Am J Gastroenterol 2017;112(10):1509–25. https://doi.org/10.1038/ajg.2017.212.
5. Syngal S, Brand RE, Church JM, et al. ACG clinical guideline: genetic testing and management of hereditary gastrointestinal cancer syndromes. Am J Gastroenterol 2015;110(2):223–63. https://doi.org/10.1038/ajg.2014.435.
6. Knudsen AL, Bülow S, Tomlinson I, et al. Attenuated familial adenomatous polyposis: results from an international collaborative study. Colorectal Dis 2010;12(10 Online):e243–9. https://doi.org/10.1111/j.1463-1318.2010.02218.x.
7. Bülow S, Bülow C, Nielsen TF, et al. Centralized registration, prophylactic examination, and treatment results in improved prognosis in familial adenomatous polyposis. Results from the Danish Polyposis Register. Scand J Gastroenterol 1995; 30(10):989–93. https://doi.org/10.3109/00365529509096343.
8. Sarvepalli S, Burke CA, Monachese M, et al. Web-based model for predicting time to surgery in young patients with familial adenomatous polyposis: an internally validated study. Am J Gastroenterol 2018;113(12):1881–90. https://doi. org/10.1038/s41395-018-0278-2.
9. Olsen KØ, Juul S, Bülow S, et al. Female fecundity before and after operation for familial adenomatous polyposis. Br J Surg 2003;90(2):227–31. https://doi.org/10. 1002/bjs.4082.
10. DE Marchis ML, Tonelli F, Quaresmini D, et al. Desmoid tumors in familial adenomatous polyposis. Anticancer Res 2017;37(7):3357–66. https://doi.org/10.21873/ anticanres.11702.
11. Elayi E, Manilich E, Church J. Polishing the crystal ball: knowing genotype improves ability to predict desmoid disease in patients with familial adenomatous polyposis. Dis Colon Rectum 2009;52(10):1762–6. https://doi.org/10.1007/DCR. 0b013e3181b5518a.
12. Warrier SK, Kalady MF. Familial adenomatous polyposis: challenges and pitfalls of surgical treatment. Clin Colon Rectal Surg 2012;25(2):83–9. https://doi.org/ 10.1055/s-0032-1313778.
13. Church J, Burke C, McGannon E, et al. Predicting polyposis severity by proctoscopy: how reliable is it? Dis Colon Rectum 2001;44(9):1249–54. https://doi.org/ 10.1007/BF02234779.
14. Slors FJ, van Zuijlen PP, van Dijk GJ. Sexual and bladder dysfunction after total mesorectal excision for benign diseases. Scand J Gastroenterol Suppl 2000;(232):48–51.

15. Günther K, Braunrieder G, Bittorf BR, et al. Patients with familial adenomatous polyposis experience better bowel function and quality of life after ileorectal anastomosis than after ileoanal pouch. Colorectal Dis 2003;5(1):38–44. https://doi.org/10.1046/j.1463-1318.2003.00413.x.

16. Sommavilla J, Liska D, Kalady M, et al. Ileal Pouch Anal Anastomosis Is More "Desmoidogenic" Than Ileorectal Anastomosis in Familial Adenomatous Polyposis. Diseases of the Colon and Rectum. 2021 Nov. https://doi.org/10.1097/dcr.0000000000002172.

17. Chittleborough TJ, Warrier SK, Heriot AG, et al. Dispelling misconceptions in the management of familial adenomatous polyposis. ANZ J Surg 2017;87(6):441–5. https://doi.org/10.1111/ans.13919.

18. Lovegrove RE, Constantinides VA, Heriot AG, et al. A comparison of hand-sewn versus stapled ileal pouch anal anastomosis (IPAA) following proctocolectomy: a meta-analysis of 4183 patients. Ann Surg 2006;244(1):18–26. https://doi.org/10.1097/01.sla.0000225031.15405.a3.

19. Ozdemir Y, Kalady MF, Aytac E, et al. Anal transitional zone neoplasia in patients with familial adenomatous polyposis after restorative proctocolectomy and IPAA: incidence, management, and oncologic and functional outcomes. Dis Colon Rectum 2013;56(7):808–14. https://doi.org/10.1097/DCR.0b013e31829005db.

20. Lee CHA, Kalady MF, Burke CA, et al. Incidence and management of rectal cuff and anal transitional zone neoplasia in patients with familial adenomatous polyposis. Dis Colon Rectum 2021;64(8):977–85. https://doi.org/10.1097/DCR.0000000000001967.

21. Thompson-Fawcett MW, Marcus VA, Redston M, et al. Adenomatous polyps develop commonly in the ileal pouch of patients with familial adenomatous polyposis. Dis Colon Rectum 2001;44(3):347–53. https://doi.org/10.1007/BF02234731.

22. Nielsen M, Morreau H, Vasen HF, et al. MUTYH-associated polyposis (MAP). Crit Rev Oncol Hematol 2011;79(1):1–16. https://doi.org/10.1016/j.critrevonc.2010.05.011.

23. Sampson JR, Dolwani S, Jones S, et al. Autosomal recessive colorectal adenomatous polyposis due to inherited mutations of MYH. Lancet 2003;362(9377):39–41. https://doi.org/10.1016/S0140-6736(03)13805-6.

24. Brosens LA, van Hattem A, Hylind LM, et al. Risk of colorectal cancer in juvenile polyposis. Gut 2007;56:965–7.

25. NCCN clinical practice Guidelines in oncology (NCCN Guidelines) peutz-jeghers syndrome screening. Version 1.2015. 2015

26. Pilarski R. PTEN hamartoma tumor syndrome: a clinical overview. Cancers (Basel) 2019;11(6):844. https://doi.org/10.3390/cancers11060844.

27. Oncel M, Church JM, Remzi FH, et al. Colonic surgery in patients with juvenile polyposis syndrome: a case series. Dis Colon Rectum 2005;48(1):49–56. https://doi.org/10.1007/s10350-004-0749-y.

28. Rosty C, Brosens LAA, Nagtegaal ID. Serrated polyposis. WHO classification of tumours. Dig Syst Tumours 2019.

29. IJspeert JE, Rana SA, Atkinson NS, et al. Clinical risk factors of colorectal cancer in patients with serrated polyposis syndrome: a multicentre cohort analysis. Gut 2017;66(2):278–84. https://doi.org/10.1136/gutjnl-2015-310630.

30. Ashburn JH, Plesec TP, Kalady MF. Serrated polyps and serrated polyposis syndrome. Clin Colon Rectal Surg 2016;29(4):336–44. https://doi.org/10.1055/s-0036-1584088.

31. Vasen HF, Mecklin JP, Khan PM, et al. The international collaborative group on hereditary non-polyposis colorectal cancer (ICG-HNPCC). Dis Colon Rectum 1991; 34(5):424–5. https://doi.org/10.1007/BF02053699.

32. Vasen HF, Watson P, Mecklin JP, et al. New clinical criteria for hereditary nonpolyposis colorectal cancer (HNPCC, Lynch syndrome) proposed by the International Collaborative Group on HNPCC. Gastroenterology 1999;116(6): 1453–6. https://doi.org/10.1016/s0016-5085(99)70510-x.

33. Leach FS, Nicolaides NC, Papadopoulos N, et al. Mutations of a mutS homolog in hereditary nonpolyposis colorectal cancer. Cell 1993;75(6):1215–25. https://doi.org/10.1016/0092-8674(93)90330-s.

34. Fishel R, Lescoe MK, Rao MR, et al. The human mutator gene homolog MSH2 and its association with hereditary nonpolyposis colon cancer [published correction appears in Cell. 1994 Apr 8;77(1):1 p following 166]. Cell 1993;75(5): 1027–38. https://doi.org/10.1016/0092-8674(93)90546-3.

35. Bronner CE, Baker SM, Morrison PT, et al. Mutation in the DNA mismatch repair gene homologue hMLH1 is associated with hereditary non-polyposis colon cancer. Nature 1994;368(6468):258–61. https://doi.org/10.1038/368258a0.

36. Papadopoulos N, Nicolaides NC, Wei YF, et al. Mutation of a mutL homolog in hereditary colon cancer. Science 1994;263(5153):1625–9. https://doi.org/10.1126/science.8128251.

37. Wijnen J, de Leeuw W, Vasen H, et al. Familial endometrial cancer in female carriers of MSH6 germline mutations. Nat Genet 1999;23(2):142–4. https://doi.org/10.1038/13773.

38. Hampel H, Frankel WL, Martin E, et al. Screening for the Lynch syndrome (hereditary nonpolyposis colorectal cancer). N Engl J Med 2005;352(18):1851–60. https://doi.org/10.1056/NEJMoa043146.

39. Rubenstein JH, Enns R, Heidelbaugh J, et al, Clinical Guidelines Committee. American gastroenterological association institute guideline on the diagnosis and management of lynch syndrome. Gastroenterology 2015;149(3):777. https://doi.org/10.1053/j.gastro.2015.07.036.

40. Dominguez-Valentin M, Sampson JR, Seppälä TT, et al. Cancer risks by gene, age, and gender in 6350 carriers of pathogenic mismatch repair variants: findings from the Prospective Lynch Syndrome Database [published correction appears in Genet Med. 2020 Sep;22(9):1569]. Genet Med 2020;22(1):15–25. https://doi.org/10.1038/s41436-019-0596-9.

41. Kobayashi H, Ohno S, Sasaki Y, et al. Hereditary breast and ovarian cancer susceptibility genes (review). Oncol Rep 2013;30(3):1019–29. https://doi.org/10.3892/or.2013.2541.

42. Møller P, Seppälä T, Bernstein I, et al. Cancer incidence and survival in Lynch syndrome patients receiving colonoscopic and gynaecological surveillance: first report from the prospective Lynch syndrome database. Gut 2017;66(3):464–72. https://doi.org/10.1136/gutjnl-2015-309675.

43. Järvinen HJ, Aarnio M, Mustonen H, et al. Controlled 15-year trial on screening for colorectal cancer in families with hereditary nonpolyposis colorectal cancer. Gastroenterology 2000;118(5):829–34. https://doi.org/10.1016/s0016-5085(00)70168-5.

44. Giardiello FM, Allen JI, Axilbund JE, et al. Guidelines on genetic evaluation and management of Lynch syndrome: a consensus statement by the US Multi-society Task Force on colorectal cancer. Am J Gastroenterol 2014;109(8): 1159–79. https://doi.org/10.1038/ajg.2014.186.

45. Herzig D, Hardiman K, Weiser M, et al. The American Society of Colon and Rectal Surgeons Clinical Practice Guidelines for the Management of Inherited Polyposis Syndromes. Dis Colon Rectum 2017 Sep;60(9):881–94.

46. Parry S, Win AK, Parry B, et al. Metachronous colorectal cancer risk for mismatch repair gene mutation carriers: the advantage of more extensive colon surgery. Gut 2011;60(7):950–7. https://doi.org/10.1136/gut.2010.228056.

47. Haanstra JF, de Vos Tot Nederveen Cappel WH, Gopie JP, et al. Quality of life after surgery for colon cancer in patients with Lynch syndrome: partial versus subtotal colectomy. Dis Colon Rectum 2012;55(6):653–9. https://doi.org/10.1097/DCR.0b013e31824f5392.

48. You YN, Chua HK, Nelson H, et al. Segmental vs. extended colectomy: measurable differences in morbidity, function, and quality of life. Dis Colon Rectum 2008; 51(7):1036–43. https://doi.org/10.1007/s10350-008-9325-1.

49. Kalady MF, Lipman J, McGannon E, et al. Risk of colonic neoplasia after proctectomy for rectal cancer in hereditary nonpolyposis colorectal cancer. Ann Surg 2012;255(6):1121–5. https://doi.org/10.1097/SLA.0b013e3182565c0b.

50. Win AK, Parry S, Parry B, et al. Risk of metachronous colon cancer following surgery for rectal cancer in mismatch repair gene mutation carriers. Ann Surg Oncol 2013;20(6):1829–36. https://doi.org/10.1245/s10434-012-2858-5.

51. Parc Y, Zutshi M, Zalinski S, et al. Preoperative radiotherapy is associated with worse functional results after coloanal anastomosis for rectal cancer. Dis Colon Rectum 2009;52(12):2004–14. https://doi.org/10.1007/DCR.0b013e3181beb4d8.

52. Wertzberger BE, Sherman SK, Byrn JC. Differences in short-term outcomes among patients undergoing IPAA with or without preoperative radiation: a National Surgical Quality Improvement Program analysis. Dis Colon Rectum 2014; 57(10):1188–94. https://doi.org/10.1097/DCR.0000000000000206.

53. Lindor NM, Rabe K, Petersen GM, et al. Lower cancer incidence in Amsterdam-I criteria families without mismatch repair deficiency: familial colorectal cancer type X. JAMA 2005;293(16):1979–85. https://doi.org/10.1001/jama.293.16.1979.

54. Shiovitz S, Copeland WK, Passarelli MN, et al. Characterisation of familial colorectal cancer Type X, Lynch syndrome, and non-familial colorectal cancer. Br J Cancer 2014;111(3):598–602. https://doi.org/10.1038/bjc.2014.309.

55. Nejadtaghi M, Jafari H, Farrokhi E, et al. Familial colorectal cancer type X (FCCTX) and the correlation with various genes-A systematic review. Curr Probl Cancer 2017;41(6):388–97. https://doi.org/10.1016/j.currproblcancer.2017.10.002.

56. Garre P, Martín L, Bando I, et al. Cancer risk and overall survival in mismatch repair proficient hereditary non-polyposis colorectal cancer, Lynch syndrome and sporadic colorectal cancer. Fam Cancer 2014;13(1):109–19. https://doi.org/10.1007/s10689-013-9683-2.

57. Lindberg LJ, Ladelund S, Frederiksen BL, et al. Outcome of 24 years national surveillance in different hereditary colorectal cancer subgroups leading to more individualised surveillance. J Med Genet 2017;54(5):297–304. https://doi.org/10.1136/jmedgenet-2016-104284.

58. Mesher D, Dove-Edwin I, Sasieni P, et al. A pooled analysis of the outcome of prospective colonoscopic surveillance for familial colorectal cancer. Int J Cancer 2014;134(4):939–47. https://doi.org/10.1002/ijc.28397.

59. Xu Y, Li C, Zhang Y, et al. Comparison between familial colorectal cancer type X and lynch syndrome: molecular, clinical, and pathological characteristics and pedigrees. Front Oncol 2020;10:1603. https://doi.org/10.3389/fonc.2020.01603.